NEUROIMAGING *in*

PSYCHIATRY

Edited by

Cynthia HY Fu MD
Clinical Research Fellow
Section of Neuroimaging
Division of Psychological Medicine
Institute of Psychiatry, King's College London
London, UK

Carl Senior BSc MSc PhD
Visiting Research Fellow, Laboratory of Brain & Cognition
National Institute of Mental Health
Bethesda, MD, USA

Tamara A Russell BSc MSc PhD
Section of Neuroscience and Emotion
Division of Psychological Medicine
Institute of Psychiatry and King's College London
London, UK

Daniel Weinberger MD
Chief, Clinical Brain Disorders Branch
National Institute of Mental health
Bethesda, MD, USA

Robin Murray MD DSc FRCP FRCPsych FMedSci
Professor of Psychiatry
Institute of Psychiatry
London, UK

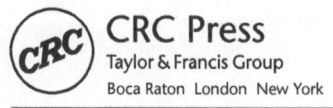
CRC Press
Taylor & Francis Group
Boca Raton London New York

CRC Press is an imprint of the
Taylor & Francis Group, an **informa** business

First published 2003 by Martin Dunitz.

Published 2023 by CRC Press
Taylor & Francis Group
6000 Broken Sound Parkway NW, Suite 300
Boca Raton, FL 33487-2742

© 2003 by Taylor & Francis Group, LLC
CRC Press is an imprint of Taylor & Francis Group, an Informa business

No claim to original U.S. Government works

ISBN-13: 978-1-84184-229-5 (pbk)

**Visit the Taylor & Francis Web site at
http://www.taylorandfrancis.com**

**and the CRC Press Web site at
http://www.crcpress.com**

Although every effort has been made to ensure that drug doses and other information are presented accurately in this publication, the ultimate responsibility rests with the prescribing physician. Neither the publishers nor the authors can be held responsible for errors or for any consequences arising from the use of information contained herein. For detailed prescribing information or instructions on the use of any product or procedure discussed herein, please consult the prescribing information or instructional material issued by the manufacturer.

A CIP record for this book is available from the British Library.

Composition by Expo Holdings, Malaysia

CONTENTS

Contributors

Peter A Bandettini BS PhD
Chief, Unit on Functional Imaging
Methods
Laboratory of Brain and Cognition
National Institute of Mental Health
Bethesda, MD, USA

Rodrigo A Bressan MD PhD
Section of Neuroscience and
Emotion
Division of Psychological Medicine
Institute of Psychiatry,
King's College London
London, UK and
Departamento de Psiquiatria
Universidade Federal de Sao Paulo
(UNIFESP)
Brazil

Wayne C Drevets MD
Senior Investigator
Chief, Section on Neuroimaging in
Mood and Anxiety Disorders
MIB/NIMH, National Institutes
of Health
Bethesda, MD, USA

Monique Ernst MD PhD
Section of Developmental and
Affective Neuroscience
MAP/NIMH/NIH/DHHS
Bethesda, MD, USA

Thomas Fahy MD MRPsych
Professor of Forensic Mental Health
Institute of Psychiatry
King's College London and
GKT School of Medicine
London, UK

Paul C Fletcher
Wellcome Senior Research Fellow
Department of Psychiatry
University of Cambridge
Addenbrooke's Hospital
Cambridge, UK

**Karl J Friston MB BS MA
MRCPsych FMedSci**
Wellcome Principal Fellow
Wellcome Department of Cognitive
Neurology
Institute of Neurology, University
College London
London, UK

Cynthia HY Fu MD
Clinical Research Fellow
Section of Neuroimaging, Division
of Psychological Medicine
Institute of Psychiatry and King's
College London
London, UK

Rebekah AE Honey PhD LlB
Research Associate
Department of Psychiatry
University of Cambridge
Addenbrooke's Hospital
Cambridge, UK

Natalia S Lawrence BSc PhD
Section of Neuroscience and
Emotion
Division of Psychological Medicine
Institute of Psychiatry, Kings
College London
London, UK

**Philip McGuire MD PhD
MRCPsych**
Professor of Cognitive
Neuroscience and Psychiatry
Head, Section of Neuroimaging,
Division of Psychological Medicine
Honorary Consultant Psychiatrist,
Lambeth Early Onset Service
Institute of Psychiatry,
King's College London, & GKT
School of Medicine
London, UK

Suzanne Munson BA
Section of Developmental and
Affective Neuroscience
MAP/NIMH/NIH/DHHS
Bethesda, MD, USA

Judith Rumsey PhD
Section of Developmental and
Affective Neuroscience
MAP/NIMH/NIH/DHHS
Bethesda, MD, USA

Tamara A Russell BSc MSc PhD
Section of Neuroscience and
Emotion
Division of Psychological Medicine
Institute of Psychiatry, King's
College London
London, UK

Sanjaya Saxena MD
Director, UCLA Obsessive-
Compulsive Disorder Research
Program
Associate Professor,
UCLA Department of Psychiatry
and Biobehavioral Sciences
UCLA Neuropsychiatric Institute
Los Angeles, CA, USA

Elliot A Stein PhD
Chief, Neuroimaging Research
Branch
National Institute on Drug Abuse
Intramural Research Program
Baltimore, MD, USA

Yaakov Stern PhD
Division Leader, Cognitive
Neuroscience Division
Professor Clinical Neuropsychology
Columbia University
New York, NY, USA

Janet Treasure PhD FRCP FRCPsych
Head, Section of Eating Disorders,
Division of Psychological Medicine
South London & Maudsley NHS
Trust Eating Disorder Unit
Institute of Psychiatry, Kings
College London
London, UK

Nigel Tunstall MB BS MRCPsych
Division of Psychological Medicine
Institute of Psychiatry,
King's College London
London, UK

Rudolph Uher MD
Section of Eating Disorders
Division of Psychological Medicine
Institute of Psychiatry, Kings
College London
London, UK

Nicholas D Walsh BSc
Clinical Research Associate
Neuroimaging Research
Institute of Psychiatry and
King's College London
London, UK

Domonick J Wegesin PhD
Assistant Professor of
Neuropsychology
G.H. Sergievsky Center, Taub
Center, Department of Neurology
Columbia University
New York, NY, USA

Fernando Zelaya PhD
Section of Neuroscience and
Emotion
Division of Psychological Medicine
Institute of Psychiatry,
King's College London
London, UK

PREFACE

Neuroimaging has developed rapidly in recent years, and has had a profound effect on fields as far apart as philosophy and linguistics. This book is an overview of the position that neuroimaging currently enjoys in psychiatry. The book is aimed at the beginner to the technique such as a student or clinician wanting to know its relevance for their patient. The idea for the book was to produce a text, which could successfully and painlessly guide a novice to a reasonable understanding of neuroimaging – both in terms of the actual techniques used and their relevance to psychiatric disorders. To meet this aim, we invited the world leaders in their various fields to contribute reviews of the most up-to-date findings from neuroimaging, to inform our understanding of schizophrenia, obsessive compulsive disorder, eating disorders, psychopathy, depression, aging, development and drug addiction.

We also wrote the book for young researchers and specialists in other areas looking to move into magnetic resonance imaging. The various neuroimaging techniques have developed at a breakneck pace – every academic journal contains glossy pictures with brain activity corresponding to a particular task emblazoned in glorious technicolour. Most medical centers have access to a number of scanners and young investigators are making increasingly imaginative use of the facilities. However, one requires a general understanding of the techniques for successful completion in any neuroimaging project. Therefore, to truly facilitate the development of neuroimaging in psychiatry a basic text with expert contributions is needed – this is what you now hold in your hands.

Cynthia HY Fu, Carl Senior, Tamara A Russel,
Daniel Weinberger, Robin Murray

1. FUNCTIONAL NEUROIMAGING: AN INTRODUCTION TO THE TECHNOLOGY, METHODOLOGY, INTERPRETATION, AND APPLICATIONS

Tamara A Russell, Fernando Zelaya, Rodrigo A Bressan, Peter A Bandettini

Introduction

Many technological advances have been seen in the neuroimaging field. These advances are allowing the investigation of new and exciting neurophysiological and pathophysiological questions. This chapter intends to provide the reader with a brief overview of the principles of MRI, fMRI, PET and SPET. Basic information on the hardware, specific applications and major limitations of the different neuroimaging techniques is provided to give the reader a perspective of what can and cannot be done with these techniques. Functional magnetic resonance imaging (fMRI) has been in existence for about 11 years.[1-3] During this time, the technique has experienced explosive growth. The reasons for this growth include the following: minimal invasiveness; the growing availability of the necessary hardware; the unique functional spatial and temporal resolution niche that it fills; its ability to map a network of substrates that intervenes in cognitive and sensory processes; and, importantly, the potential that it promises for the investigation of abnormal brain function. Figure 1.1 is an attempt to graphically illustrate a timeline of the advancement of many, but certainly not all, significant aspects of functional imaging technologies.

Although the use of this tool has increased exponentially, it is still quite difficult for the average end-user, perhaps a psychologist or psychiatrist, to come to grips with the basic principles and physics of MR. The aim of the first section of this chapter is to provide an overview of these basic principles. Subsequent sections will describe aspects of the hardware used in the MRI environment, and advances and developments that are being made in

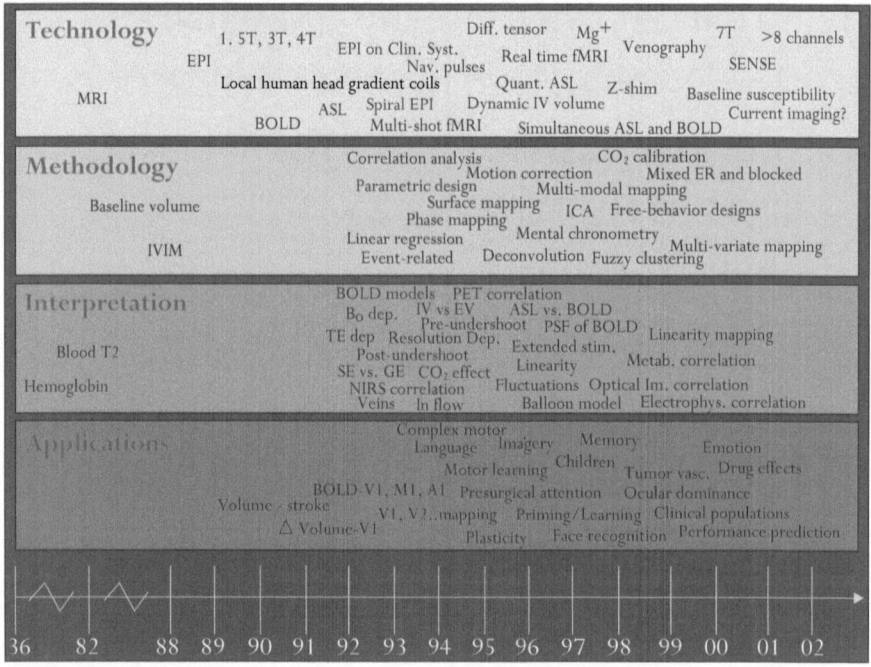

Figure 1.1 *Growth and progression of neuroimaging techniques. A1, auditory cortex; ASL, arterial spin labeling; B_0, external field; BOLD, blood oxygenation-level dependent; EPI, echo planar imaging; ER, event related; EV, extravascular; fMRI, functional magnetic resonance imaging; GE, gradient echo; ICA, independent component analysis; IV, intravenous; IVIM, intravoxel incoherent motion; IV v EV, intravascular versus extravascular; M1, motor cortex; MRI, magnetic resonance imaging; NIRS, near infrared spectroscopy; PSF, point spread function; SE, spin echo; SENSE, sensitivity encoding for fast MRI; T, tesla; V1, visual area 1; V2, visual area 2.*

this area. Additionally, some discussion of the neuronal information extracted from the blood oxygenation-level-dependent (BOLD) signal will be discussed. Lastly, the applications of this tool are briefly outlined.

Basic principles of functional magnetic resonance imaging (fMRI)

fMRI is a new application of an existing technology (i.e. MRI). This section will attempt to introduce, in a basic way accessible to the novice, the elements involved in the production of the MRI signal. It will cover basic principles relating to the nuclei of hydrogen atoms (which is where most of the

MR signal comes from) and their properties when an external magnetic field is applied. Precession and resonance will be described, as will the mechanisms by which protons can be excited and relaxed. By necessity, in order to provide a brief introduction to this area, some aspects of this explanation may be deemed by the more experienced reader as oversimplified. It is stressed at this point that the purpose of this chapter is to provide an introductory overview to the novice neuroimager, providing a level of understanding that will demystify some of the principles and terminology used, not to provide an in-depth understanding of all the physics involved in MRI.

Nucleus of the hydrogen atom

Hydrogen atoms give rise to most of the signal in an MR image. The nucleus of the hydrogen atom consists of one proton and no neutrons. This gives the hydrogen atom a positive charge and an atomic number of 1, as there is only one proton in its nucleus. Hydrogen atoms are abundant in the human body: approximately 70% of the body is made up of water (containing two hydrogen atoms and one oxygen atom). In the brain, gray matter has approximately a 70% water content, blood approximately a 93% water content and white matter (glial cells) approximately an 85% water content. The large quantity of hydrogen atoms in the human body and the large magnetic moment (see below) of the single proton in the nucleus of the atom are responsible for the large MR signal they produce when compared with those of other nuclei.

Magnetic moment

Some atomic nuclei have the property of 'spin'. This means that they have a *net* angular momentum, i.e. they can be seen as 'rotating' around their main axis. The spinning protons combined with their net electric charge create what is called a net magnetic moment, as if they were a small magnet with a north and a south pole.

External magnetic fields

In the absence of any external magnetic field, proton magnetic moments are randomly orientated and (as a group) are considered to have a net magnetization of zero. When an external magnetic field is applied to an object, the spin axes of all the nuclei in the object line up with the magnetic field. The nuclei can either align *parallel* to the magnetic field or *anti-parallel* to it (i.e. in the opposite direction). Factors which influence the direction of orientation include the thermal energy of the atoms and the strength of the external magnetic field. High-energy protons are strong enough to be able to align

3

themselves anti-parallel to the external magnetic field while those with low energy will align in a direction parallel to the magnetic field. In reality, the number of protons that align parallel and anti-parallel with the field is not the same. This difference produces a net magnetization of the whole sample (in our case, the human brain). With increases in magnetic field strength, this difference increases, therefore enhancing the net magnetization of the sample.

For simplicity, it is easier to consider from here onwards only the *net* magnetization of the sample. As you may have realized, this net magnetization has a definite orientation, i.e. in the direction of the excess of protons that align parallel with the field. Therefore, it is represented as a vector quantity, which is termed the *net magnetization vector* (NMV) or *M*.

Precession

Because of their intrinsic angular momentum (described above), protons do not align with the external field (parallel or anti-parallel) in a 'straight' line. Instead, they behave just like a spinning top does as it starts to fall. *Precession* is the term used to describe the way in which protons 'wobble' around their axes. When an external magnetic field is applied, the protons precess in line with it, but wobble in a conical manner that is similar to the spinning top rotating around a vertical axis. *Precessional frequency* is a term used to describe the rate (or speed) at which the protons or the NMV precesses.

Resonance and the Larmor frequency

When exposed to an external magnetic field, all hydrogen protons will precess at the same frequency. This frequency is determined by the gyro-magnetic ratio of the particular protons and the strength of the magnetic field. It is described by a very simple equation called the Larmor equation, which states that the frequency of precession (ω) is given by the product of the gyromagnetic ratio of the protons (γ) times the strength of the external field (B_0):

$$\omega = \gamma B_0$$

The gyromagnetic ratio of hydrogen is 42.57 MHz/tesla (T) and all hydrogen protons will precess at this same frequency when exposed to an external magnetic field of 1 T. The strength of the magnetic field (from the scanner) is measured in tesla (T) or gauss (G): 1 T is equivalent to 1×10^4 G (about 20,000 times stronger than the earth's magnetic field).

As can be seen, this equation determines the frequency at which the protons will resonate. The resonant frequency is also referred to as the *precessional frequency* or the *Larmor frequency*. The equation also demonstrates that the higher the magnetic field, the greater the precessional frequency.

The strength of the magnetic field will usually increase the intensity of the signal because the net magnetization will be larger. It is also worth noting that fMRI contrast also increases approximately linearly with field strength.[4–6] Field strength drives both the frequency of precession of protons and the fMRI contrast in a linear fashion. The drive for an increased signal:noise ratio (S:N; i.e. the height of the signal of interest compared to the background noise) and for increased functional contrast has been respons ible for the proliferation of higher field strength magnets for human fMRI, from typically 1.0 T in 1984 to the present day where scanners in the range of 4–7 T are being developed for human use. Field strengths as high as 12 T are being developed for animal use. The majority of scanners in use in academic centers are in the range of 1.5–4 T. Higher field magnets cost more to build and maintain, and create their own techni-cal hurdles. Some of the advantages and disadvantages of high field strength are outlined in Table 1.1.

But what actually is *resonance*? Resonance refers to the property of a body (in this case the nucleus of an atom) to absorb energy at a characteristic, natural frequency. In MR, the natural frequency for resonance absorption is given by the Larmor equation. A condition of resonance can be achieved by placing the protons within a strong external field and exciting them with a second, alternating magnetic field [in the form of radiofrequency (RF) waves, see below]. When resonance occurs, not only do the magnetic moments of the protons change their angle of rotation, but all the protons begin to precess in phase with each other (referred to as *phase coherence*).

Protons can absorb energy from external sources but also give off energy when they try to change their alignment back to their initial configuration in the magnetic field. These two types of processes form the basis of how the MR signal is created and how it disappears.

Noll[7] has described the resonance phenomena using the analogy of a guitar string. With a guitar, the frequency varies according to how much tension is applied to the string by the fingers [similar to the strength of the magnetic field (B_0)]. The string is most often plucked in order to excite it and create resonance (in the form of acoustic waves), however, it can also be excited by holding up a loudspeaker near to the string and playing a note *at the same frequency* as the string. This is similar in manner to the way in which nuclear spins are excited by the application of RF waves (a second, alternating magnetic field of the correct frequency).

Table 1.1 Advantages and disadvantages of high field strength functional magnetic resonance imaging (fMRI)

Advantages	Disadvantages
Signal to noise (S:N) is linearly proportional to field strength	In fMRI what matters is temporal signal to noise, which does not scale with field strength at typical (low) resolutions since physiologic fluctuations, independent of field strength, contribute significantly. This will blunt external field (B_0)-based gains in S:N ratios and functional contrast to noise
Functional contrast to noise increases with B_0, allowing comparisons of more subtle signal changes or for shorter scans for similar quality functional maps	Baseline T2* and T2 also decrease with B_0, therefore lowering the time interval between the radiofrequency (RF) pulse and the middle echo (TE) at which optimal contrast is obtained, reducing the gain in functional contrast to noise somewhat
High S:N ratio allows higher resolutions to be obtained	To achieve high resolutions, one needs a longer readout window (difficult at higher field strengths) or multishot imaging (time consuming and more temporally unstable)
Blood T1 increases, increasing functional contrast for arterial spin labeling (ASL) perfusion imaging techniques. It is thought that at just above 7 T, perfusion and blood oxygenation-level dependent (BOLD) functional contrasts are similar	At typical fMRI resolutions, signal dropout is greater at higher field strengths, requiring better shimming techniques and/or smaller voxel sizes
At field strengths ≥ 3 T, vein T2* becomes much less than gray matter T2*, making the creation of venograms a simple matter of collecting a high-resolution T2* scan	RF power deposition issues are more significant at higher field strengths, therefore limiting continuous ASL techniques and high-resolution fast spin-echo imaging.
At field strengths ≥ 9T, the intravascular contribution is zero, therefore enabling more precise functional localization	It is more difficult to create a homogeneous RF power deposition at higher field strengths

The term *excitation* is used to describe the delivery of energy to the protons at their characteristic frequency. As the proton resonates it moves out of alignment with the external magnetic field (B_0), to attempt to align with the second, alternating magnetic field. The NMV is now also changing out of alignment with B_0. This alternating magnetic field is delivered in the form of a pulse. The length of the pulse will determine the *flip* angle (in degrees) by which the net magnetization is tilted away from B_0. If a pulse is applied to produce a rotation of 90° then, eventually, all the protons that were aligned with B_0 will change their alignment so that they are precessing in what is called the *transverse plane* (at 90° to B_0). Similarly, if a flip angle of 180° is used, then the precession and alignment of the protons will eventually be anti-parallel to the original magnetization direction. Maximum detection is obtained with a flip angle of 90°.

Once the protons have been 'flipped' by the external energy source (in this case RF pulse) and the pulse is terminated, the protons will start to relax and begin to attempt to realign with B_0. This process will take a finite period of time and will evolve with a time constant referred to as T1. T1 is dependent on the physical and chemical properties of the environment in which the protons are residing. The time between successive RF pulses (TR) will determine the optimum flip angle for the experiment. For a given value of TR, the shorter T1, the larger the flip angle which can be used between successive excitations.

Relaxation of excited protons

In general terms, T1 is the time constant with which protons will reach their equilibrium magnetization. As mentioned above, T1 is roughly the time it takes for the protons to change their alignment from the transverse plane back to the original direction B_0. This is also called longitudinal relaxation. As T1 occurs, another separate, but simultaneous, phenomena called T2 occurs. This is the transverse relaxation time, or T2 decay, which is the natural decay of the signal in the transverse plane. It is also referred to as T2 relaxation time, T2 decay or 'spin–spin relaxation time'. It is observed that when the RF pulse is terminated, those protons precessing in the transverse plane will gradually begin to realign with B_0 and, at the same time, the signal will decay. The decay is caused by both the return to equilibrium and the transverse relaxation (with a time constant of T2). Like T1, T2 decay is also dependent on the interactions the spins have with each other and with their microenvironment, i.e. the tissue that they are in, e.g. fat or water. Some spins might decay more quickly than others. The longer TR is, the more the protons in the transverse plane decay and begin to lose phase coherence (i.e. they will no longer be spinning at the same frequency or in the same plane). An important concept to note is that, strictly speaking, the term T2* is the term used to describe the time constant with which the detected signal decays. This reduction of signal in the transverse plane is primarily caused by the fact that the magnetic field is not precisely the same in all parts of the sample, i.e. the field is inhomogeneous. From the Larmor equation, it can be seen that since these differences in field will give rise to differences in the Larmor frequencies at each point in space, the precession of protons at different rates will make them lose phase coherence, thus destroying the signal. Therefore T2* is shorter than the natural decay, T2.

Tissue contrast

Signals given out over the course of manipulations with RF pulses depend on the local microenvironment surrounding the proton; e.g. hydrogen nuclei in fats transmit different radio signals compared to those in water. This property allows the signal obtained to be used to distinguish between different tissues in the body, or create contrast. Due to the T1 and T2 relaxation properties, it is possible to differentiate between various tissues in the body: this is called *contrast*.

Fat nuclei have a slow molecular motion and longitudinal relaxation (T1) occurs rapidly. Therefore, the time it takes for the NMV to realign with B_0 in fat is short. In contrast, water molecules have a high mobility, which means that the proton–proton interactions between water nuclei (which also contribute to the decay of the signal) are averaged towards zero, and hence it takes longer for them to realign with B_0, i.e. they have a long T1. With respect to T2 decay, fat has a very efficient energy exchange with its surrounding tissue and therefore it can very quickly give up the energy it has absorbed to neighboring cells, leading to a short T2. Water, on the other hand, is less efficient and has a longer T2.

The concept of contrast can also be extended to other types of differentiations between proton signals. One of the reasons for the widespread use of MRI is the fact that it can also be used to differentiate between healthy and pathologic tissue by examining their differences in mobility, composition, etc. As will be seen later, in fMRI these concepts are used to create contrast between active and less active sites of brain activity.

Summary
- Protons (i.e. the nuclei of hydrogen atoms) are randomly aligned in the body.
- An applied external magnetic field (B_0), measured in tesla (T), comes from the magnet of the scanner.

- Protons align either parallel or anti-parallel to B_0, and the difference between these two populations gives the net magnetization vector (NMF).
- Protons precess or wobble around the axis of this magnetic field.
- A radiofrequency (RF) pulse at the Lamor frequency for hydrogen is applied, which causes protons to tilt away from the direction of the applied field.
- The duration of the RF pulse will determine the angle by which the protons will tilt away from the field.
- The MR signal is detected by tilting the magnetization towards the direction of a receiver coil.
- When the RF is terminated, protons de-phase and lose their coherence, and try to realign with B_0.
- Proton realignment (T1) and longitudinal (T2) relaxation occur simultaneously.

Magnetic resononance imaging hardware

The section above has attempted to describe, in a simply way, some of the basic principles behind the MR signal and how it is obtained. To a certain extent, these principles are invariant, i.e. they are physical facts that cannot be manipulated. In order to gain optimum use of the natural contrast that occurs as the result of magnetization of the human brain, certain tools or hardware are used and manipulated by MR physicists. It is here that a degree of variation can be introduced in order to optimize the signal that is received.

This section describes some of the tools at the disposal of the physicist and, additionally, some of the new directions that can be taken with various manipulations to take fMRI forward, e.g. gradient coils, different pulse sequences and RF receiver coils.

Gradient coils

The component of the imaging system that allows the spatial localization of the protons is a set of *magnetic field gradients*, set up by magnetic coils which are turned on and off. Coils are used to apply magnetic field gradients within the larger magnetic field of the scanner magnet. Their purpose is to make the Larmor frequencies of the sample proportional to their position in space.

How is a slice selected?

A magnetic field gradient along the z-axis, also called the slice-select gradient, is normally turned on at the same time that the first RF pulse is applied. For example, with a 2 T system, a gradient of 0.1 T/cm may be set up along the z-axis. This would mean that, at the center of the magnet, the amplitude of the magnetic field was 2 T. But, along the z-direction, the value of the magnetic field (B_0) will increase or decrease by 0.1 T/cm. This gradient causes hydrogen nuclei at one end of the magnet to precess at a higher frequency (more than the Larmor frequency) and those at the other end (weaker magnetic field) to precess at a lower frequency (less than the Larmor frequency). Remember (as described earlier under Resonance and the Larmor frequency) that resonance only occurs when protons are excited at their own frequency, as determined by the Larmor equation. For example, if a gradient was set up that caused protons to precess at 63 MHz at one end of the magnet (this could be at the feet of the subject) up to 65 MHz at the other end (the head of the subject), then a 65 MHz RF pulse would excite nuclei in a slice near the head of the subject but not near the feet; conversely, a 63 MHz pulse would excite nuclei near the feet of the subject and not at the head. Thus, a single 'slice' of the gradient can be excited depending on the frequency at which the RF pulse is delivered. Only the protons in that slice will be excited. Other slices can be excited by shifting either the frequency of the RF pulse up or down, or by shifting the overall magnetic field up or down. This gradient will, however, only give spatial information in one dimension.

The width of the selected slice will be given by the particular characteristics of the RF pulse that is employed, and the magnitude of the slice-select gradient. 'Shaped' pulses (where the RF envelope has a special shape) are employed which select only a band of frequencies. The amplitude of the gradient then determines the spatial thickness that the band of frequencies corresponds to.

Encoding the information in the plane of the image

The previous section showed how to select a 'slice' of protons anywhere in the volume of the magnet, but what is wanted is the anatomical detail in the plane of the image. In other words, the Larmor frequencies of the protons of the slice in the remaining two dimensions (if the slice was selected across the z-direction, then the plane of the slice would be in the xy-plane) need to be encoded.

This is done by using two additional field gradients, one that linearly varies the Larmor frequencies along x-plane and the other that does the same thing along the y-plane. The actual manner in which this process of frequency encoding is done can be made in literally hundreds of ways. For simplicity, described here is the simplest scenario. In this context, the situation is similar to that described above, i.e. the frequencies of the protons will depend on their position along x by turning on a linear gradient along the x-axis (hence, protons at one end of the x-axis of the magnet will precess faster than protons at the other end).

The important distinction from the process of slice selection is that in this part of the acquisition process we will actually *detect* the MR signal in the presence of the x-gradient. This means that the signal captured contains contributions from *all* of the protons in the selected slice, but the individual frequencies that contribute to it have a signature of where they come from in the x-direction by virtue of the gradient applied. This is what is meant by frequency encoding along x. Note that all that has been achieved so far is to select a slice and to give that slice an amount of frequency encoding, there is still not enough information to create an image. All we have is a projection of all the points of the slice along the x-axis.

What about the other dimension (i.e. y)? This second dimension could be encoded in exactly the same manner, i.e. in principle, two linear gradients could be turned on along x and y simultaneously, and the signal captured in the presence of both of them. The resulting signal would correspond to a projection of the entire slice along a line defined by the vector sum of the x- and y-gradients. This could be repeated many times for various values of the x- and y-gradients until enough frequency information for the entire sample was defined. Indeed, this is how MRI was first performed in 1973, when it was called projection reconstruction.[8]

However, a more efficient way of encoding the second dimension is to do the process in two stages. Firstly (after selecting the slice), a gradient is turned on in the y-dimension for a finite amount of time, but the MR signal is *not* detected in its presence; some quantity of frequency encoding to the protons have simply been assigned depending on their position along y. Some time after the y-gradient pulse, a gradient is turned on in the x-direction, but this time the signal is detected in the presence of the x-gradient. So, the signal detected carries contributions from the frequencies of all protons according to their position in x but, because of the preceding y-gradient pulse, their relative phase is different depending on their position along y. The y-gradient has therefore achieved the function of *phase encoding* the signals and the x-gradient has provided the role of *frequency encoding*.

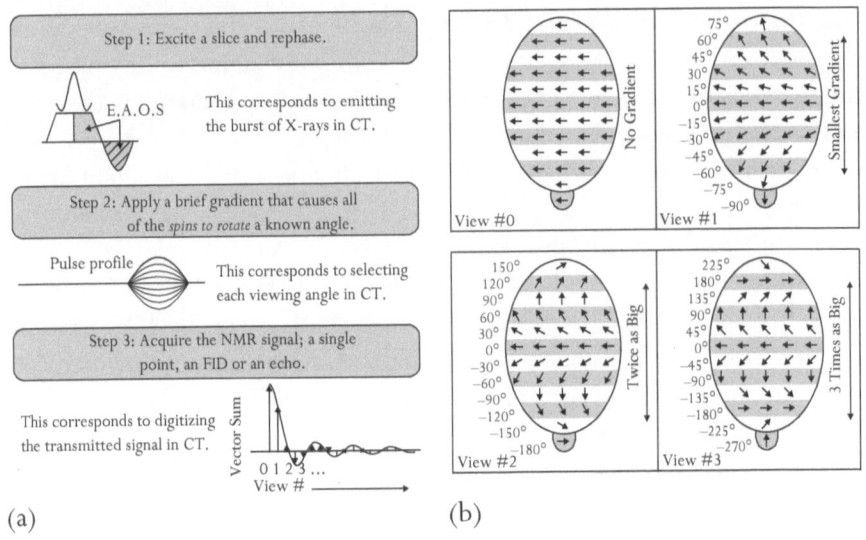

Figure 1.2 (a) Schematic representation of the principle of 'spin–warp' phase encoding. In Step 2, a different magnitude of the phase encoding gradient is applied for each 'view'. This makes all the spins in the sample rotate by a known angle. In Step 3, the signal that is captured immediately has a relative phase difference which is directly proportional to the amplitude and duration of that gradient. (b) The effect of the phase encoding gradient on each one of the 'views'. The signal acquires a relative phase evolution along the vertical direction which is dependent upon its position. Notice that along the horizontal direction all spins possess the same phase angle. (Reproduced from NessAiver. All you need to know about MRI physics, University of Maryland, Medical Centre with permission from Moriel NessAvier, Simply Physics.)

In practice, the process detailed above is repeated several times for different values of the y-gradient until all the frequency encoding (see Figure 1.2) in both dimensions has been achieved.

Decoding the signal

Although the processes leading to the complete encoding of three-dimensional information on the MR signal have been described, the issue of how this information is decoded in order to produce the two-dimensional image has not been addressed.

In order to achieve this, an operation called Fourier transformation (FT) is used. This literally transforms the signals from the time domain in which they are acquired to a frequency domain, which, as has been shown, is equivalent to their position in space because the magnitude of frequency encoding applied along the x- and y-directions is known. The FT gives, for each signal, the spectrum of frequencies that make up that signal. In simple terms, once it is known which signal amplitudes correspond to which frequencies, then the frequency is converted to spatial coordinates from the magnitude of the applied gradient.

Fourier transformation is one of various types of transform operations that can take us from one domain to another, in this case from time to frequency (i.e. space). FT is performed because there are readily available algorithms which allow most computers to perform this function very quickly.

Nowadays, there are literally hundreds of schemes for frequency and phase encoding. The ones of interest for functional imaging are those which can be performed very quickly, so as to provide good temporal resolution in the evaluation of cognitive and sensory processes. The fast imaging method of choice is echo planar imaging (EPI), a technique in which *all* the necessary frequency and phase encoding information is generated from a single excitation. This means that one complete two-dimensional slice can be collected in approximately 100 ms. (As will be seen later, the second criterion for choosing an imaging modality for functional studies is the manner in which the *contrast* of the image is tailored to reflect the differences between states of activity.)

Different acquisition techniques

The rate of image acquisition is primarily limited by how rapidly the gradients can be switched on and off, and how long the signal lasts whilst it is being digitized.

From the point of view of how all the information necessary to construct the image is collected, MRI can be divided into *single-shot* and *multishot* techniques. In single-shot techniques, all the data necessary for creation of an image are collected (read) in one single time window, or in a series of small time windows within the same repetition time. The information arises only from samples of longitudinal magnetization. As mentioned above, EPI is one such single-shot technique in that one 'plane' of data is collected after the application of a single RF pulse (gradient-echo EPI) or two RF pulses (spin-echo EPI).

The temporal domain in which signals are collected (in the presence of the frequency-encoding gradient) is often called the k-space, a term that arose because of the similarities between MRI and diffraction (and crystallography[9]). The k-space is simply a convenient coordinate system in which the raw data is represented, but it also has the property that it corresponds to the inverse space of the object. So, in order to collect all the information to make the image, we simply have to collect the minimum number of k-space points needed to be inverted by FT (mentioned above) to generate the image of the object.

In single-shot EPI, all the k-space points that make the image are collected in one repetition time. In multishot EPI, various parts of k-space are collected sequentially in different repetition times. Higher image quality is obtained in this manner but a large penalty is paid in terms of acquisition time, which is why multishot techniques are not generally used for functional imaging studies.

In multishot MRI, a single 'line' (in k-space) of raw data is acquired with each excitation pulse. Because of the relatively slow rate at which the magnetization returns to equilibrium following excitation (determined by T1 of the particular tissue), a certain amount of time is required between shots, otherwise the signal would rapidly be saturated. Because of this required recovery time (at least 150 ms for gray matter protons at 1.5 T), multishot techniques are typically slower than single-shot techniques. For a 150 ms TR (elapsed time between successive RF excitation pulses), a multishot image with 128 lines of raw data would take 150 ms $\times$ 128 = 19.2 s.

In the case of EPI, the entire data set for a single plane is typically acquired in about 20–40 ms. For an fMRI experiment, the time interval between the RF pulse and the measurement of the middle echo (TE) is about 40 ms. Along with some additional time for applying other necessary gradients, the total time for an image to be acquired is about 60–100 ms, allowing 10–16 images to be acquired in 1 s (one image in 100 ms = 10 images in 1000 ms). Improvements in digital sampling rates and gradient slew rates (how fast a gradient can be turned on and off to different field strengths) will allow further gains in this number, but, essentially, this is about the upper limit for imaging humans.

In the context of an fMRI experiment with EPI, the typical image acquisition rate (for the whole brain volume) is also determined by how many slices can temporally fit into TR. For whole brain imaging, approximately 20 slices (5 mm thickness) are typically required to cover the entire brain. This would allow a TR of about 1.5–2 s at minimum. This image sampling rate is often adequate to capture most of the details of the slow and dispersed activation-related hemodynamic response, which takes about 12 s to completely evolve. The basic dynamics of the signal are shown in Figure 1.3.

Image *spatial* resolution is also primarily determined by the gradient strength, the digitizing rate, and the time available. For multishot imaging, higher resolution images can be achieved at the expense of prolonged imaging times. But note that these techniques become unsuitable for *functional* imaging studies since, in most instances, we want to improve the temporal resolution of the functional examination and, as is the case in

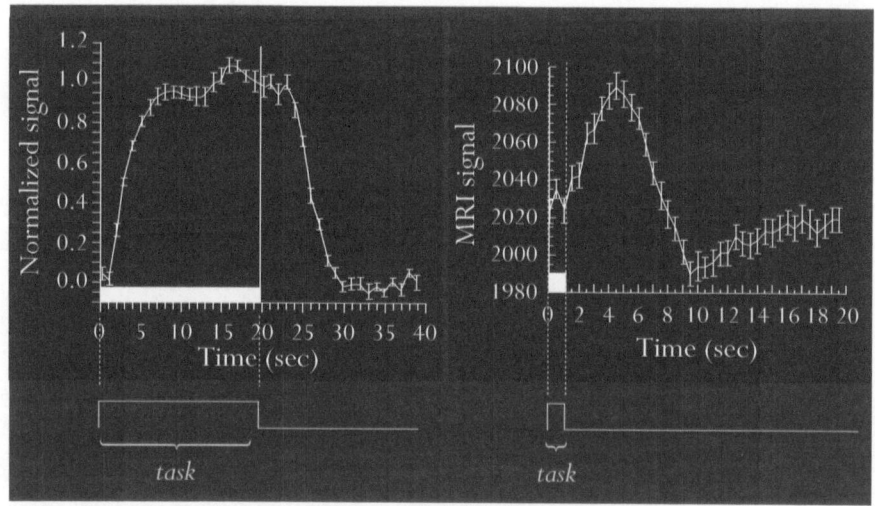

Figure 1.3 *Basic dynamics of the magnetic resonance imaging (MRI) signal.*

event-related investigations, preserve the ability to assign at least one volume to every stimulus that is presented.

In EPI, all the gradient pulses necessary to define the image matrix in two dimensions are applied following a single excitation (i.e. one RF pulse). The frequency encoding is achieved by successive reversals of one of the gradients (normally called the *read* gradient). In other words, the gradient waveform looks like a series of positive and negative lobes. This gives rise to a series of gradient echoes in the middle of each one of the lobes, and each echo is used to encode one line of k-space along the read (frequency-encoding) direction.

Prior to each frequency gradient lobe, a small gradient (a blip) is applied along the other (orthogonal) direction of the image, which effectively shifts the position of each one of the lines traced by the read gradient along the second dimension. In essence, the resultant trajectory in k-space resembles a zig-zag raster, which eventually covers the desired area.

For example, to create a typical image with 64 × 64 pixels in plane, a frequency-encoding gradient waveform with 64 lobes (32 negative and 32 positive ones, alternatively) needs to be applied, which should happen well within the time of one signal decay. Gradient switching therefore has to happen extremely quickly, and with sufficient stability so that the image does not suffer from artefacts. With typical current technology, it takes approximately 25–40 ms to perform 64 spatial encoding steps (in a classic 64 × 64 acquisition matrix). This limit is determined partly by the physical limits of the scanner and partly by the biological limits of the subject. If the rate of change and the magnitude of the frequency-encoding gradient field are too high, currents may be induced in the peripheral nerves, creating the sensation of twitching, which is not dangerous but neither is it desirable.

Three methods exist for switching the gradients rapidly.[10] One is to have extremely high-powered gradient amplifiers – a brute force approach. Another is to create gradient waveforms that match the characteristic frequency of the amplifiers and the gradient coils – providing less flexibility in adjusting the gradient readout parameters. A third is to use a low-inductance gradient coil which does not require a large amount of power to create a rapidly switched and strong gradient. For imaging humans, the first systems used for EPI were either the resonant type (e.g. Massachusetts General Hospital NMR Center) or standard clinical systems equipped with home-built low-inductance gradient coils (e.g. Medical College of Wisconsin Biophysics Research Institute). The use of local gradient coils, while cheap, does not offer much room for patients or for stimulus delivery. The introduction of EPI on clinical scanners – using the brute force high-powered gradient amplifier approach – was critical in the explosive growth in fMRI applications. This allowed users to simply buy a system for doing EPI rather than relying on the development of a system by a local team of physicists. Currently, hundreds of such systems are in operation, whereas, in 1992, only a small handful of centers could perform EPI. It should be noted that although EPI is a very fast method, it generally has poorer spatial resolution than conventional MRI techniques. However, the gain obtained in the speed of acquisition is substantial, and without its implementation, the proliferation of fMRI would not have taken place.

Pulse sequences

MRI pulse sequences are the programs that control the timings of the magnetic field gradients, RF pulses, and RF receivers. Essentially, a pulse sequence is a computer program giving a list of instructions to the MRI scanner to control all the elements that go into obtaining an image. For example, one pulse sequence might conceptually be as shown in Figure 1.4, demonstrating the application of the RF pulse (at a 90° flip angle) and the switching on and off of the gradients in three dimensions (x, y and z). Note that TE is the time between the RF pulse and the measurement of the signal. This process is repeated 128 times in order to obtain the image and increase detection of the signal.

MR physicists spend some of their time optimizing the parameters of the pulse program to tailor the sequences to the desired application. Different

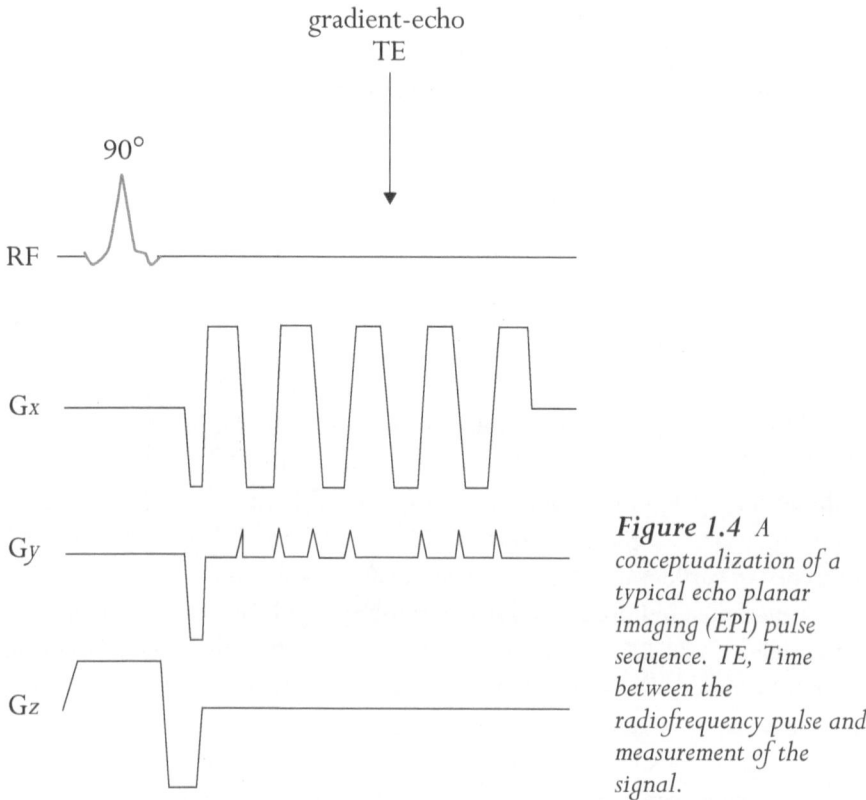

Figure 1.4 A conceptualization of a typical echo planar imaging (EPI) pulse sequence. TE, Time between the radiofrequency pulse and measurement of the signal.

types of manipulations (e.g. number of gradient switches, length of RF pulse, frequency of RF pulse or the echo time) can alter the signal that is received, and can be used to obtain images with different characteristics (both temporal and spatial). Other modifications of the pulse sequence program may be carried out to alter the contrast of the images in order to address specific neuronal and/or physiologic information (discussed in more detail in Extracting neuronal and physiologic information, see later).

RF receivers and coils

Gradient coils are used to vary the magnitude of the magnetic field gradient in a linear fashion along varying axes. A different type of coil is used to receive the RF signals that are emitted from the protons when excitation ceases. These are the coils that read the incoming signal. Decoding the signal (see earlier) described the nature of the incoming signal and how it is mapped from *k*-space to real (subject) space, and transformed into the MR image; this section describes the hardware that is used to collect the signal.

For whole brain imaging, a quadrature 8–12 RF coil is typically used. This coil, which in many systems is brought over the head and face of the subject as they lie in the scanner, is used both to send RF pulses to excite the protons and to receive the incoming signals. Most clinical RF coils are sensitive to signals from the entire head and upper neck area, and are therefore not ideal for fMRI of the brain. This is because they work better when they are tailored to produce a homogeneous RF field over a smaller region of space. Furthermore, the main magnetic field is also more homogeneous over a smaller volume. Gains typically in the range of 30% in the S:N ratio can be obtained by using an RF coil that is closer to the head and has a reception field that does not extend beyond the base of the brain. One should be aware that, again, while a gain of 30% in the S:N ratio is good, the temporal S:N ratio is what really matters in fMRI. At typical voxel volumes ($3 \times 3 \times 5$ mm^3), a gain of 30% in the S:N ratio will likely translate to no more than a gain of about 10% in the temporal S:N ratio, given the presence of cardiac and respiratory fluctuations over time.

It is desirable to improve the spatial resolution of fMRI and, hence, smaller and smaller voxel sizes are currently used. This has the advantage of reducing partial volume effects. Furthermore, in voxels that contain gray matter parenchyma, it maximizes the amount of signal change due to functional contrast, since there is less contamination from other tissue types where there is no blood oxygenation-level dependent (BOLD)-related signal change, such as white matter and cerebrospinal fluid (CSF). However, this gain is partly counteracted by a loss in the S:N ratio of each voxel, as the number of protons in the voxel volume decreases. Therefore, at each field strength there is an optimum voxel size that maximizes these two competing mechanisms.[11]

If very high resolution is required over a specific and highly localized region of interest (e.g. the visual or motor cortex), then surface coils can been used. This means that a small RF coil is placed over the region of interest. The S:N ratio in this region is a function of the coil size – the smaller the coil, the greater the S:N ratio. One problem with surface coils, however, is that they do not have a homogeneous reception or excitation field. This is a problem for reception in that the sensitivity drops off rapidly. It is a larger problem for excitation since the excitation energy is inhomogeneously distributed, meaning that in one part of the brain spins receive an excitation of 90° (flip angle) and, in another region, different flip angles might be excited (flip angles are discussed in Resonance and the Larmor frequency, see earlier). To create a homogenous flip angle distribution, it is necessary to use either specialized excitation pulses or a larger coil for excitation. Typically, at 1.5 T, whole body

RF coils are typically used for excitation, therefore obviating this problem. At field strengths > 3 T, whole body coils are not yet feasible. A workable strategy has been to use an intermediate-sized coil for excitation and smaller coils inside the large coil for reception. In this case, a large excitation coil gives a homogeneous distribution of RF power and the surface receiver coil focuses on a specific region for high resolution and/or a high S:N ratio fMRI.

Surface coils can be combined into arrays to increase the S:N ratio and brain coverage. In addition, specific pulse sequences involving RF sensitivity encoding are being designed to make use of independent surface coil arrays to increase the S:N ratio, imaging speed and resolution. Significant advancements in this area are expected in the near future.

Extracting neuronal and physiologic information

Several types of physiologic information can be mapped using fMRI. This information includes baseline cerebral blood volume (CBV),[12, 13] changes in blood volume,[14] baseline and changes in cerebral perfusion,[15–19] and changes in blood oxygenation.[1,3,20–24] Recent advances in fMRI pulse sequence and experimental manipulation have allowed quantitative measures of oxygen extraction fraction,[25] cerebral metabolic rate of oxygen ($CMRO_2$) changes[26–29] and dynamic non-invasive measures in blood volume[30] with activation. It is beyond the scope of this chapter to review all of these methods. Similarly, the exact mechanisms of the change in blood oxygenation that occur with brain activity are not completely understood, and more detailed discussion on this point can be found in Arthurs and Boniface[31] and Attwell and Iadeola.[32] Below, a brief overview of the role of blood oxygenation in brain function is given, the most common method to obtain activity-related contrast; fMRI relies directly on this parameter. Some advantages and disadvantages of this method are discussed, as is the issue of hemodynamic specificity. Lastly, a particularly interesting emerging method to detect $CMRO_2$ changes directly will be briefly considered.

Blood oxygenation

Cerebral blood flow (CBF), and the rate of oxygen consumption by cells, as a result of oxidative phosphorylation, are directly coupled to neuronal activity. Oxygen consumed by neurons is supplied by the blood, where oxygen is bound to hemoglobin. Arteries carry hemoglobin which is fully oxygenated.

Table 1.2 Summary of the practical advantages and disadvantages of pulse sequences that have contrast based on blood oxygenation-level dependent (BOLD), perfusion, volume, and cerebral metabolic rate of oxygen (CMRO$_2$) signals

	Advantages	Disadvantages
BOLD	Highest functional activation contrast by a factor of two to four over perfusion Easiest to implement Multislice trivial Can use very short times between radiofrequency pulses (TR)	Complicated non-quantitative signal No baseline information Susceptibility artifacts
Perfusion	Unique and quantitative information Baseline information Easy control over observed vasculature Non-invasive No susceptibility artifacts	Low functional activation contrast (up to 7 T) Longer TR required Multislice is difficult Slow mapping of baseline information
Volume	Unique information Baseline information Multislice is trivial Rapid mapping of baseline information	Invasive Susceptibility artifacts Requires separate rest and activation runs
CMRO$_2$	Unique and quantitative information	Semi-invasive (requires CO$_2$ inhalation) Low functional activation contrast Susceptibility artifacts Processing intensive Multislice is difficult Longer TR required

When cells are 'working' they need to extract this oxygen in the blood supply and, consequently, in the veins, most of the hemoglobin becomes deoxygenated. As early as the 1930s it was known that deoxyhemoglobin was paramagnetic (susceptible to magnetization) and oxyhemoglobin was diamagnetic.[33] In 1982, it was discovered that changes in blood oxygenation changed T2 of blood, but it was not until 1989 that this knowledge was used to image *in vivo* changes in blood oxygenation.[34] The BOLD contrast (a term coined by Ogawa et al[2]) was used to image the activated brain for the first time in 1991. The basic concept behind this endogenous contrast mechanism is that increases in brain activity are almost invariably accompanied by increases in blood flow. This localized increase in blood flow causes an increase in blood oxygenation which exceeds the metabolic need (i.e. far more oxygen is delivered than is actually required).

Because the supply of oxygen exceeds demand, the excess oxygen is returned by the veins, causing a sudden increase in the amount of oxygenated hemoglobin of the venous return. The original (baseline) levels of deoxyhemoglobin in the blood would normally cause T2* and T2 to be decreased. (Remember, T2 is the natural decay of protons precessing in the transverse plane and T2* is the same decay within an inhomogeneous magnetic field.) Following the increase in the relative concentration of oxygenated hemoglobin of the venous blood (and the corresponding decrease in the amount of deoxyhemoglobin), T2* and T2 increase, leading to a small signal increase in T2- and T2*-weighted images. Although the relative sensitivity of this effect is low (the signal change is of the order of 1–3% at 1.5 T), the advent of rapid imaging techniques such as EPI have simplified its implementation, and BOLD contrast using gradient-echo imaging has emerged as the most commonly used fMRI method.

Advantages in BOLD contrast imaging

With BOLD contrast, several distinct advantages exist. First, it is, of course, completely non-invasive. Second, the functional contrast to noise is at least a factor of two to four greater than that seen in perfusion or in CBV-based imaging techniques. Third, it is easiest to implement since it only requires, typically, a gradient-echo sequence with an echo time (TE) of 30–40 ms. Fourth, the technique is fast enough to incorporate multislice, whole brain echo acquisition. All that is required is that the repetition time (TR) is long enough to accommodate all of the slices in each volume. Typically, with a TE of about 40 ms, the total time for acquiring a single-shot EPI is about 60–100 ms, which translates to a rate of 10–16 slices/s. This is a massive improvement in temporal resolution when compared with other techniques such as positron emission tomography (PET) or single photon emission computed tomography (SPECT). If a reduced number of slices is allowed, then a very short TR can be utilized for fine temporal mapping of the dynamics of the BOLD signal change.

Disadvantages in BOLD contrast imaging

Several disadvantages exist in regard to BOLD contrast imaging. First, the nature of the BOLD contrast is extremely complicated, involving the interplay of perfusion, $CMRO_2$ and blood volume changes, and is modulated by the heterogeneity of the vasculature and neurovascular coupling over time and space. This problem leads to limits of interpretation of the location, magnitude, linearity, and dynamics of the BOLD contrast signal. In addition, it makes across-population comparisons, clinical mapping and pharmacologic-effect mapping extremely challenging. This is because it is assumed that all these parameters hold true across brains and this may not necessarily be the case in the diseased brain. Second, when it comes to pharmacology, it is difficult to establish what effect the medication taken by the clinical populations may be having on CBF, neurovascular coupling, or both. Also, unlike the perfusion and volume mapping methods, no baseline oxygenation information can, as yet, be obtained, since resting state T2* and T2 times are dominated by tissue type rather than oxygenation state. However, progress is being made.[35] If resting state oxygenation information is implied, considerable assumptions have to be made regarding blood volume and vessel geometry, among other things. Another problem with BOLD contrast in general is that the same susceptibility weighting that allows for the observation of the functional contrast also contributes to many of the artifacts in the images used. These artifacts include signal dropout at tissue interfaces and at the base of the brain. This dropout occurs because the interfaces of tissues have different magnetic susceptibilities; the protons precess at different frequencies and begin to cancel each other out, and the loss of phase coherence occurs more rapidly. The problem becomes greater at higher field strengths.

Hemodynamic specificity

With the BOLD technique described above, the precise type of observable cerebrovascular information can be more finely delineated. While the information described below is typically more than most fMRI users are primarily concerned with, it is useful to have an abbreviated summary of how specific MRI can be. Please refer to Figure 1.5 for a schematic depiction of pulse sequence sensitization to specific vascular components and the heterogeneity of the vasculature across voxels. It shows intravascular and extravascular signals. If the specific vessel type is filled in (red, arteries; blue, veins), then there exists a contribution from intravascular effects (protons spinning in blood vessels). If the region around the vessel is filled in, then there are extravascular spins (water spins that are in the tissue); extravascular susceptibility gradients contribute to the functional contrast.

Regarding susceptibility contrast imaging, spin-echo sequences are more sensitive to small susceptibility compartments (capillaries and red blood

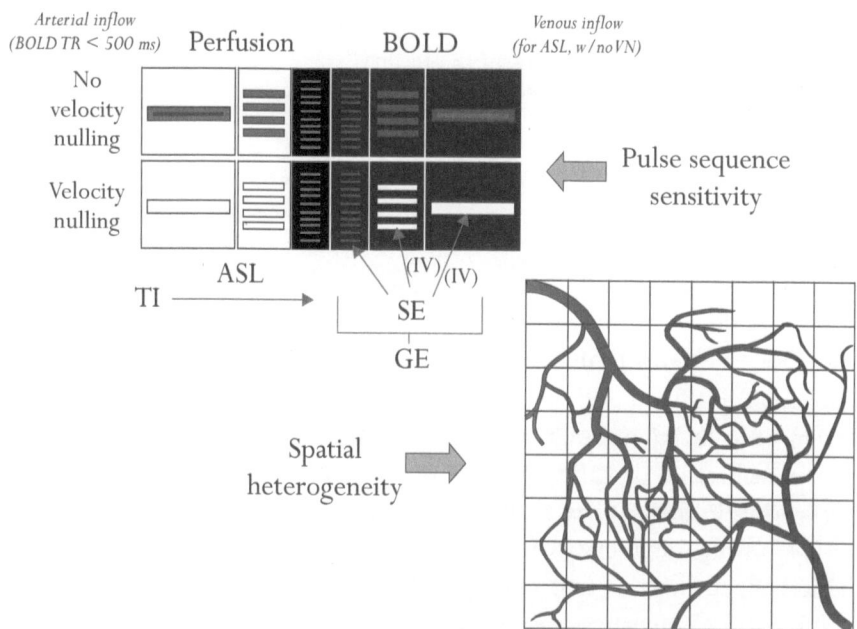

Figure 1.5 A schematic depiction of pulse sequence sensitization to specific vascular components and the heterogeneity of the vasculature across voxels ASL, Arterial spin labeling; BOLD, blood oxygenation-level dependent; GE, gradient echo; IV, intravascular; SE, spin echo; T1, a time constant; TR, time between successive radiofrequency pulses; VN, velocity nulling.

cells) and gradient-echo sequences are sensitive to susceptibility compartments of all sizes.[36–40] A common mistake is to assume that spin-echo sequences are sensitive to capillaries only. Since red blood cells are also small compartments, spin-echo sequences are selectively sensitive to intravascular signals arising from small and large vessels.[41] Since BOLD contrast is highly weighted by the resting state blood volume that happens to be in the voxel, it is likely that many voxels having pial vessels running through them will have at least 50% blood volume. These voxels are therefore likely to show the largest gradient-echo and spin-echo signal changes. At field strengths approaching 9 T, intravascular spins may no longer contribute since T2* and T2 of blood becomes extremely short.

Performing BOLD contrast fMRI at high field strengths has the same effect as diffusion weighting in the context of susceptibility-based contrast because T2* and T2 of venous blood become increasingly shorter than T2* and T2 of gray matter as field strength increases, therefore less signal will arise from intravascular space at higher field strengths.[4] This unique characteristic of imaging at high field strengths can be put to use in the creation of high-resolution *venograms* (vein maps of the brain).[4]

Mapping of $CMRO_2$ – advances in imaging

Recently, significant advances in mapping activation-induced changes in $CMRO_2$ using fMRI have emerged.[26,28,29,42] The basis for this method is the realization that the BOLD signal change between two levels of brain activity (baseline and some active state) can be modeled by an expression which combines the effect of the change in $CMRO_2$ and the change in CBF. The dependence of this BOLD signal change on CBF alone can be mapped by allowing subjects to perform the same task while breathing at least two different concentrations of CO_2 (hypercapnia).

Normalization or calibration using a hypercapnia stress (increasing the CO_2 levels in the air) has evolved to be a method for reducing the number of unknown parameters to allow for mapping of changes in $CMRO_2$.[26] The basic concept here is that when the brain is activated, increases in flow, volume and oxygenation are accompanied by an increase in $CMRO_2$. When a subject (at rest) is undergoing a hypercapnic stress [5% CO_2, i.e. the subject is breathing in a gas with a small proportion (1–5%) of CO_2 in it], only the CBF and CBV will change without an accompanying increase in $CMRO_2$. Therefore, less oxygen is extracted from the blood, allowing the blood oxygenation change, relative to the perfusion change, to be greater than with brain activation. The change in BOLD signal and the change in blood flow are separately measured at each level of hypercapnia.

If the change in the BOLD signal is plotted versus the measured change in blood flow, curves of constant $CMRO_2$ are obtained. When subjects performed the desired tasks, the measured changes in the BOLD signal and the CBF generate curves that travel between the iso-$CMRO_2$ contours. By comparing the ratio of the (simultaneously measured) perfusion and the BOLD signal changes during hypercapnia, and during brain activation, $CMRO_2$ information can be derived. The information is derived either by fitting the data to the model using the iso-$CMRO_2$ contours obtained in the first part of the experiment or by numerically interpolating the data.

Methods for extraction of baseline $CMRO_2$ are on the immediate horizon.[43] The key to these techniques is the more precise extraction of hemodynamic information, such as blood volume and blood oxygenation, and the use of appropriate calibration procedures.

$CMRO_2$ change mapping is still a work in progress. Its big potential is that the information is unique and perhaps most associated with neuronal activity. Of course, to derive this information, several still-unresolved assumptions about the hemodynamic changes with CO_2 stress, and about the perfusion and BOLD signal itself, have to be made. Since this method for mapping $CMRO_2$ changes uses techniques that simultaneously map perfusion and BOLD signals, it has all of the disadvantages of both techniques, and at least one more. The additional disadvantage is that it typically requires the subject to breathe a gas mixture of elevated CO_2 for at least 2 min. This is slightly uncomfortable for the motivated volunteer and may even be lethal to a patient. However, the data collected so far shows excellent agreement with data collected by alternative means. Furthermore, the models employed so far appear to be very robust and relatively insensitive to variations in the value of the empirical constants employed in the model.

Advancements in understanding the blood oxygenation-level-dependent (BOLD) signal

For many users, the issues involved in determining the precise neural underpinnings of BOLD contrast may seem an esoteric after > 10 years of successful implementation of fMRI. It is clear that changes in BOLD contrast-derived maps, for the most part, correlate well with maps derived using other techniques. BOLD is successful for these reasons. While the success of BOLD contrast has, of course, allowed new insights into human brain function to be derived, the technique can certainly have much more potential in regard to spatially resolved quantification of neuronal activity. We, as users, would love to use it for ever more applications: for more precise comparison of subject populations, parametric manipulations, and extraction of transient neuronal activity; for better understanding networked activity; for understanding coupling variations in disease and healthy subjects, and for deriving maps of resting state activity.

In this section, the specific characteristics, including location, latency, magnitude, and linearity of the fMRI signal, will be described in more detail. Emphasis will be placed on how this understanding relates to practical implementation of fMRI.

Location
In the resting state, hemoglobin oxygen saturation is about 95% in arteries and 60% in veins. The increase in hemoglobin saturation with activation is

25

largest in veins, changing in saturation from about 60–90%. Likewise, capillary blood changes from about 80–90% saturation. Arterial blood, already near saturation, shows no change.

The second reason why the strongest BOLD effect is seen in draining veins is that activation-induced BOLD contrast is highly weighted by blood volume in each voxel. Since capillaries are much smaller than a typical imaging voxel, most voxels, regardless of size, will likely contain about 2–4% capillary blood volume. In contrast, since the size and spacing of draining veins is on the same scale as most imaging voxels, it is likely that veins dominate the relative blood volume in any voxel that they pass through. Voxels that pial veins pass through can have 100% blood volume, while voxels that contain no pial veins may have only 2% blood volume. This stratification in blood volume distribution strongly determines the magnitude of the BOLD signal.

As illustrated in Figure 1.5, different RF pulse-sequence weightings can give different locations of activation. For instance, in regard to imaging perfusion and BOLD contrast, while much overlap is seen, the hot spots vary by as much as 10 mm. The perfusion change map is sensitive primarily to *capillary* perfusion changes, while the BOLD contrast activation map is weighted mostly by *veins*. A potential worry regarding fMRI location is that venous blood, flowing away from the activated area, may maintain its elevated oxygen saturation as far as 1 cm away. When observing brain activation on the scale of centimeters, this has not been of major concern; however, with increased spatial resolution this will likely become an important issue.

Latency

One of the first observations made regarding fMRI signal changes is that, after activation, the BOLD signal takes about 2–3 s to begin to deviate from baseline.[23,44] This is often referred to as the hemodynamic delay. This can be seen in the right-hand panel of Figure 1.2, where approximately 2 s elapse after stimulus presentation (at time 0) prior to an increase in the MRI signal. Since the BOLD signal is highly weighted towards venous oxygenation changes, with a flow increase, the time for venous oxygenation to start to increase will be about the time that it takes blood to travel from arteries to capillaries and draining veins – 2–3 s. The hemodynamic impulse response function has been effectively used to characterize much of the BOLD signal change dynamics[45–47] and has been derived empirically by delivering very brief and well-controlled stimuli. Additionally, it can be derived by deconvolving the stimulus input from the measured hemodynamic response.[48,49]

This type of analysis assumes that the BOLD response behaves in a manner that can be completely described by linear systems analysis, which is still an open issue.

If task onset or duration is modulated, the accuracy with which one can correlate the modulated input parameters (stimuli) to the measured output signal depends on the variability of the signal within a voxel or region of interest. In a study by Savoy et al,[50] addressing this issue, variability of several temporal sections of a stimulus-induced response were determined. Six subjects were studied and, for each subject, 10 activation-induced response curves were analyzed. The relative onsets were determined by finding the latency with which the correlation coefficient was maximized with each of three reference functions, representing three parts of the response curve – the entire curve, the rising section, and the falling section. The standard deviation (SD) of the whole curve, rising phase, and falling phase were found to be 650, 1250, and 450 ms, respectively.[51] Across-region differences in the onset and return to baseline of the BOLD signal during primary visual activation[52] and cognitive tasks have been observed.[53] For example, during a visually presented, event-related, word-stem completion task, Buckner et al[53] reported that the signal in the visual cortex increased about 1 s before the signal in the left anterior prefrontal cortex. One might argue that this observation makes sense from a cognitive perspective, since the subject first observes the word stem then, after about 1 s, generates a word to complete this task. Others would argue that the neuronal onset latencies should not be > 200 ms. Can inferences of the cascade of brain activation be made on this timescale from fMRI data? Without a method to constrain, or work around, the intrinsic variability of the onset of the BOLD signal over space, such inferences should not be made in temporal latency differences < 4 s. Combined techniques, such as fMRI with electroencephalography (EEG), are currently under development to address these issues.

Lee et al[54] were the first to observe that the fMRI signal change onset within the visual cortex during simple visual stimulation varied from 6 to 12 s. These latencies were also shown to correlate with the underlying vascular structure. The earliest onset of the signal change appeared to be in gray matter and the latest onset appeared to occur in the largest draining veins. Similar latency dispersions in the motor cortex have been observed. In one study, latency differences, detected in the visual cortex using the Hilbert transform, did not show a clear correlation of latency with evidence for draining veins.[55]

Magnitude

The magnitude of the fMRI signal change is influenced by variables which can vary across subjects, neuronal systems, and voxels.[39] To make a complete and direct correlation between neuronal activity and the fMRI signal change magnitude, in a single experiment, all the variables which influence these changes must be characterized on a voxel-wise basis. Because of these primarily physiologic variables, brain activation maps typically show a range of BOLD signal change with magnitudes of 1–5% (at 1.5 T, GE sequence, TE = 40 ms), and higher with greater field strengths (up to 15% at 4 T). In the past several years, considerable progress has been made in characterizing the magnitude of the fMRI signal change with underlying neuronal activity. Figure 1.6 shows a flow chart roughly outlining both the complicating factors behind the fMRI signal as well as the richness of information contained within it.

First, it was clear that areas that showed significant BOLD signal change were in the appropriate neuronal area corresponding to specific well-characterized tasks. Second, inferred neuronal modulation was carried out by systematically varying some aspect of the task. Clear correlations

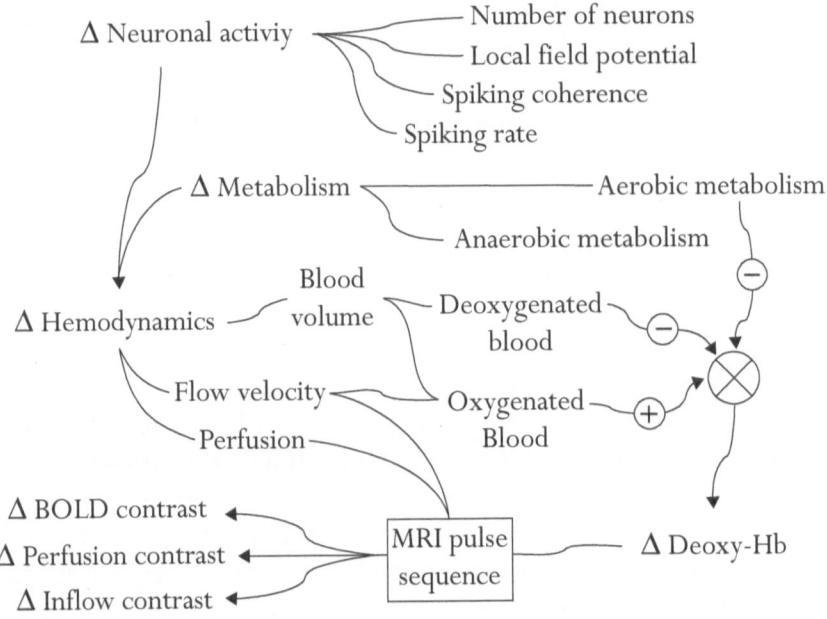

Figure 1.6 Flow chart outlining both the complicating factors behind the functional magnetic resonance imaging (fMRI) signal as well as the richness of information contained within it.

between BOLD signal change magnitude and visual flicker rate, contrast, word presentation rate, and finger-tapping rate were observed.[3,56–58]

Recently, several studies have emerged correlating measured neuronal firing rate with well-known stimuli in animals[59] and humans,[60,61] demonstrating a high correlation between BOLD signal change and electrophysiological measures. A recent article by Logothetis et al[62] described the simultaneous measurement of electrical activity and BOLD contrast in primate visual cortex, and revealed a linear relationship between neuronal activity and stimuli contrast, albeit with one caveat – the lower the level of neuronal activity, the more BOLD contrast overestimated the degree of neuronal activity. In other words, BOLD contrast does indeed change in proportion to the degree of neuronal activity, but the relative rate at which it changes with neuronal activity is generally less. Results from this article have not only impacted how fMRI signal changes are interpreted in terms of magnitude of change with a change in a task but have also shed light on some issues regarding the dynamics of fMRI contrast, as described below.

Linearity

Understanding the relationship between fMRI signal change magnitude and neuronal firing rate is critically important for both the clearer interpretation of experimental results and also for experimental design. Described above was the relationship between BOLD signal change magnitude and neuronal activity at a steady state, or after several seconds of continuous activity. Described in this section is the relationship between BOLD contrast and neuronal activity over time during very brief neuronal stimulation. Does the BOLD signal change increase in a manner that is directly linear with stimulus duration? It has been found that, with very brief stimulus durations, the BOLD response shows a larger signal change magnitude than expected from a linear system.[63,64] This greater than expected BOLD signal change is generally specific to stimuli durations < 3 s. Reasons for a greater than expected event-related response may be neuronal, hemodynamic, and/or metabolic in nature. The neuronal input may not be a simple boxcar function. Instead, an increased neuronal firing rate at the onset of stimulation (neuronal 'bursting') may cause a slightly larger amount of vasodilatation that later plateaus at a lower steady state level. Results from Logothetis et al[62] have demonstrated clearly this 'bursting' at the onset of visual stimulation. In the visual cortex, this effect has been extremely well characterized in past literature describing single unit recordings.

BOLD contrast is highly sensitive to the interplay of blood flow, blood volume, and oxidative metabolic rate. If, with activation, any one of these variables changes with a different time constant, the fMRI signal may show fluctuations until a steady state is reached.[65,66]

It is clear that, in spite of the widespread use of fMRI and the success that the method has had in the study of brain function, there are still a lot of unanswered questions about the specific manner in which physiological, metabolic, and vascular aspects interact in response to increased neuronal activity, and how they manifest themselves in the BOLD response. However, the elucidation of these questions constitutes one of the most interesting aspects of this field, and current investigations are encouraging.

Positron emission tomography (PET) and single photon emission computed tomography (SPECT)

Since Langley's (1878) hypothesis of 'receptive substances' involved in the response to pharmacological agents, much work has been done to reach the current concept of neuroreceptors.[67] They consist of large protein or glyco-protein molecules commonly located on the cell surface, which are responsible for mediating the action of both endogenous neurotransmitters and exogenous pharmacologic agents in the nervous system. Several neurotransmitters and respective receptors have been characterized and implicated in brain physiology.

Using radioactive-labeled ligands and autoradiographic techniques, it is possible to visualize the distribution of several kinds of neuroreceptors *in vitro* and *ex vivo*. The same principles have now been applied to allow the visualization and measurement of neuroreceptors *in vivo*. PET and SPECT provide a unique means to investigate neurochemical abnormalities in neuro-psychiatric conditions, as well as to study the mechanisms of action of drugs.[68] This section will briefly review some basic aspects of PET and SPECT neuroreceptor imaging as a basis for understanding data presented in the following chapters of this book.

Basic principles of PET and SPECT

Emission tomography techniques are based on the *in vivo* administration of radioisotope-labeled tracers or ligands (radiotracer/radioligand) with affinity for the target structures (e.g. neuroreceptors and enzymes). The radioisotopes are unstable (proton-rich nuclides) and decay to a more stable state emitting gamma (γ) rays in the process. PET or SPECT cameras are able to detect the emitted γ-rays and provide a tomographic image of the distribution of the tracer in different regions of the body.

PET tracers are labeled with radioisotopes such as ^{11}C, ^{18}F and [76]Br, that emit positrons (β[+] particles), which, after travelling a short distance in tissue, collide with surrounding electrons to form a positronium.[69] Almost instantaneously, the positronium annihilates, forming two photons (γ-rays) of 511 keV, which are released in opposite directions at 180° (Figure 1.7a). Detection of the photons is based on the trajectory and the timing of impact on the camera's detector. The photons are detected or counted if both hit the detector (so-called coincidence detection).[69] The 180° geometry permits good accuracy for localizing the source of the energy along a straight line.

SPECT radiotracers are labeled with photon-emitter isotopes such as ^{123}I and technetium-99m (Tc-99m). Photon-emitter isotopes have unstable nuclei due to a deficiency in the number of neutrons and may, as an alternative to positron emission, capture an orbiting electron into the nuclei.[70] The captured electron transforms a proton into a neutron, emitting a cluster of photons (γ-ray) in the process. Emissions of photons occur randomly and in 360° geometry (Figure 1.7b). Each emitted photon is singular and independent in

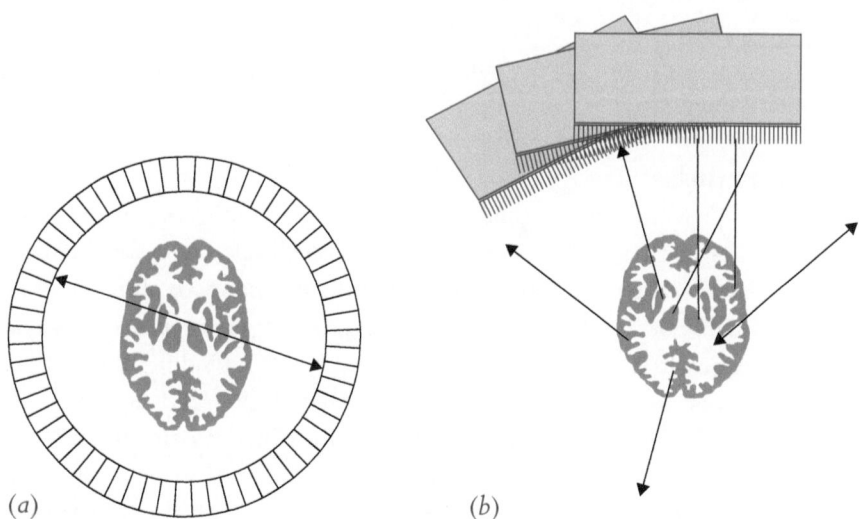

(a)   (b)

Figure 1.7 (a) Positron emission tomography (PET) (adapted from Meikle and Dahlbom[69]); (b) single photon emission computed tomography (SPECT) (adapted from Distance Assisted Training Program for Nuclear Medicine Technologists, 2000, http://casino.cchs.usyd.edu.au/mrs/iaea/)

nature, hence single photon.[71,72] In brain SPECT the detectors rotate around the subject's head and the data are acquired over 360°.

PET and SPECT gamma cameras detect the emitted γ-rays when they hit crystals in the surrounding detectors. The light energy generated in the crystals is converted to an amplified electrical pulse through the photomultiplier tubes, which allows the computer to map different intensities of energy onto a frequency map in three dimensions, where energy is characterized according to intensity with a pulse height analyzer.[73]

SPECT cameras use collimators (lead sheets with thin holes) to prevent photons outside the line of a particular plane from impacting on the detectors (Figure 1.5b). Any photon that reaches the detector is assumed to originate from a particular plane in the subject directly beneath and parallel to the holes in the collimator. Although collimators are crucial for SPECT imaging, they are also the limiting factor for sensitivity (number of photons that pass through the collimator) and resolution (number of photons excluded to minimize detection of scatter and attenuated photons).[71]

PET imaging has generally higher sensitivity and resolution due to the 180° coincidence event, which eliminates the need for physical collimation. Problems such as scatter (γ-rays impacting on the detector away from their line of trajectory) and attenuation (γ-rays slowed by progress through the tissues) are minimized in PET. However, new SPECT cameras and computational methods for scatter and attenuation correction have significantly improved the quality of SPECT images, narrowing the gap with PET imaging.[74]

Radioligands

In order to provide accurate binding estimates the radioligands need to fulfil several criteria.[75] High affinity (nM range) and high selectivity for the target receptor are essential. Minimal lipophilicity is necessary to allow easy and rapid crossing of the blood–brain barrier, but high lipophilicity is not desirable since it is associated with high non-specific binding. Insignificant metabolism is desirable, such that labeled metabolites do not cross the blood–brain barrier to interact with the target binding site during data acquisition. Lack of pharmacological effect at tracer doses (< 100 pmol) and safety for intravenous (IV) injection is necessary. Finally, the labeling process has to be amenable so that the scans can proceed within the time constrains of the radioisotope's half-life.[68]

The development of radioligands that match the above requisites is not an easy process. Radioligands are the limiting factor in the investigation of neuroreceptor systems. There are PET and SPECT tracers for some receptor systems, such as dopamine (D1, D2, and dopamine transporter), serotonin [(5-hydroxytryptamine) $5HT_{1A}$, $5HT_{2A}$, and serotonin transporter], gamma-aminobutyric acid [(GABA) $GABA_A$], opiate, cholinergic (muscarinic and nicotinic) and for the enzyme amino acid decarboxylase (AADC).[76] Many interesting targets are lacking appropriate radioligands for *in vivo* investigation. Work is in progress towards developing suitable radioligands for neurotransmitter systems that are highly relevant for neuropsychiatric disorders, but hitherto have not been investigated *in vivo*, such as the glutamatergic system [N-methyl-D-aspartate (NMDA), AMPA, kainate and metabotropic receptors].

Data acquisition

Dynamic imaging protocols are currently preferred to obtain PET and SPECT receptor binding data. These involve the acquisition of sequential images of the same regions over time after radioligand administration. The region-of-interest (ROI) approach is the most commonly employed for analysing receptor images. Regions of interest are defined around brain areas of interest, and regional measures of radioligand uptake obtained in different moments. This process allows the generation of radiotracer uptake and washout.

In vivo neuroreceptor quantification

Basic principles

The principles of *in vivo* neuroreceptor imaging are based on *in vitro* receptor pharmacology, with the advantage that they investigate functional receptors in living brains, preserving the receptor's natural environment.

The outcome measures most commonly used in *in vitro* pharmacology are the equilibrium dissociation constant (K_D) and the receptor density (B_{max}).[77] K_D is the ratio of the rate of association constant (K_{on}) and the rate of dissociation constant (K_{off}) at equilibrium. K_D describes inverse binding affinity of the ligand for a determined receptor (the lower K_D the greater the binding affinity). B_{max} is the density of receptors (receptor number per tissue volume) and corresponds to the ligand concentration specifically bound to the receptor at saturation point.

In vitro receptor pharmacology is not easily applied to neuroreceptor imaging. The general principle underlying neuroreceptor imaging is that the regional uptake of the radiotracer will be related to the number of receptors for which the tracer exhibits selective affinity.[78] Unlike *in vitro* studies where radioligand concentration is tightly controlled, many variables determine radioligand availability *in vivo*, including: (1) blood–brain barrier permeability;

33

(2) non-specific binding in the brain; (3) regional CBF (rCBF); (4) rate of peripheral clearance; (5) binding to plasma proteins; (6) potential penetration of radiolabeled metabolites; (7) concentration of endogenous competitor; and (8) partial voluming and cross-scattering from adjacent brain regions.[78,79] These variables have to be taken into account otherwise binding parameters may only remotely relate to the receptor concentration.

The methods to evaluate receptor parameters *in vivo* with SPECT and PET can be divided in two, *quantitative* and *semiquantitative*. The most commonly used outcome measures are the binding potential (*BP*) and the total volume of distribution (V_T). *BP* is the total number of receptors multiplied by their affinity for the radioligand ($BP = B_{max}/K_D$). VT, which is defined as the equilibrium ratio of the total concentration of tracer in tissue to the total concentration of parent tracer in plasma. VT represents the volume of tracer from the plasma that is extracted by the tissue, thus it expressed in mL plasma/mL tissue. This is a robust parameter, for reversible kinetics, proportional to the specific binding in a brain region and independent of blood flow.

Semiquantitative methods
Among the semiquantitative methods, the *ratio method* is the most commonly used, calculated by the formula: $BP' = (R_R - R_T)/R_R$, where R_T (target region) is the concentration of activity in the brain regions that are rich in receptors and R_R (reference region) is the concentration of activity in the brain area devoid of receptors. R_T and R_R are defined based on receptor concentrations from post-mortem autoradiography studies. The activity in the target region represents non-specific uptake plus free ligand (C_{NS}) and specific binding (C_S), whereas in the reference region it represents only C_{NS} (Figure 1.6). The reference region is used to subtract C_{NS} of the target region in order to measure C_S. This ratio method provides an approximation to the saturable component of binding (BP'), and is therefore linearly proportional to B_{max} when calculated at equilibrium. There are problems in determining equilibrium in these studies, and the ability of semiquantitative methods to provide an accurate value for *BP* needs to be validated by model-based methods.[79]

Quantitative methods
Model-based methods were developed to provide *in vivo* quantitative estimates of receptor number and affinity. These methods can be divided into *kinetic modeling* and *equilibrium methods*. The *BP* value calculated with quantitative methods incorporates measurements of local radioactivity in the brain tissue and the radioligand input to the brain (arterial concentration) as a

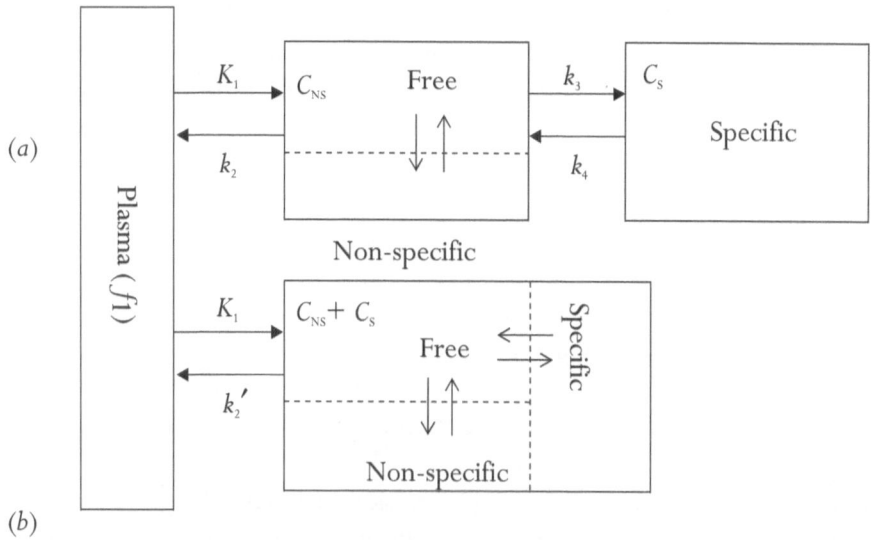

Figure 1.8 *Compartment models. (a) Graphic representation of the two-tissue compartment model (2-TC), where the plasma compartment is the input function and f_1 is the free fraction of the tracer. The C_{NS} compartment represents non-specific and free tracer, and the C_S compartment represents specific binding. (b) Graphic representation of the one-tissue compartment model (1-TC), which has the same input function from the plasma compartment, but C_{NS} and C_S are combined in one compartment.*

function of time.[79] Mintun et al[77] introduced a compartmental *kinetic model* to measure neuroreceptor ligand binding, in which mathematical models try to characterize the kinetics of the radiotracer between plasma, brain and receptor compartments by estimating the rate constants (K) (Figure 1.8).

Two compartmental models are commonly described – a two-tissue compartment model (2-TC model; Figure 1.8a) and a one-tissue compartment model (1-TC model; Figure 1.8b). The 2-TC model assumes that the free and non-specifically bound compartments equilibrate rapidly and may then be considered as a single compartment yielding the following parameterization: K_1 (plasma to tissue influx constant), k_2 (tissue to plasma efflux constant), $k_3 = f_2 k_{on} B_A$ (k_3' pseudo first-order association rate constant, f_2 is the tissue-free fraction of the tracer, k_{on} is the first-order bimolecular association rate constant and B_A is the concentration of available binding sites); $k_4 = k_{off}$ (disassociation rate constant). The 1-TC model assumes that the free, non-specifically bound and specifically bound compartments all equilibrate rapidly, and may then be considered as a single compartment yielding the following parameterization; K_1 (plasma to tissue influx constant) and k_2'

[tissue to plasma efflux constant: $k_2' = k_2/(1 + k_3/k_4)$]. The compartmental model estimates BP using the rate constants obtained in the compartmental analysis, where $BP = K_1k_3/k_2k_4f_1$ (f_1 is the plasma-free fraction of the tracer). Quantitative estimation of BP has been widely used in PET, and has been successfully incorporated to SPECT studies.[80,81] Different model-based methods using on this formulation have been validated to estimate binding parameters including *kinetic analysis*,[77] *graphic models*,[82] and the *reference tissue model*.[83]

The *equilibrium method* is a model-based analysis performed when radioligand distribution is at equilibrium, i.e. when receptor–ligand association and dissociation rates are equal.[80,84,85] Equilibrium is obtained through a bolus plus constant infusion of the radioligand. This paradigm simplifies receptor quantification. It allows the estimation of V_T, defined as the ratio at true equilibrium of total tissue concentration to a reference concentration (e.g. free metabolite-corrected plasma concentration). BP is calculated using the ratio of V_T measurements from regions with specific and non-specific uptake, under the assumption of uniform non-specific binding.[86] Equilibrium studies with constant infusion and can provide a stable baseline for pharmacological challenge experiments.[87]

Specific technical issues

Many factors can influence the quality of receptor imaging data, e.g. the specific sensitivity of the PET and SPECT cameras, accurate and reliable delineation of ROI, duration of the scan, patient motion between scans, and general suitability of analytical imaging techniques. Careful procedures should be implemented to address these problems, such as the use of fiducial markers (i.e. little sticks containing a tiny bit of radiation that are placed on the subjects head), which help in improving post-acquisition data realignment; head fixation with masks; anatomically guided ROI analysis, ideally guided by a structural MRI of the same subject or via spatial normalization to standard templates; and use of validated model-based analysis.

A major advantage of these radiotracer techniques is extraordinary high sensitivity (about 10^{-9}–10^{-12} M), many orders of magnitude greater than the sensitivities available with MRI (about 10^{-4} M) or MR spectroscopy (about 10^{-3}–10^{-5} M).[68] In terms of spatial resolution, the gap between PET and SPECT has been narrowing. Given ideal imaging conditions, 4–5 mm full width at half maximum (FWHM) is achievable with PET while 8–10 mm FWHM is achievable with SPECT.[3] Progress has recently been made with animal-dedicated PET devices achieving resolutions of about 1–2 mm.

Emission tomography scans implicate exposure to ionizing radiation, which restricts its use under some conditions. Exposition to radiation is a potential risk for the fetus, so pregnancy has to be checked before each scan. Previous exposition to ionizing radiation can be a contraindication to scans. The number of research scans that can be conducted in 1 year is generally limited to two, sometimes four. This is a potential problem for longitudinal studies, such as follow-up studies evaluating the effects of treatment on neuroreceptors. Studies evaluating acute pharmacological challenges can either be performed in a two-scan protocol (baseline and challenge), or in a one-scan protocol using bolus plus constant infusion of the radiotracer. Each radiotracer allows the investigation of one receptor system, and exposure to radiation limits the receptor systems that can be checked in the same subject. Although emission tomography techniques have molecular sensitivity, the number of conditions that can be tested in each study is infinitely inferior to fMRI studies.

Methodology

The preceding sections have provided an introduction to the principles behind the information contained in the MR signal. A description of how and what is acquired with PET and SPECT has also been provided. The hardware used to acquire and process the signal, and some advances in these systems, have also been described.

A further aspect in the understanding of functional neuroimaging is the methodology used by the researcher. Methodology is defined here as the strategies by which the technology and the understanding of the signal are brought to bear on specific applications. While this definition can be quite broad, covering everything including subject handling, subject interface, data processing, and data pooling, the focus in this section is primarily concerned with how neuronal activation paradigms can be designed. A schematic summary of these strategies is shown in Figure 1.9. A description of each of these is given below.

Block design

Block design paradigms are the classical paradigm used in fMRI and are widely reported in the current literature. Essentially adapted from PET paradigm designs, a block design requires a subject to perform a task for

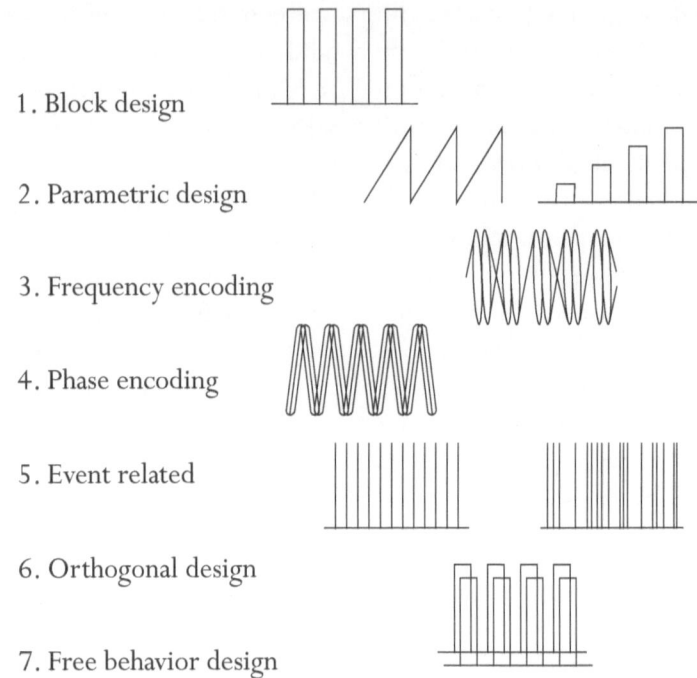

1. Block design

2. Parametric design

3. Frequency encoding

4. Phase encoding

5. Event related

6. Orthogonal design

7. Free behavior design

Figure 1.9 *Various neuronal input strategies.*

at least 10 s (to reach a hemodynamically steady state), alternated for a similar amount of time with one (AB) or multiple (ABC or ABCD, for example) control tasks. The control task might be something as simple as a fixation cross or more complex. The central tenet of this method is that experimental condition A contains identical cognitive elements to control task B with the addition of the cognitive process of interest. For example, in a study looking at the perception of fear in facial expressions, one control condition might be a face expressing no emotion (neutral) or a different emotion (happy), which would be contrasted with the experimental condition, i.e. a face expressing fear. In this example, all the elements of the experimental condition are also in the control condition (attending to and processing a complex facial stimulus), and only the experimental condition contains what is of interest, i.e. the element of fear. Within each block it is advisable to present your stimulus as many times as possible as it is thought that an increase in the S:R ratio can be obtained with repeated presentation. The drawback of this design is that it is based on a model of pure insertion,[88] which assumes that there are no interactions between the cognitive components of the two conditions.

This may be a useful way of conceptualizing cognitive processes at a behavioral level but neuroimaging investigations suggest that the brain is a highly non-linear system and thus the pure insertion model may not necessarily be appropriate.

There are several reasons to use a block design paradigm. There is an increased S:R ratio over multiple presentations of the stimulus, analysis and interpretation are relatively simple, and it is a useful technique for measuring a physiological state that is sustained over a fairly long (about 1–2 min) period. There are also, however, some limitations which should be borne in mind at the design stage. There may be potential confounds from maintaining attentional and cognitive set, e.g. boredom, reduced attention, habituation or fatigue. This type of design may not be suitable for questions pertaining to cognitive processes that operate on a very short time-scale. Lastly, it is not possible to randomize the presentation of items within each block, although counterbalancing presentation across subjects can, to a certain degree, overcome this problem.

Parametric designs

Parametric designs make the assumption that neuronal activity is a function of stimulus strength or intensity. It was observed that the fMRI signal increases with the level of intensity of the stimulus and therefore by varying the intensity of the stimulus it is possible to characterize how the brain responds to these changes.[3,56,57] The essential aspect of parametrically designed experiments is that the task itself is varied in some systematic fashion and the corresponding changes in the brain are compared, rather than simply the magnitudes themselves against a single control task. Taking the example from above (see Block design section above), one might compare faces displaying 50 or 100% expressions of fear. The results from tasks such as these are more directly interpretable in that if only two conditions are compared (as in a block design). When the task is systematically varied (as with parametric designs), and the slopes compared on a voxel-wise basis, the spatial variations in blood volume and other physiologic factors not related to brain activation are controlled to some degree. Parametric designs can involve continuous variation of the stimuli or can be set up in a blocked fashion, with each block involving a different degree or intensity of stimulation. As an example of the latter, taking the fearful faces experiment as an example, you might have one block of neutral faces, a second block of mildly fearful faces (50%) and a third block of prototypically (100%) fearful faces.

Frequency encoding

Frequency encoding is probably the least common of task designs but perhaps lends itself optimally to very specific types of stimuli. The method involves designating a specific on–off frequency for each type of stimulus used. Using Fourier analysis to analyze the data reveals the maximum power under a specific spectral peak corresponding to the brain area specific to the particular on–off frequency. The utility of this method has been demonstrated in the mapping of left and right motor cortex by cueing the subject to perform a finger-tapping task at different on–off rates for each hand.[89,90] In general, the goal of any paradigm design is to encode as much information as possible into a single time series. This allows more precise comparisons since a primary source of error is variation across time series due to scanner instabilities or subject movement. Keeping as many comparisons as possible in one time series is one method to reduce the effects of these variations.

Phase encoding

Phase encoding the stimulus input involves varying some aspect of the stimuli in a continuous and cyclic manner. This strategy has been most successfully used in performing retinotopic mapping.[91–93] In this type of study, a visual stimulus ring is continuously varied in eccentricity then, after the most extreme eccentricity is reached, the cycle is repeated again. The data are then typically analyzed using Fourier analysis, mapping out the areas that show a signal change temporal phase that correlates with the stimulus phase. This is a powerful technique since it makes use of the entire time series in that there are no 'off' states. This method also lends itself to Fourier analysis, and has also been used for somatotopic[94], and tonotopic mapping.[95]

Event-related designs

Increasingly, researchers are beginning to use event-related designs in fMRI. Before 1995, a critical question in event-related fMRI was whether a transient cognitive activation could elicit a significant and usable fMRI signal change. In 1996, Buckner et al[53] demonstrated that, in fact, event-related fMRI lent itself quite well to cognitive neuroscience questions. In their study, a word-stem completion task was performed using a block-design strategy and an event-related strategy. Robust activation in the regions involved with word generation were observed using both methodologies. The advantages of event-related activation strategies are many:[96] tasks can be better randomized,[97–99] fMRI analysis can be conducted based on measured behavioral responses to individual trials,[100] and there is the option to incorporate overt responses into a time series (e.g. a verbal response by the subject). Practice and habituation effects can also be minimized.

One disadvantage of event-related designs is the fact that since (as pointed out above) the BOLD signal change is measured from a single stimulus, many more trials have to be repeated to obtain sufficient S:N ratios. Since the responses need to be singularly and unambiguously assigned to each event, the interstimulus time needs to be at least as long as the typical width of the BOLD response curve (8–10 s). Therefore, these experiments need to be very long, and become prohibitively long for certain subject populations such as children and the elderly.

When using a constant interstimulus interval (ISI), such as might be used in a block-design paradigm, the optimal ISI is about 10–12 s. Dale[101] showed that responses to visual stimuli, presented as rapidly as once every 1 s, can be adequately separated using overlap correction methods. Overlap correction methods are only possible if the ISI is varied during the time series. These results appear to demonstrate that the hemodynamic response is sufficiently linear, or at least additive, to apply deconvolution methods to extract overlapping responses. Burock et al[102] has demonstrated that remarkably clean activation maps can be created using an average ISI of 500 ms. Assuming the hemodynamic response is essentially a linear system, there appears to be no obvious minimum ISI when trying to estimate it. Dale[101] suggested that an exponential distribution of ISI, having a mean as short as is psychophysically possible, is optimal for estimation of the individual hemodynamic responses of each stimulus. One rate-limiting factor in stimulus presentation depends on the study being performed. Many cognitive tasks may require a slightly longer average presentation rate. Additionally, it is possible that for very short ISI (e.g. < 50 ms) there may be logistical difficulties in physically presented stimuli at that speed due to slower refresh rates on presentation screens.

Recent studies by Liu et al[103] and Birn at al[104] have helped to determine the optimal timing parameters to use when performing variable ISI event-related studies. It turns out that the optimal design depends on the question being asked. If one is interested in simply making the most robust map of activation, the longer the stimulation duration the better, and the optimal ISI is such that the average ISI is the stimulus duration, resulting in a 50/50 distribution of on versus off time. If one is interested in creating the most accurate estimate of the hemodynamic response, say for comparisons of subtle changes in activation in a predetermined region, then the shorter the task duration the better.

Orthogonal designs

Orthogonal task design is a powerful extension of block-design studies. The basic concept is that if one designs two different task timings that would create BOLD responses that are orthogonal to each other (i.e. their vector product is zero), then these tasks can be performed simultaneously during a single time series collection with no cross-task interference, making comparison much more precise. This technique was first demonstrated by Courtney et al.[105] In their study, six orthogonal tasks were designed into a single time series. This type of design also lends itself to event-related studies. For example, in a study looking at auditory and visual processing simultaneously, the same time series can be used to collect information from both 'studies', as they elicit orthogonal BOLD responses (they have no temporal correlation with each other).

Free behavior designs

For many types of cognitive neuroscience questions, it is not possible to precisely constrain the timing or performance of a task. It is necessary then to allow the subject to perform the task 'freely' and take a continuous measurement of the performance (e.g. SCR or change in blood pressure), then use this other measurement as a reference function for subsequent time series analysis. Examples of this type of design are emerging. As an example, changes in skin conductance are difficult to predict or control. In a study by Patterson et al,[106] skin conductance was simultaneously recorded during an array of tasks and during a rest period. The skin conductance signal change was then used as a reference function in the fMRI time series analysis. Several cortical and subcortical regions were shown to have signal changes that were highly correlated with the skin conductance changes. Similarly, this type of design has been used successfully to reveal areas of the brain that are active in patients with schizophrenia during hallucinations. McGuire and colleagues[107] asked subjects to indicate with a button press when they were hearing voices throughout the scanning session, and these responses were later used as an input function in the analysis stage.

Applications

Over the past decade, applications of fMRI have expanded as the technology, methodology, and interpretation has improved. Two primary areas of application have included basic research – understanding the organization of the healthy human brain – and clinical research.

Basic research has involved describing, with greater precision and robustness, the functional anatomy of systems in the developing and adult brain, including motor, visual, auditory, tactile, taste, language, attention, emotion, learning, priming, plasticity, and memory.

Clinical research has involved two primary avenues. The first is towards robust daily clinical application. This depends on the creation of a means by which all types of patients can be rapidly and reproducibly scanned for the purposes of presurgical mapping, perfusion assessment or vascular reserve assessment. Using fMRI in the clinic requires the implementation of a method by which immediate feedback is provided to the user to ensure quality control, accurate functional localization, sufficient brain coverage, and implementation of methods by which regions of activation are rapidly registered to useful anatomical landmarks that can then be used as guides in the context of neurosurgical procedures. The second clinical application has been towards understanding the neural correlates of specific neurological and psychiatric disorders. This can include testing the integrity of basic sensory systems in various disorders (such as visual or auditory) up to exploring far more complicated brain responses to particular symptoms (as in a symptom challenge study). Reviews of the current neuroimaging literature for psychiatric disorders are provided in the following chapters. Steady progress is being made towards using fMRI to better understand human brain organization, and on a meaningful temporal and spatial scale. The advantage of being able to scan individuals repeatedly over time has addressed questions of etiology and disease progression. Similarly, particular patterns of brain activity over time can inform particular predictors of response to certain medications.

Applications of neuroreceptor imaging

The main applications of neuroreceptor imaging are to investigate the pathophysiology of neuropsychiatric disorders and to evaluate interactions of pharmacological agents with receptor systems.[67] In the pathophysiology of neuropsychiatric conditions, these techniques can investigate issues such as regional abnormalities of receptor density, correlations between receptor-binding parameters and clinical variables, neurotransmitter concentrations, and response to pharmacological challenges. In psychopharmacology, these techniques are useful to investigate the receptor-binding profile of drugs, potency of psychotropic drugs (displacement studies), the dose–receptor-occupancy relationship, receptor occupancy and outcome variables, clinical efficacy and side effects, and in therapeutic drug development (radiolabeling of the drugs allows determination of blood–brain barrier penetration, brain distribution, receptor binding and dosing).

The future possibilities of radiotracer imaging are broad and exciting, going beyond neuroreceptors to include transporters, enzymes, signal transduction and gene expression. For this broader perspective, PET and SPECT methodologies have been described as '*in vivo* molecular imaging', which promises to help answer new scientific questions.[68]

Conclusions

The aim of this chapter was to provide the reader with a brief overview of the principles of MRI, PET and SPECT. Furthermore, it is hoped that some understanding of the hardware used in the neuroimaging environment has been obtained, along with insight into how these technologies are developing in order to better address specific research questions. The goal was that the reader come away with a better perspective of what can be done, as well as what may be possible with MRI, fMRI, PET and SPECT. These techniques have developed considerably since the first noisy signals were observed over a decade ago, yet significant developments are required technologically, and in methodology, interpretation and applications.

References

1. Bandettini PA, Wong EC, Hinks RS, Tikofsky RS, Hyde JS. Time course EPI of human brain function during task activation. *Magn Reson Med* 1992; **25:** 390–7.
2. Ogawa S, Tank DW, Menon R et al. Intrinsic signal changes accompanying sensory stimulation: functional brain mapping with magnetic resonance imaging. *Proc Natl Acad Sci USA* 1992; **89:** 5951–5.
3. Kwong KK, Belliveau JW, Chesler DA et al. Dynamic magnetic resonance imaging of human brain activity during primary sensory stimulation. *Proc Natl Acad Sci USA* 1992; **89:** 5675–9.
4. Menon RS, Ogawa S, Tank DW, Ugurbil K. 4 tesla gradient recalled echo characteristics of photic stimulation – induced signal changes in the human primary visual cortex. *Magn Reson Med* 1993; **30:** 380–6.
5. Turner R, Jezzard P, Wen H et al. Functional mapping of the human visual cortex at 4 and 1.5 tesla using deoxygenation contrast EPI. *Magn Reson Med* 1993; **29:** 277–9.

6. Gati JS, Menon RS, Ugurbil K, Rutt BK. Experimental determination of the BOLD field strength dependence in vessels and tissue. *Magn Reson Med* 1997; **38:** 296–302.

7. Noll D. A primer on MRI and functional MRI (Version 2.1, 6/21/01). http://www.bme.umich.edu/~dnoll/primer2.pdf.

8. Lauterbur PC. Imager formation by induced local interactions. Examples employing nuclear magnetic resonance. *Nature* 1973; **242:** 190–1.

9. Mansfield P, Grannell PK. Diffraction and microscopy in solids and liquids by NMR. *Phys Rev B* 1975; **12:** 3618–34.

10. Cohen MS, Weisskoff RM. Ultra-fast imaging. *Magn Reson Imaging* 1991; **9:** 1–37.

11. Howseman AM, Grootoonk S, Porter DA et al. The effect of slice order and thickness on fMRI activation data using multislice echo-planar imaging. *Neuroimage* 1999; **9:** 363–76.

12. Rosen BR, Belliveau JW, Aronen HJ et al. Susceptibility contrast imaging of cerebral blood volume: human experience. *Magn Reson Med* 1991; **22:** 293–9.

13. Rosen BR, Belliveau JW, Chien D. Perfusion imaging by nuclear magnetic resonance. *Magn Reson Quart* 1989; **5:** 263–81.

14. Belliveau JW, Kennedy DN, McKinstry RC et al. Functional mapping of the human visual cortex by magnetic resonance imaging. *Science* 1991; **254:** 716–19.

15. Williams DS, Detre JA, Leigh JS, Koretsky AS. Magnetic resonance imaging of perfusion using spin-inversion of arterial water. *Proc Natl Acad Sci USA* 1992; **89:** 212–16.

16. Detre JA, Leigh JS, Williams DS, Koretsky AP. Perfusion imaging. *Magn Reson Med* 1992; **23:** 37–45.

17. Kwong KK, Chesler DA, Weisskoff RM, Rosen BR. Perfusion MR imaging. In: Proceedings of SMR, 2nd Annual Meeting, San Francisco, 1994.

18. Wong EC, Buxton RB, Frank LR. Implementation of quantitative perfusion imaging techniques for functional brain mapping using pulsed arterial spin labeling. *NMR Biomed* 1997; **10:** 237–49.

19. Kim S-G. Quantification of relative cerebral blood flow change by flow-sensitive alternating inversion recovery (FAIR) technique: application to functional mapping. *Magn Reson Med* 1995; **34:** 293–301.

20. Ogawa S, Lee TM, Kay AR, Tank DW. Brain magnetic resonance imaging with contrast dependent on blood oxygenation. *Proc Natl Acad Sci USA* 1990; **87:** 9868–72.

21. Turner R, LeBihan D, Moonen CTW, Despres D, Frank J. Echo-planar time course MRI of cat brain oxygenation changes. *Magn Reson Med* 1991; **22:** 159–66.

22. Ogawa S, Lee TM. Functional brain imaging with physiologically sensitive image signals. *J Magn Reson Imaging* 1992; **2 (Suppl):** S22.

23. Frahm J, Bruhn H, Merboldt K-D, Hanicke W, Math D. Dynamic MR imaging of human brain oxygenation during rest and photic stimulation. *J Magn Reson Imaging* 1992; **2:** 501–505.

24. Haacke EM, Lai S, Reichenbach JR et al. In vivo measurement of blood oxygen saturation using magnetic resonance imaging: a direct validation of the blood oxygen level-dependent concept in functional brain imaging. *Hum Brain Mapping* 1997; **5:** 341–6.

25. vanZijl PCM, Eleff SM, Ulatowski JA et al. Quantitative assessment of blood flow, blood volume, and blood oxygenation effects in functional magnetic resonance imaging. *Nature Med* 1998; **4:** 159–60.

26. Davis TL, Kwong KK, Weisskoff RM, Rosen BR. Calibrated functional MRI: mapping the dynamics of oxidative metabolism. *Proc Natl Acad Sci USA* 1998; **95**: 1834–9.

27. Kim S-G, Ugurbil K. Comparison of blood oxygenation and cerebral blood flow effects in fMRI: estimation of relative oxygen consumption change. *Magn Reson Med* 1997; **38**: 59–65.

28. Hoge RD, Atkinson J, Gill B, Crelier GR, Marrett S, Pike GB. Investigation of BOLD signal dependence on cerebral blood flow and oxygen consumption: the deoxyhemoglobin dilution model. *Magn Reson Med* 1999; **42**: 849–63.

29. Hoge RD, Atkinson J, Gill B, Crelier GR, Marrett S, Pike GB. Stimulus-dependent BOLD and perfusion dynamics in human V1. *Neuroimage* 1999; **9**: 573–85.

30. Liu TT, Luh W-M, Wong EC, Frank LR, Buxton RB. A method for dynamic measurement of blood volume with compensation for T2 changes. In: Proceedings of ISMRM 8th Annual Meeting, Denver, 2000.

31. Arthurs, OJ, Boniface, S. How well do we understand the origins of the fMRI BOLD signal? *Trends Neurosci* 2002; **25**: 27–31

32. Attwell D, Iadeola C. The neural basis of functional brain imaging signals. *Trends Neurosci* 2002; **25**: 621–5.

33. Pauling L, Coryell CD. The magnetic properties and structure of hemoglobin, oxyhemoglobin, and carbonmonoxyhemoglobin. *Proc Natl Acad Sci USA* 1936; **22**: 210–16.

34. Thulborn KR, Waterton JC, Matthews PM, Radda GK. Oxygenation dependence of the transverse relaxation time of water protons in whole blood at high field. *Biochim Biophys Acta* 1982; **714**: 265–70.

35. Yablonskiy DA. Quantitation of intrinsic magnetic susceptibility-related effects in a tissue matrix. Phantom study. *Magn Reson Med* 1998; **39**: 417–28.

36. Ogawa S, Menon RS, Tank DW et al. Functional brain mapping by blood oxygenation level-dependent contrast magnetic resonance imaging: a comparison of signal characteristics with a biophysical model. *Biophysical J* 1993; **64**: 803–12.

37. Boxerman JL, Hamberg LM, Rosen BR, Weisskoff RM. MR contrast due to intravascular magnetic susceptibility perturbations. *Magn Reson Med* 1995; **34**: 555–66.

38. Kennan RP, Zhong J, Gore JC. Intravascular susceptibility contrast mechanisms in tissues. *Magn Reson Med* 1994; **31**: 9–21.

39. Bandettini PA, Wong EC. Effects of biophysical and physiologic parameters on brain activation-induced R2* and R2 changes: simulations using a deterministic diffusion model. *Int J Imaging Sys Technol* 1995; **6**: 134–52.

40. Weisskoff RM, Zuo CS, Boxerman JL, Rosen BR. Microscopic susceptibility variation and transverse relaxation: theory and experiment. *Magn Reson Med* 1994; **31**: 601–10.

41. Boxerman JL, Bandettini PA, Kwong KK et al. The intravascular contribution to fMRI signal change: Monte Carlo modelling and diffusion-weighted studies in vivo. *Magn Reson Med* 1995; **34**: 4–10.

42. Kim SG, Rostrup E, Larsson HB, Ogawa S, Paulson OB. Determination of relative $CMRO_2$ from CBF and BOLD changes: significant increase of oxygen consumption rate during visual stimulation. *Magn Reson Med* 1999; **41**: 1152–61.

43. An H, Lin W, Celik A, Lee YZ. Quantitative measurements of cerebral metabolic rate of oxygen utilization using MRI: a volunteer study. *NMR Biomed* 2001; **14:** 441–7.

44. Bandettini PA et al. Functional MRI using the BOLD approach: dynamic characteristics and data analysis methods. In D LeBihan (Ed) Diffusion and Perfusion: Magnetic Resonance Imaging (New York: Raven Press 1995) 335–49.

45. Friston KJ, Josephs O, Rees G, Turner R. Nonlinear event-related responses in fMRI. *Magn Reson Med* 1998; **39:** 41–52.

46. Josephs O, Turner R, Friston K. Event-related fMRI. *Hum Brain Mapping* 1997; **5:** 243–8.

47. Cohen MS. Parametric analysis of fMRI data using linear systems methods. *Neuroimage* 1997; **6:** 93–103.

48. Glover GH. Deconvolution of impulse response in event-related BOLD fMRI. *Neuroimage* 1999; **9:** 416–29.

49. Dale AM, Buckner RL. Selective averaging of rapidly presented individual trials using fMRI. *Hum Brain Mapping* 1997; **5:** 329–40.

50. Savoy RL, O'Craven KM, Weisskoff RM, Davis TL, Baker J, Rosen B. Exploring the temporal boundaries of fMRI: measuring responses to very brief visual stimuli. In: Book of Abstracts, Society for Neuroscience 24th Annual Meeting; Miami, 1994.

51. Savoy RL, Bandettini PA, Weisskoff RM et al. Pushing the temporal resolution of fMRI: studies of very brief visual stimuli, onset variablity and asynchrony, and stimulus-correlated changes in noise. In: Proceedings of SMR, 3rd Annual Meeting, Nice, 1995.

52. Saad ZS, Ropella KM, Cox RW, DeYoe EA. Analysis and use of FMRI response delays. *Hum Brain Mapping* 2001; **13:** 74–93.

53. Buckner RL, Bandettini PA, O'Craven KM et al. Detection of cortical activation during averaged single trials of a cognitive task using functional magnetic resonance imaging. *Proc Natl Acad Sci USA* 1996; **93:** 14,878–83.

54. Lee AT, Glover GH, Meyer CH. Discrimination of large venous vessels in time-course spiral blood-oxygen-level-dependent magntic-resonance functional neuroimaging. *Magn Reson Med* 1995; **33:** 745–54.

55. Saad ZS, DeYoe EA. Time delay estimates of FMRI signals: efficient algorithm & estimate variance. In: Proceedings of the 19th annual international conference of IEEE/EMBS, Chicago, 1997.

56. Binder JR, Rao SM, Hammeke TA, Frost JA, Bandettini PA, Hyde JS. Effects of stimulus rate on signal response during functional magnetic resonance imaging of auditory cortex. *Cognitive Brain Res* 1994; **2:** 31–8.

57. Rao SM, Bandettini PA, Binder JR et al. Relationship between finger movement rate and functional magnetic resonance signal change in human primary motor cortex. *J Cereb Blood Flow Metab* 1996; **16:** 1250–4.

58. Tootell RB, Reppas JB, Kwong KK et al. Functional analysis of human MT and related visual cortical areas using magnetic resonance imaging. *J Neurosci* 1995; **15:** 3215–30.

59. Disbrow EA, Slutsky DA, Roberts TP, Krubitzer LA. Functional MRI at 1.5 tesla: a comparison of the blood oxygenation level-dependent signal and electrophysiology. *Proc Natl Acad Sci USA* 2000; **97:** 9718–23.

60. Rees G, Friston K, Koch C. A direct quantitative relationship between the functional properties of human and macaque V5. *Nat Neurosci* 2000; **3:** 716–23.

61. Heeger DJ, Huk AC, Geisler WS, Albrecht DG. Spikes versus BOLD: what does neuroimaging tell us about neuronal activity? *Nat Neurosci* 2000; **3:** 631–3.

62. Logothetis N, Pauls J, Augath M, Trinath T, Oeltermann A. Neurophysiological investigation of the basis of the fMRI signal. *Nature* 2001; **412:** 150–7.

63. Boynton GM, Engel SA, Glover GH, Heeger DJ. Linear systems analysis of functional magnetic resonance imaging in human V1. *J Neurosci* 1996; **16:** 4207–21.

64. Vazquez AL, Noll DC. Nonlinear aspects of the BOLD response in functional MRI. *Neuroimage* 1998; **7:** 108–18.

65. Buxton RB, Wong EC, Frank LR. A biomechanical interpretation of the BOLD signal time course: the balloon model. In: Proceedings of the ISMRM, 5th Annual Meeting, Vancouver, 1997.

66. Frahm J, Krüger G, Merboldt K-D, Kleinschmidt A. Dynamic uncoupling and recoupling of perfusion and oxidative metabolism during focal activation in man. *Magn Reson Med* 1996; **35:** 143–8.

67. Busatto GF, Pilowsky LS. Neuroreceptor imaging with PET and SPET: research and clinical applications. In: (Kerwin R, ed) *Neurobiology and Psychiatry – Neuroimaging.* (Cambridge University Press: Cambridge, 1995) 111–24.

68. Fugita M., Innis RB. In vivo molecular imaging: ligand development and research application. In: (Davis KL, Charney D, Coyle JT, Nemeroff CB, eds) *Psychopharmacology: the Fifth Generation of Progress.* (Raven Press Ltd: New York, 2002) 411–25.

69. Meikle SR, Dahlbom M. Positron emission tomography. In: (Murray IPC, Ell PJ, eds) *Nuclear Medicine in Clinical Diagnosis and Treatment.* (Churchill Livingstone: London, 1998) 1603–16.

70. Walker B, Jarrit P. Basic physics of nuclear medicine. In: (Murray IPC, Ell PJ, eds) *Nuclear Medicine in Clinical Diagnosis and Treatment.* (Churchill Livingstone: London, 1998) 1445–58.

71. Reba RC. PET and SPECT: opportunities and challenges for psychiatry. *J Clin Psychiatry* 1993; **54:** 26–32.

72. Mallison RT. Positron and single photon emission tomography. In: (Bloom FE, Kupfer DJ, eds) *Psychopharmacology: the Fourth Generation of Progress.* (Raven Press Ltd: New York, 1994) 865–79.

73. Eberl S, Zimmerman RE. Nuclear medicine imaging instrumentation. In: (Murray IPC, Ell PJ, eds) *Nuclear Medicine in Clinical Diagnosis and Treatment.* (Churchill Livingstone: London, 1998) 1559–69.

74. Westera G, Buck A, Burger C, Leenders KL, von Schulthess GK, Schubiger AP. Carbon-11 and iodine-123 labelled iomazenil: a direct PET–SPET comparison. *Eur J Nucl Med* 1996; **23:** 5–12.

75. Pike VW. Positron-emitting radioligand for studies in vivo – probes for human psychopharmacology. *J Psychopharmacol* 1993; **7:** 139–58.

76. Halldin C, Gulyas B, Langer O, Farde L. Brain radioligands – state of the art and new trends. *Q J Nucl Med* 2001; **45:** 139–52.

77. Mintun MA, Raichle ME, Kilbourn MR, Wooten GF, Welch MJ. A quantitative model for the in vivo assessment of drug binding sites with positron emission tomography. *Ann Neurol* 1984; **15:** 217–27.

78. Laruelle M. The role of model-based methods in the development of single scan techniques. *Nucl Med Biol* 2000; **27**: 637–42.

79. Carson RE. Precision and accuracy considerations of physiological quantitation in PET. *J Cereb Blood Flow Metab* 1991; **11**: A45–A50.

80. Laruelle M, Abi-Dargham A, al Tikriti MS et al. SPECT quantification of [123I]iomazenil binding to benzodiazepine receptors in nonhuman primates: II. Equilibrium analysis of constant infusion experiments and correlation with in vitro parameters. *J Cereb Blood Flow Metab* 1994; **14**: 453–65.

81. Laruelle M, Baldwin RM, Rattner Z et al. SPECT quantification of [123I]iomazenil binding to benzodiazepine receptors in nonhuman primates: I. Kinetic modeling of single bolus experiments. *J Cereb Blood Flow Metab* 1994; **14**: 439–52.

82. Logan J, Volkow ND, Fowler JS et al. Effects of blood flow on [11C]raclopride binding in the brain: model simulations and kinetic analysis of PET data. *J Cereb Blood Flow Metab* 1994; **14**: 995–1010.

83. Lammertsma AA, Hume SP. Simplified reference tissue model for PET receptor studies. *Neuroimage* 1996; **4**: 153–8.

84. Carson RE, Channing MA, Blasberg RG et al. Comparison of bolus and infusion methods for receptor quantitation: application to [18F]cyclofoxy and positron emission tomography. *J Cereb Blood Flow Metab* 1993; **13**: 24–42.

85. Farde L, Hall H, Ehrin E, Sedvall G. Quantitative analysis of D2 dopamine receptor binding in the living human brain by PET. *Science* 1986; **231**: 258–61.

86. Carson RE. PET physiological measurements using constant infusion. *Nucl Med Biol* 2000; **27**: 657–60.

87. Innis RB, al Tikriti MS, Zoghbi SS et al. SPECT imaging of the benzodiazepine receptor: feasibility of in vivo potency measurements from stepwise displacement curves. *J Nucl Med* 1991; **32**: 1754–61.

88. Friston KJ, Price CJ, Fletcher P, Moore C, Frackowiak RSJ, Dolan RJ. The trouble with cognitive subtraction. *Neuroimage* 1996; **4**: 97–104.

89. Bandettini PA, Jesmanowicz A, Wong EC, Hyde JS. Processing strategies for time-course data sets in functional MRI of the human brain. *Magn Reson Med* 1993; **30**: 161–73.

90. Bandettini PA. *Magnetic resonance imaging of human brain activation using endogenous susceptibility contrast.* PhD Thesis, Milwaukee: Medical College of Wisconsin, 1995.

91. Engel SA, Glover GH, Wandell BA. Retinotopic organization in human visual cortex and the spatial precision of functional MRI. *Cerebral Cortex* 1997; **7**: 181–92.

92. Sereno MI, Dale AM, Reppas JR et al. Functional MRI reveals borders of multiple visual areas in humans. *Science* 1995; **268**: 889–93.

93. DeYoe EA, Carman G, Bandettini P et al. Mapping striate and extrastriate areas in human cerebral cortex. *Proc Natl Acad Sci USA* 1996; **93**: 2382–6.

94. Servos P, Zacks J, Rumelhart DE, Glover GH. Somatotopy of the human arm using fMRI. *Neuroreport* 1998; **9**: 605–9.

95. Talavage TM, Ledden PJ, Sereno MI, Benson RR, Rosen BR. Preliminary fMRI evidence for tonotopicity in human auditory cortex. *Neuroimage* 1996; **3**: S355.

96. Zarahn E, Aguirre G, D'Esposito M. A trial-based experimental design for fMRI. *Neuroimage* 1997; **6**: 122–38.

97. Clark VP, Maisog JM, Haxby JV. fMRI study of face perception and memory using random stimulus sequences. *J Neurophysiol* 1998; **79:** 3257–65.

98. Dale A, Buckner R. Selective averaging of individual trials using fMRI. In: Third International Conference on Functional Mapping of the Human Brain, Copenhagen, 1997.

99. McCarthy G, Luby M, Gore J, Goldman-Rakic P. Infrequent events transiently activate human prefrontal and parietal cortex as measured by functional MRI. *J Neurophysiol* 1997; **77:** 1630–4.

100. Schacter DL, Buckner RL, Koutstaal W, Dale AM, Rosen BR. Late onset of anterior prefrontal activity during true and false recognition: an event-related fMRI study. *Neuroimage* 1997; **6:** 259–69.

101. Dale AM. Optimal experimental design for event-related fMRI. *Hum Brain Mapping* 1999; **8:** 109–14.

102. Burock MA, Buckner RL, Woldorff MG, Rosen BR, Dale AM. Randomized event-related experimental designs allow for extremely rapid presentation rates using functional MRI. *Neuroreport* 1998; **9:** 3735–9.

103. Liu TT, Frank LR, Wong EC, Buxton RB. Detection power, estimation efficiency, and predictability in event-related fMRI. *Neuroimage* 2001; **13:** 759–73.

104. Birn RM, Cox RW, Bandettini PA. Detection versus estimation in event-related fMRI: choosing the optimal stimulus timing. *Neuroimage* 2002; **15:** 252–64.

105. Courtney SM, Ungerleider LG, Keil K, Haxby JV. Transient and sustained activity in a distributed neural system for human working memory. *Nature* 1997; **386:** 608–11.

106. Patterson J, Bandettini P, Ungerleider LG. Simultaneous skin conductance measurement and fMRI during cognitive tasks: correlations of skin conductance activity with ventromedial prefrontal cortex (PFC) and orbitofrontal cortex (OFC) activity. In: Proceedings of Human Brain Mapping, San Antonio, 2000.

107. Shergill SS, Bullmore E, Simmons A, Murray R, McGuire P. Functional anatomy of auditory verbal imagery in schizophrenic patients with auditory hallucinations. *Am J Psychiatry* 2000; **157:** 1691–3.

2. UPDATE ON FUNCTIONAL NEUROIMAGING IN CHILD PSYCHIATRY

Monique Ernst, Judith Rumsey, Suzanne Munson

Introduction

Advances in neuroimaging make it possible to non-invasively detect and measure brain activity and neurochemistry *in vivo* in children. Although pediatric functional neuroimaging research presents both practical and ethical challenges, the knowledge gained from this type of research has enormous potential for informing the detection, prevention, and treatment of childhood-onset disorders. Functional neuroimaging holds promise not only for pediatric illnesses but also for the understanding of adult-onset disorders, whose geneses lie in early development. Nuclear medicine imaging techniques [i.e. positron emission tomography (PET) and single photon emission computed tomography (SPECT)], functional magnetic resonance imaging (fMRI) and magnetic resonance spectroscopy (MRS) are the main tools used for this research. Alternatives such as optical imaging and magnetic electroencephalography (MEG) have not been exploited systematically in pediatric research. A comprehensive review of functional neuroimaging in child psychiatry, including research through 2000, is available in an edited volume by Ernst and Rumsey.[1] The current chapter describes the most up-to-date findings in child neuroimaging studies with specific reference to psychiatric childhood disorders.

Issues specific to imaging children

Practical considerations
Experimental accommodations are needed to image children. Children cannot remain immobile for long periods of time. Therefore, studies need to be short (e.g. 30 min for children younger than 8 years of age, 45 min for

children up to 12 years of age), and special training ought to be provided to teach them when and how to remain still.

Medical environments are usually more anxiogenic for children than for adults. Children should get to know the research staff and MRI facilities prior to scanning. Institutions that study children often have an MRI simulator which matches the physical characteristics of the operational MRI scanner so that training does not demand expensive time on the operational MRI scanner.

Cognitive abilities change qualitatively (cognitive strategies) and quantitatively (cognitive load) with brain maturation. These changes are not linear with age and tend to occur in spurts. For studies involving activation, experimental paradigms need to be carefully adapted to the cognitive level of the children, and adequate training should be provided to ensure the understanding of task demands and adequate performance. Tasks developed for use in imaging studies of adults need to be tested in children behaviorally before being used in a scanner to determine levels of performance and identify age-related problems. For example, children may experience difficulty in executing manual responses when unable to see their fingers.

Brain maturation raises both technical and scientific issues. Developmental changes in the characteristics of brain tissue, such as in volume, ratio of white to gray matter, vascularization, and synaptic density all can affect functional neuroimaging signals. While there is little reason to believe that the physiology underlying the blood oxygenation-level dependent (BOLD) fMRI response differs substantially between children and adults, minor differences in reactivity may hold implications for the statistical thresholds used to identify activations. In very young children, i.e. infants/neonates, vascular responses to stimulation may result in a decrease rather than an increase in the fMRI signal.[2,3] Physical differences between children and adults, e.g. in head size, skull thickness, and cardiopulmonary cycle, may also impact imaging studies attempting to address developmental issues.[4] More needs to be learned about the trajectories of these changes in children from infancy through adolescence and early adulthood, such that mathematical models can be developed to adjust for these changes. Differences in the sizes of brain structures can introduce errors in functional imaging measures. Algorithms developed to correct for small volumes in PET research (partial volume correction)[5] might be adapted for studies of young children. Finally, the widespread use of an adult brain template[6] to coregister functional and anatomic scans of children may compromise the validity of the measures. Alternative approaches include the use of separate anatomic templates for different age groups or the application of mathematical models with age or with markers of brain structural maturation as determinant variables.

Taken together, these caveats highlight the critical importance of carefully accounting for maturational changes in size, shape and composition of brain tissue in pediatric neuroimaging to avoid misinterpreting the resulting functional signals. Although normative data are becoming available,[7,8] it is without question that support for normative studies of brain structural maturation is key for the future of functional neuroimaging in children. The dire need for normative studies is highlighted by the absence of any of the above-mentioned corrective measures in the most recent studies reviewed in this chapter.

Ethical considerations

Ethical issues specific to pediatric research stem from the classification of minors as a 'vulnerable population'. Special legal and ethical regulations protect children from the risks of research.[9] In the USA, federal research safeguards for children [45 Code of Federal Regulation (CFR), Subtitle A, Part 46, Subpart D, 10–1–91 edition] indicate that parents' or guardians' permission for research involving their children as subjects may not be solicited or accepted for research with substantially greater than *minimal risk* unless there is direct benefit to the child with a benefit:risk ratio at least as good as available clinical alternatives. Hence, the concept of minimal risk is central to the debate on whether to include children, especially healthy children, in research protocols.

The threshold defining minimal risk can vary greatly among institutional review boards (IRB) because of its ambiguous meaning. The 45 CFR, Subtitle A, Part 46, Subpart A, 46.102(g) 10–1–91 edition defines minimal risk as '. . . the risks of harm anticipated in the proposed research [that] are not greater, considering probability and magnitude, than those ordinarily encountered in daily life or during the performance of routine physical or psychological examinations or tests'. Whereas the inclusion of children in fMRI studies does not usually raise significant concerns, PET studies in minors are controversial.[10]

Most of the debate is centered on the level of risk associated with low-level radiation exposure. Although no adverse effects have been detected at the doses used in PET studies, most IRB consider such studies to represent greater than minimal risk and prohibit healthy children from participating. Indeed, to date, no studies have systematically examined normal brain development in healthy minors using PET. Ernst et al[11] have provided a thorough review of the potential health consequences of exposure to low-level radiation to help assist researchers and IRB in determining the level of risk associated with PET studies.

Studies of children with psychiatric disorders

The emergence of MR techniques, particularly fMRI, has begun to expand functional neuroimaging in child psychiatry, a trend that is certain to continue for some time. Because child fMRI studies date back only 5–6 years, studies of child psychiatric disorders prior to the mid to late 1990s made use primarily of techniques such as PET and SPECT. Because of the ethical concerns, these studies most often involved adults with childhood-onset psychiatric disorders and children with substantial impairments and/or significant comorbid medical conditions. Surprisingly, the present review emphasizing the past 3 years of neuroimaging research in child psychiatry still includes a large number of nuclear medicine studies (PET or SPECT) relative to the total number of published studies despite the radiation exposure associated with these techniques. These recent studies are listed in Table 2.1, which includes age, gender, size and other characteristics of study samples.

Models of cerebral dysfunction have been proposed for most psychiatric disorders. The studies described below attempt to test these models while adding a developmental perspective. This review will address only the psychiatric disorders that have been the object of functional neuroimaging studies in children over the past 3 years. For the sake of space, developmental reading disorder, which has been investigated in several pediatric studies[12–18] and would require a chapter on its own, has been excluded. The disorders considered below have been associated with hypothesized dysfunction of the following neural structures or circuits, which often overlap across disorders. Attention deficit hyperactivity disorder (ADHD), Tourette's syndrome (TS) and obsessive-compulsive disorder (OCD) are proposed to result from dysfunction of cortico–striato–thalamo–cortical loops and to involve dopaminergic (ADHD and TS) and serotonergic systems (OCD). Autistic disorder and Asperger's syndrome are associated with limbic, prefrontal and cerebellar dysfunction, and have been associated with dopaminergic and, to a lesser extent, serotonergic abnormalities.

Table 2.1 Studies of pediatric functional imaging in child psychiatry (except for reading disorders) published between 1999 and present*

Disorder	Method	Patient sample	Comparison sample(s)	Authors (ref)
ADHD	SPECT	28 ADHD (m/f 24/4; ages 6–11, mean 9.0±1.6)	–	Gustafsson et al (113)
ADHD	SPECT	32 ADHD (m/f 32/0; ages 7–14, mean 10.6±5.6; r/l 32/0) before and after treatment with MPH	–	Kim et al (32)
ADHD	SPECT	Nine ADHD [m/f 6/3, mean 9.8(2.3)] before and after MPH	–	Ilgin et al (41)
ADHD	SPECT	20 ADHD (m/f 20/0, ages 8–12, mean 10.2)	Four healthy (m/f 4/0, ages 8–12, mean age 10.2)	Langleben et al (31)
ADHD	fMRI	11 ADHD (m/f 11/0; mean 9.3±1.6)	Six healthy (m/f = 6/0; mean 10.2±1.5)	Teicher et al (38)
ADHD	fMRI	Seven ADHD (m/f 7/0; ages 12–18, mean 15.7)	Nine healthy (m/f 9/0; ages 12–17, mean 15.01)	Rubia et al (29)
ADHD	MRS	12 ADHD (m/f 12/0, ages 10–16, mean 13.0) before and after MPH	10 healthy (m/f 10/0, ages 11–15, mean 13.0)	Jin et al (42)
ADHD	PET	10 ADHD (m/f 8/2; ages 12–17; mean 13.8±1.9; r/l 9/1)	10 healthy controls (m/f 7/3; ages 12–17; mean 14.8±1.7; r/l 2/8)	Ernst et al (23)
OCD	MRS	11 psychotropic medication-naïve OCD (m/f 4/7; ages 8.2–15.6, mean 11.2±2.5; r/l 11/0)	11 healthy (m/f 4/7; ages 8–17, mean 11.6±2.4; r/l 11/0)	Rosenberg et al (55)
OCD	MRS	11 OCD (m/f 4/7; ages 8–17, mean 11±3; r/l 11/0)	11 healthy (m/f 4/7; ages 9–17, mean 12±2; r/l 11/0	Fitzgerald et al (59)
OCD	MRS	11 OCD (m/f 4/7; ages 8–17, mean 11.2±2.5; r/l 11/0)	11 healthy (m/f 4/7; ages 8–17, mean 11.6±2.4; r/l 11/0	Rosenberg et al (60)

Table 2.1 Studies of pediatric functional imaging in child psychiatry (except for reading disorders) published between 1999 and present* – *Continued*

Disorder	Method	Patient sample	Comparison sample(s)	Authors (ref)
TS	PET	11 TS (m/f 8/3; ages 12–17, mean age 15.2±1.9; r/l 10/1)	10 healthy (m/f 7/3; ages 12–17, mean age 14.8±1.7; r/l 8/2)	Ernst et al (73)
Asperger's syndrome	fMRI	Nine Asperger's syndrome (ages 7–17, mean 12.0±3.1)	Eight controls from pediatric clinic (ages 8–16, mean 11.0±2.5)	Oktem et al (88)
Autism	SPECT	23 autistic and MR (m/f 19/4, ages 2–13, mean 6.5)	26 non-autistic MR (m/f 21/5, ages 2–13, mean 6.5)	Ohnishi et al (94)
Autism	SPECT	30 autistic and MR (9% female, mean 11.1±7.0)	14 non-autistic MR (5% female, mean 11.2±4.3)	Starkstein et al (96)
Autism	SPECT	18 autistic (m/f 14/4, ages 3–11, mean 6.13±1.99)	11 non-autistic (m/f 6/5, ages 2–11, mean 6.5±3.39)	Kaya et al (95)
Autism	PET	21 autistic and MR (m/f 17/4, ages 5–13, mean 8.4), and a replication group of 12 autistic and MR (m/f 11/1, ages 5–13, mean 7.4)	10 non-autistic MR (m/f 8/2, ages 5–13, mean 8.1)	Zilbovicius et al (89)
Autism (TSC and epilepsy)	PET	Nine autistic and TSC (4.1±3.0)	Nine MR TSC (5.5±1.8) Eight relatively normal intelligence non-autistic TSC (5.7±2.9)	Asano et al (90)
Autism	MRS	Nine autistic (m/f 8/1, ages 3–12, mean 5.7±2.5)	Five healthy siblings (m/f 4/1; ages 6–14 mean 9±3)	Chugani et al (84)
Autism	PET	30 autistic (m/f 24/6, ages 2.3–15.4, mean 6.4±3.3)	Eight healthy siblings (m/f 6/2, ages 2.1–14.4, mean age 9.2±3.4) 16 with epilepsy (m/f 9/7, ages 3 months–13.4 years, mean 5.7±3.6)	Chugani et al (81)

Table 2.1 Studies of pediatric functional imaging in child psychiatry (except for reading disorders) published between 1999 and present* – Continued

Disorder	Method	Patient sample	Comparison sample(s)	Authors (ref)
Depression	SPECT	31 depressed (m/f 22/9, mean 13.5±2.5)	10 not depressed (m/f 5/5, mean 12.2±2.9)	Dahlstrom et al (103)
Depression	SPECT	10 depressed (m/f 6/4 females, mean age 15.5±1.6; r/l 10/0)	Seven healthy controls (age and gender matched)	Kowatch et al (105)
Depression	MRS	17 depressed (m/f 14/3 males, mean 15.8±1.6)	28 healthy (m/f 10/18, mean 14.5±1.7)	Steingard et al (106)
Depression/ anxiety	fMRI	12 GAD/PD (m/f 7/5, ages 8–16, mean age 12.8±2.1) Five MD (m/f 0/5, ages 8–16, mean 12.3±2.7)	12 healthy (m/f 7/5, mean 12.2±2.6)	Thomas et al (112)

* Missing data reflect that the information was not reported for the given samples. ADHD, Attention deficit hyperactivity disorder; age, in years; fMRI, functional magnetic resonance imaging; GAD/PD, generalized anxiety disorder or panic disorder; MD, major depression; mean, mean age ± standard deviation; m/f, male/female; MPH, methylphenidate; MR, mentally retarded; MRS, magnetic resonance spectroscopy; OCD, obsessive-compulsive disorder; r/l, right/left handed; SPECT, single photon emission computed tomography; TS, Tourette's syndrome; TSC, tuberous sclerosis complex.

Mood disorders have been associated with limbic and paralimbic deficits, affecting primarily the hippocampus, amygdala, orbitofrontal cortex and anterior cingulate. Biochemical underpinnings of mood disorders currently emphasize serotonergic involvement, although noradrenergic and dopaminergic systems have also been implicated.

Functional neuroimaging can provide essentially three types of measures: (1) a pattern of basal neural activity [e.g. regional cerebral glucose metabolism (rCMRglu) with PET and [^{18}F]fluorodeoxyglucose; regional cerebral blood flow [rCBF] with SPECT and ^{133}Xe]; (2) neurotransmitter function [e.g. PET and dopamine transporter ligands (DAT)]; (3) biochemical integrity with MRS; and (4) cognitive activation (e.g. PET, ^{15}O H$_2$O or fMRI). These approaches address anatomofunctional, biochemical and neuropsychological models, respectively.

Disorders of cortico–striato–thalamo–cortical loops

Attention deficit hyperactivity disorder (ADHD)

ADHD is defined by persistent inattention and/or situationally excessive motor activity and impulsive behavior. Symptoms must appear before 7 years of age and be present for at least 6 months.[19] In the USA, ADHD affects about 4% of the school-age population, ranging from 3 to 11% depending on the source of the sample. Boys are 2.5–9 times more likely than girls to be diagnosed with ADHD.[20] Although the recognition of ADHD dates back half a century, its neural mechanisms remain unclear. Functional neuroimaging combined with molecular genetics are now the most promising approaches for elucidating the biological causes of ADHD and contributing to the development of focused treatment strategies.

Neuropsychophysiological models of ADHD are drawn from neuropsychology, psychopharmacology, neuroelectrophysiology and animal models. However, across these models, there is agreement on a role of prefrontal, cingulate and parietal cortices, and dopaminergic structures. Convergence of findings from studies of the general pattern of *basal* cerebral synaptic activity suggest: (1) reduced synaptic activity associated with ADHD symptoms, consistently in the prefrontal cortex and less so in the striatum; (2) possibly greater cerebral abnormality in females than males; (3) evolution of functional abnormalities from discrete in ADHD adolescents toward more generalized in ADHD adults; and (4) only few isolated regional metabolic changes associated with stimulant effects (see Ernst and Torta[21]).

At present, neurotransmitter studies in ADHD have been restricted to the dopaminergic system, particularly to its presynaptic component. Studies of dopamine synthesis have shown prefrontal dopaminergic reduction in adults,[22] in contrast to enhanced midbrain dopaminergic activity in children.[23] DAT density in the striatum has been consistently found to be higher in adults with ADHD than in healthy controls.[24–26] The most compelling interpretation of these findings in adults is an overall decreased dopamine synthesis and dopamine release in both prefrontal and striatal regions, which would be compensated by an increased number of dopaminergic terminals in the striatum (resulting in increased density of DAT). However, in children, the absence of reduced prefrontal dopamine synthesis may reflect the peripubertal dendritic pruning process[27] that later may unmask a deficit in dopamine synthesis in the prefrontal cortex. The abnormally high dopamine synthesis in the midbrain (the site of dopaminergic cell bodies in the substantia nigra and ventral tegmentum) of adolescents with ADHD suggests the possibility that reduced dopamine synthesis in cell terminals may occur as a compensatory response to the excessive dopaminergic activity in the cell bodies. Finally, four cognitive–behavioral domains, i.e. attention,[28] response inhibition,[29] motor timing[29] and working memory,[30] have been explored with functional neuroimaging (PET and fMRI) in ADHD individuals. Although these studies all showed abnormally low cerebral activation in the ADHD groups, particularly in the prefrontal cortex, findings are not yet integrated into a single pathophysiological model of ADHD.

Several studies evaluated ADHD children and adolescents in unmedicated states. In one fMRI study, prefrontal cortical dysfunction was investigated in ADHD male adolescents who showed lower activation in the right mesial prefrontal cortex during two tasks requiring motor inhibition (stop task) and motor timing (delay task).[29] In addition, hypoactivation was also noted in the right inferior prefrontal cortex and the left caudate nucleus during the motor inhibition task (stop task). Task performance did not differ significantly between groups on both tasks. The authors proposed the theory of a maturational lag of frontal lobes as a cause of ADHD. Another SPECT study[31] explored abnormalities in functional hemispheric asymmetry in ADHD children using SPECT and technetium-99m (Tc-99m)-ethyl cysteinate dimmer (ECD) during the performance of a go no-go task. Relative right hypofrontality was observed in the most severe hyperactive boys, supporting right prefrontal functional deficits.

Stimulant treatment effects on brain function were addressed by the following studies. Kim et al[32] used SPECT and Tc-99m-d,l-hexamethyl-propyleneamineoxime (HMPAO) to assess changes in rCBF after an 8-week stimulant treatment [methylphenidate (MPH) 0.7 mg/kg/day] of 32 boys with ADHD. Findings included significant clinical improvement, and increased rCBF in caudate, frontal and thalamic regions, predominantly in the right hemisphere. These findings are at odds with the paucity of effects of MPH treatment on rCMRglu in adults with ADHD.[33–35] This discrepancy may be due to an age effect, different experimental conditions (no attention task in this particular study compared to the use of a continuous performance task in previous work), or the different indices of neural activity employed (rCBF versus rCMRglu). Notwithstanding, the cerebellum, which is becoming a region of prime interest in the pathophysiology of ADHD,[36,37] showed no rCBF changes upon MPH treatment. A placebo arm would have controlled for a potential order effect.

Teicher et al[38] addressed a similar question using fMRI with a new technique, fMRI T2 relaxometry, which permits the measurement of absolute rCBF. This technique, devoid of radiation exposure, allowed the authors to include healthy children as controls. Healthy children were scanned once at rest and did not receive MPH, and ADHD children were scanned twice, once during placebo and 1 week after MPH treatment (1–3 h post-administration of MPH 1.5 mg/kg/day). A region-of-interest (ROI) analysis sampled the caudate nuclei, putamen and thalamus. Only the putamen differed between groups. rCBF was lower in ADHD children (during placebo) compared to controls. Regarding treatment effect in the ADHD group, MPH significantly altered rCBF in the putamen, and the direction of this effect depended on unmedicated activity state, i.e. increased perfusion in the most hyperactive subjects and decreased perfusion in less active subjects. These findings are consistent with reports of different effects of MPH in ADHD and control children.[39] The differential effects of MPH on indices of neural activity as a function of basal behavioral and neural measures was also noted in ADHD adults by Volkow et al,[40] who reported MPH induced increased frontotemporal rCMRglu in adults with high D2 receptor availability and decreased rCMRglu in adults with low D2 receptor availability.

Finally, the dopamine hypothesis was evaluated by Ernst et al,[23] who compared dopamine accumulation in ADHD adolescents and healthy adolescents. This work, part of a larger study that contrasted dopamine function among several disorders, permitted the use of healthy siblings of research participants with disorders other than ADHD to serve as healthy controls. Dopamine activity in ADHD adolescents was significantly higher in the right midbrain and tended to be lower in the prefrontal cortex compared to controls. Figure 2.1 shows this increased dopaminergic activity in a 13-year-old ADHD boy compared to a 13-year-old healthy control on an axial (horizontal) view of the brain at the midbrain level. Previous findings in ADHD adults showed significantly lower prefrontal dopamine activity but no differences in subcortical areas compared to control adults.[22] Taken together, these studies suggest a developmental evolution of dopaminergic deficits from childhood into adulthood.

Ilgin et al[41] compared D2 receptor availability before and after 3-month treatment with MPH (0.5–1.5 mg/kg/day) in ADHD children, between the ages of 7 and 14, using SPECT and [^{123}I]iodobenzamide (IBZM). Striatal D2 receptor availability was up to 30% lower in the post-treatment phase than in pretreatment, possibly reflecting downregulation. Compared to published values in young adults and its expected age-related decrease, D2 receptor availability appears to be higher than expected in these ADHD children. These findings are important and warrant a replication in young

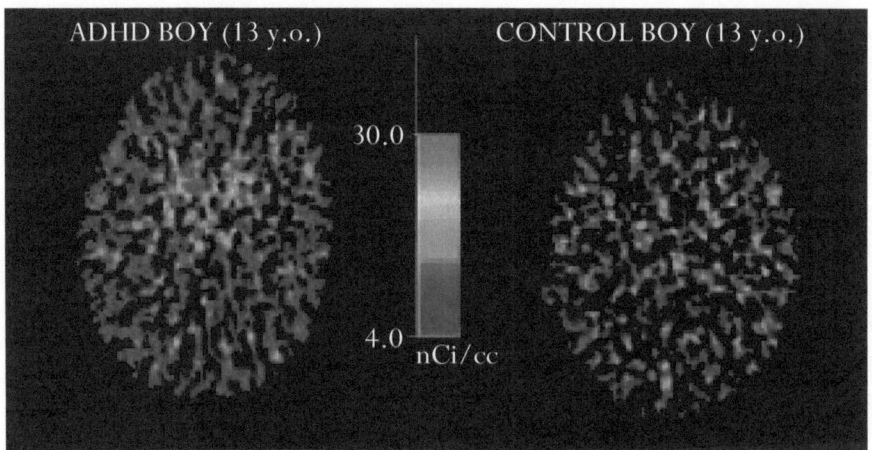

Figure 2.1 *Axial slices of positron emission tomography (PET) scans with [^{18}F]dopa at the level of the midbrain of a 13-year-old attention deficit hyperactivity disorder (ADHD) boy on the left and a 13-year-old healthy adolescent on the right. The color bar identified high activity (red) and low activity (purple). Enhanced activity is apparent in midbrain of the ADHD boy relative to the control boy. (Courtesy of Dr Ernst)*

adults with ADHD and a matched healthy control group, perhaps using a more sensitive neuroimaging technique.

Another study suggested abnormalities of the neuronal integrity in the globus pallidus of ADHD children based on the findings of abnormally low N-acetyl-aspartate (NAA)/(creatine/phosphocreatine) (Cr) ratio in unmedicated ADHD children compared to healthy children.[42] The reasons for selecting the globus pallidus as the structure of interest, rather than other dopaminergic structures such as the caudate nucleus or the putamen, were not addressed.

Obsessive-compulsive disorder (OCD)

OCD is a severe and chronically disabling disorder characterized by repetitive, ritualistic thoughts, impulses and behaviors over which individuals have little control. Its lifetime prevalence is 2–3%,[43,44] with as many as 80% of all cases of OCD having their onset in childhood and adolescence.[45] The mean age of onset of OCD in referred children and adolescents ranges from 9[46] to 10.7 years of age.[47]

Functional neuroimaging studies in adult patients with childhood-onset OCD have demonstrated abnormally high metabolic activity in the ventral prefrontal cortex and the head of the caudate nucleus.[48–54] Based on animal studies, the following explanation has been proposed for the therapeutic efficacy of serotonergic agents in OCD. Selective serotonin reuptake inhibitors (SSRI) increase prefrontal serotonin release, which stimulates gamma-aminobutyric acid (GABA) interneurons, which, in turn, inhibit glutamate projections to the striatum. Thus, an end-effect of SSRI treatment may be to decrease glutamate in the caudate, which could be detected using MRS techniques. Differential clinical responses to SSRI may reflect variations in the sensitivity of this modulatory system, in which case MRS studies might provide markers of treatment response.

To explore this possibility, Rosenberg et al[55] used ^{1}H MRS to measure glutamatergic compounds in the caudate nucleus of drug-naïve children and adolescents with OCD, both pre- and post-effective pharmacotherapy with the SSRI paroxetine. Figure 2.2 shows the spectra acquired from a control adolescent and from an adolescent with OCD. Among the five components of the

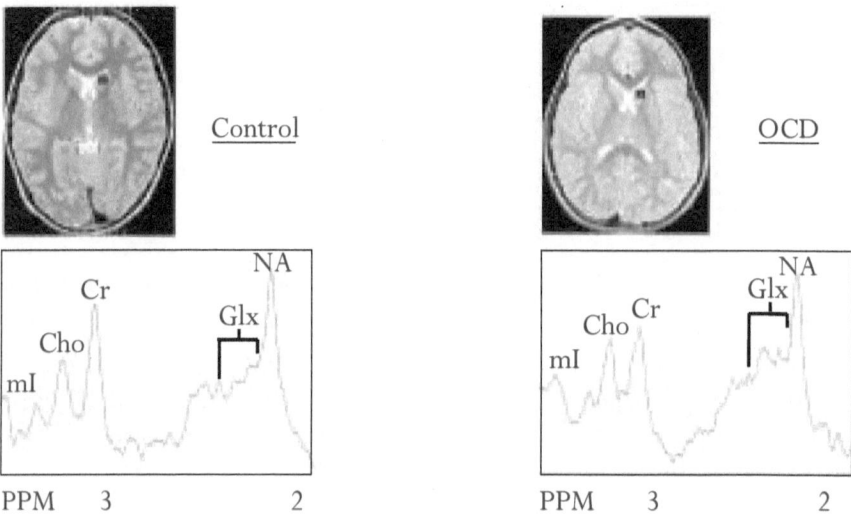

mI = myo-inositol
Cho = choline compounds
Glx = glutamate/glutamine/GABA
Cr = creatine/phosphocreatine
NA = N-acetylasparate

Figure 2.2 Proton magnetic resonance spectrum from the head of the left caudate (0.7 ml volume) of a healthy control adolescent and an adolescent with obsessive-compulsive disorder (OCD). The larger glutamate/glutamine gamma-aminobutyric acid (GABA) (Glx) peak in the OCD adolescent compared to the control adolescent is highlighted. (Courtesy of Dr Rosenberg)

^{1}H MRS spectra which were anaylzed, i.e. Glx (glutamine, glutamate and GABA), NAA, Cr (creatine/phosphocreatine), Ch (choline compounds) and mI (myoinositol), only Glx measures differed between the groups at baseline (OCD > controls). After a 12-week open-label treatment with paroxetine (20–60 mg daily), OCD symptoms were significantly improved and Glx levels in the OCD group decreased to the controls' levels. Despite the caveats of the limited specificity of Glx measure, the open-trial nature of the treatment, the psychiatric comorbidity in the OCD sample (only four of 11 children were free of comorbidity), and the single regional measurement, these findings are consistent with reports in OCD adults of abnormally high rCMRglu in caudate nuclei, which normalized after effective SSRI treatment.[48]

The role of the thalamus as a key sensory gate to the cortex may hold a special place in OCD pathology. Consistent with this observation, volumetric[56] and metabolic[48] abnormalities of the thalamus have been reported in adults with OCD. Regionally based functional specialization has been proposed for the thalamic nuclei. Medial thalamic regions, which have been implicated in affective and motivational processes, are more likely to be involved in OCD than are lateral thalamic regions, which may contribute predominantly to motor functioning.[57,58]

Two MRS studies of the same samples have examined four thalamic regions, left and right medial and lateral areas, using two different analyses.[59,60] Using concentration ratios as the outcome variables, Fitzgerald et al[59] found reduced NAA/Ch levels in the left and right medial, but not lateral, thalamus in treatment-naïve pediatric OCD patients. Rosenberg et al[60] examined absolute concentrations (mmol) of these compounds and found abnormally high cytosolic Ch levels in the right and left medial, but not lateral, thalamic regions of the OCD children. Although the origin of the Ch spectra is known (glycerophosphocholine and phosphocholine metabolites of phosphotidylcholine, a membrane lipid),[61,62] its exact functional significance is not entirely clear. Nonetheless, these studies provide support for thalamic and striatal involvement in the pathophysiology of OCD.

Tourette's syndrome (TS)

TS is characterized by chronic, fluctuating motor and vocal tics that affect 4–10 times more males than females.[63–66] The most efficacious treatment of TS remains dopamine-receptor blocking agents. Peterson and Thomas[67] provide an excellent discussion of the potential confounds of pediatric functional neuroimaging research in general, which includes, in the case of TS, the high rate of comorbid illness and the effects on brain function of active inhibition of tics during imaging. *In vivo* PET and SPECT studies of regional neural activity (rCBF and rCMRglu) generally report hypometabolic cortical and subcortical brain regions in adults with TS (see Peterson and Thomas[67]). The functional significance of these findings is unclear because they can reflect a primary causal mechanism, a secondary adaptive process, or voluntary inhibition of tics during the scanning procedures. In fact, Peterson et al[68] observed in an fMRI study of adults with TS that tic suppression was associated with more a widely spread decreased signal than increased signal in the subcortex. Neurotransmitter studies in adults with TS initially reported no dopaminergic abnormalities,[69,70] but a later SPECT study reported elevated DAT densities.[71] D2 dopamine receptor density has also been found to be elevated with severity of TS symptomatology.[72]

These findings in adults differ from those reported by Ernst et al[73] in adolescents. The Ernst et al[73] study compared dopamine activity in children diagnosed with TS and healthy age- and sex-matched controls using PET and [18F]dopa. Regional accumulation of [18F]dopa was abnormally high in the left caudate nucleus and the right midbrain of the TS group. While consistent with growing evidence implicating the right caudate nucleus in TS pathophysiology (see Peterson and Thomas[67]), the regionally specific increase in the [18F]dopa signal may reflect a larger number of dopaminergic synapses or enzyme upregulation. The prior findings in adults of increased presynaptic transporter in TS singletons[71] and increased postsynaptic D2 receptor availability in more severely affected monozygotic co-twins[72] could both be consistent with reduced levels of extracellular dopamine leading to upregulation of dopa decarboxylase and increased [18F]dopa accumulation. Alternatively, normal developmental changes in the dopaminergic system may alter the pattern of abnormalities in TS and result in different findings in children and adults with this disorder. However, taken together, the above findings are consistent with abnormal dopamine function in both adolescents and adults with TS.

Limbic, prefrontal and cerebellar dysfunction
Pervasive developmental disorders
Autistic disorder and Asperger's syndrome share impairments in reciprocal social interaction and a restricted repertoire of activities and interests as core symptoms, but are differentiated by the presence of language impairments in autism and that of motor incoordination in Asperger's syndrome. In general, patients with Asperger's syndrome are of average or nearly average intelligence in contrast to the extreme heterogeneity of intellectual

function in autism. Whether Asperger's syndrome and autism in high-functioning individuals are etiologically related is unknown. Most cases of autistic disorder and Asperger's syndrome are idiopathic, i.e. lack an identifiable medical etiology. However, autism has been associated with infectious, metabolic and genetic conditions [e.g. prenatal exposure to rubella, phenylketonuria, Fragile X, tuberous sclerosis complex (TSC)] (see Ciaranello and Ciaranello[74]). In addition, approximately 25% of autistic patients have seizures.[19] These medical conditions have in themselves been associated with abnormal neuroimaging findings, suggesting that studies of autistic patients with such comorbid conditions require appropriate non-autistic medical contrast groups.

Neuroimaging studies of these disorders, to date, have primarily included relatively high-functioning adults or lower functioning children with frequent comorbid mental retardation, epilepsy and medical illness. Brain morphometric studies of autism suggest an abnormal increase in brain volume.[75,76] Some MRI studies of autism have also reported altered cerebellar morphology.[76] In a recent comprehensive review of functional neuroimaging in these disorders, covering the period between 1985 and 2000, Rumsey and Ernst[77] concluded that single-state studies of blood flow and metabolism have failed to yield consistent findings, and that samples of patients with idiopathic (primary) autism are less likely to show abnormalities than are patients with comorbid illness or epilepsy. Activation studies[78–80] have begun to suggest alterations in brain organization for language and cognition that include reduced activation of the prefrontal cortex and amygdala. Neurotransmitter studies using PET suggest abnormalities of serotonergic[81,82] and dopaminergic function,[83] while MRS studies[84–87] document metabolic deficits in the frontal cortex and the cerebellum.

An fMRI study of nine children with a diagnosis of Asperger's syndrome and eight medical controls examined changes in fMRI signal intensity elicited by social reasoning.[88] Subjects were instructed to think over their answers to questions obtained or modified from the comprehension subtest of the Wechsler Intelligence Scale for Children Revised (WISC-R) (e.g. 'What is the thing to do if your friend has lied?'), on which Asperger's patients perform poorly. All controls ($n = 8$) but only five of nine Asperger's patients showed neural changes in the frontal cortex (either activation or deactivation), with or without parietal activation. While the lack of quantification and performance measures limit the interpretations that can be made, this study represents a preliminary exploration of the social cognitive deficits characteristic of pervasive developmental disorders.

65

In contrast to the study of Asperger's syndrome, the following studies focused on the other end of the pervasive developmental disorder (PDD) spectrum, i.e. autistic patients with mental retardation[89] and with comorbid medical conditions (e.g. epilepsy, mental retardation, TSC).[81,84,90]

In the largest rCBF PET studies of autistic children (33 children with primary autism and 10 children with idiopathic mental retardation), Zilbovicius et al[89] reported hypoperfusion in the associative auditory and adjacent multimodal temporal cortex (superior temporal gyrus), which was bilateral but more extended in the right hemisphere. Seizure disorder was an exclusion criterion for both the autistic and non-autistic groups, and the level of mental retardation was matched between groups. Children were off psychotropic medications for 1 month prior to the study. Methodological limitations included the use of two different PET scanners and that children were scanned during sleep induced by premedication with 4 mg/kg of pentobarbital sodium. The findings are consistent with the reported association of early abnormalities in the temporal lobe in secondary autism,[91,92] as well as the animal model of autism produced by neonatal temporal lesions in non-human primates.[93] These results were replicated by an independent group using SPECT and Tc-99 m ECD.[94] The authors also found deactivation of the superior temporal gyrus in a group of children with primary autism and mental retardation compared to children with idiopathic mental retardation. Additional deactivation was shown in the bilateral insula, and the left inferior and middle frontal gyrus in the autistic group compared to the control group. In this study, sedation was given after the administration of the tracer and thus did not affect SPECT measures. Two other SPECT studies of rCBF in similar diagnostic groups reported hypoperfusion associated with autism, including areas of the temporal cortex such as the basal and inferior temporal regions rather than the superior temporal gyrus.[95,96] Functional cerebral deactivation consistently reported in autistic children suggests the presence of functional (e.g. excessive inhibitory processes, abnormal connectivity leading to failure to activate neuronal pathways) or structural deficits resulting in reduced synaptic density. Neurotransmitter studies may permit to shed some light on this issue.

Chugani and her group investigated three different aspects of autism: serotonergic,[81] metabolic[84] and neurochemical characteristics, using PET and $\alpha[^{11}C]$methyltryptophan ([^{11}C]AMT),[97] PET and [18F]fluorodeoxyglucose (FDG), and ^{1}H MRS, respectively.

Asano et al[90] used PET with FDG and [^{11}C]AMT to assess regional cerebral dysfunction associated with the presence of autism and mental retardation in TSC. TSC is an autosomal dominant genetic disorder occurring sporadically in 65% of cases. It is characterized by tissue growths (tubers) in multiple organs including the brain. Autism is diagnosed in 17–61% of individuals with this disorder. Tubers in the temporal lobes are present in 43–100% TSC cases associated with autism. The findings of Asano et al[90] revealed lower rCMRglu levels in lateral temporal gyri, higher rCMRglu levels in deep cerebellar nuclei, and increased serotonin synthesis in the caudate nuclei of the autistic group compared to the mentally-retarded non-autistic group. Due to the difficulty in conducting these types of studies, the experimental design tended to be suboptimal. Concerns include the small sample sizes (six or seven participants per group), the wide age range of the subjects, the difficulty in diagnosing autism in young mentally retarded children ($n = 4 < 2$ years of age), the presence of epilepsy and antiepileptic polydrug treatment, and sedation at the time of scanning [intravenous (IV) nembutal or midazolam]. However, the findings corroborate evidence of temporal lobe,[93,98] cerebellar[99] and serotonergic[81,82] deficits in autism.

Chugani et al[84] also reported deficits in the neuronal integrity of the cerebellum of autistic children compared to their healthy siblings using ^{1}H MRS. In this study, NAA was abnormally low in the cerebellum of the autistic group but did not differ from control values in the frontal and temporal lobes. The wide age range of the sample and the use of siblings of the affected subjects remain caveats in the interpretation of the results. Issues related to a wide age range in pediatric research are illustrated in the following PET study.

Global brain values for serotonin synthesis capacity were obtained for autistic children, healthy siblings of autistic participants and children with medically intractable seizures, using PET and [^{11}C]AMT.[81] All subjects except for four controls were sedated with nembutal or midazolam. In the non-autistic groups, serotonin synthesis capacity was more than twice the adult values until the age of 5 and then declined toward adult levels. These normative developmental data must be regarded with caution because of the suboptimal nature of the control group (children with intractable seizures and siblings of affected subjects). In autistic children, serotonin synthesis capacity increased gradually between the ages of 2 and 15 to values 1.5 times the adult normal values. These data suggest that humans undergo a period of high brain serotonin synthesis capacity during childhood and that this developmental process is disrupted in autistic children. In a previous study, serotonin synthesis capacity values were found to be significantly higher in autistic men compared to healthy men,[97] suggesting that the trend toward abnormally high serotonergic activity in adolescents of 15 years of age is maintained into adulthood. The changes in serotonergic activity from relatively low in young autistic children to abnormally elevated in autistic adults may explain the age-related differences in treatment response to serotonergic agents, effective in adults[56,97,100] but not in children.[101] Because of differences between affected and non-affected children in the developmental trajectories of the serotonergic system throughout childhood, it is important to study the pediatric population within a relatively narrow range.

Depression

Primary candidate structures involved in depression include limbic and paralimbic regions known to modulate emotion. Among these structures, the hippocampus, amygdala, and anterior cingulate have been most consistently implicated by structural and functional neuroimaging studies of depressed adults. Dysfunction in the noradrenergic, serotonergic, and dopaminergic neurotransmitter systems, neuroendocrinological and neuroimmunological systems all have been shown in depression. Most recently, impairments in signaling pathways that regulate neuroplasticity and cell survival have been proposed.[102]

Dahlstrom et al[103] studied serotonin transporter (SET) and DAT densities in 41 drug-naïve children and adolescents (7.7–17.4 years of age, mean 13.2) with diagnoses of depression, bipolar disorder, anxiety, conduct disorder, and/or pervasive developmental disorders. The ligand [^{123}I]CIT binds to both SET and DAT, and thus can provide measures of transporter densities. The serotonergic versus dopaminergic origin of the SPECT signal can be separated spatially because of different relative concentrations of SET and DAT in different brain structures. For example, DAT predominates in the striatum, whereas DAT and SET are present approximately equally in the midbrain. The sample was divided into subjects with ($n = 31$) and without ($n = 10$) a current depressive disorder. Region-of-interest (ROI) included the striatum, thalamus, prefrontal cortex and hypothalamus/midbrain (i.e. raphe nuclei, substantia nigra and colliculi). The occipital ROI was used as a reference region for non-specific activity. DAT–SET binding in the hypothalamic/midbrain area was higher in the depressed group than in the non-depressed group. DAT binding in the striatum did not differ across groups. These findings are difficult to interpret because of the lack of a control group and the significant psychiatric comorbidity present in this sample. Associations between symptom severity and SPECT measures were not explored. The presence of other disorders, such as conduct disorder, may have contributed to the SPECT signal, particularly in view of the known association of low serotonin activity with aggressive behavior. Overall, when compared to reduced [^{123}I]CIT signals in depressed adults,[104] the findings of this study suggest developmental changes in SET or DAT in depressive disorders, perhaps representing the development of a compensatory adaptation to a chronic deficit of synaptic serotonin in adulthood.

Using SPECT with Tc-99 m-HMPAO, Kowatch et al[105] conducted the first study of basal neural activity in adolescents with depression. Resting state rCBF was measured in 17 depressed adolescents and 28 healthy adolescents. Compared to healthy controls, depressed adolescents showed elevated normalized rCBF (ratio of rCBF to whole brain CBF) in the right mesial temporal cortex (including the amygdala), the right superior–anterior temporal lobe, and the left inferolateral temporal lobe. Decreased relative rCBF in the depressed group relative to the control group was localized to the left parietal lobe, the anterior thalamus and the right caudate. The discrepancy in the direction of temporal rCBF abnormality [low in adult major depressive disorder (MDD) and high in adolescent MDD] suggests developmental differences in the neurobiology of adolescent MDD versus adult MDD.

Based on the adult literature implicating the orbitofrontal cortex in depression, Steingard et al[106] examined biochemical concentrations in this region in depressed adolescents using ^{1}H MRS. Figure 2.3 shows a typical image of the location of the region of interest and of the MRS spectra. Compared to healthy adolescents, depressed adolescents showed higher Ch/Cr ratios and normal Cho/NAA ratios in the orbitofrontal cortex. These findings, similar to those reported in depressed adults, may reflect alterations in cholinergic neurotransmission in the orbitofrontal cortex in patients with affective disorders.[107] An abundant literature exists on the relationship between cholinergic neurotransmission and the clinical expression of mood disorders (e.g. as reviewed by Dilsaver[107] and Fritze[109]). However, the relationship between Ch-containing compounds, as detected by ^{1}H MRS, and cholinergic activity is not straightforward, because Ch is used for multiple purposes within cells and the total cellular Ch pool is quite large. Nonetheless, these findings are consistent with the involvement of orbitofrontal cortex as a primary locus of dysfunction present early in the expression of the disorder, probably through its role in affect modulation and integration of thought and emotion.[110,111]

Finally, the role of the amygdala in depression and anxiety in children was investigated in an fMRI study using a cognitive activation paradigm

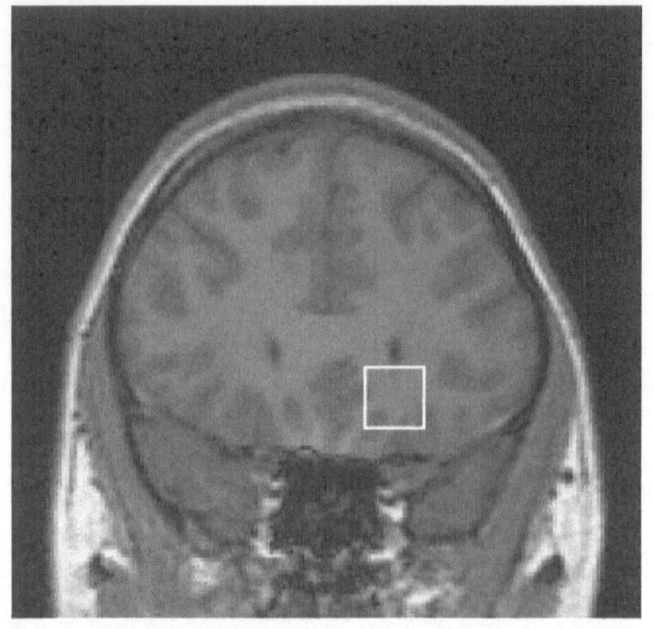

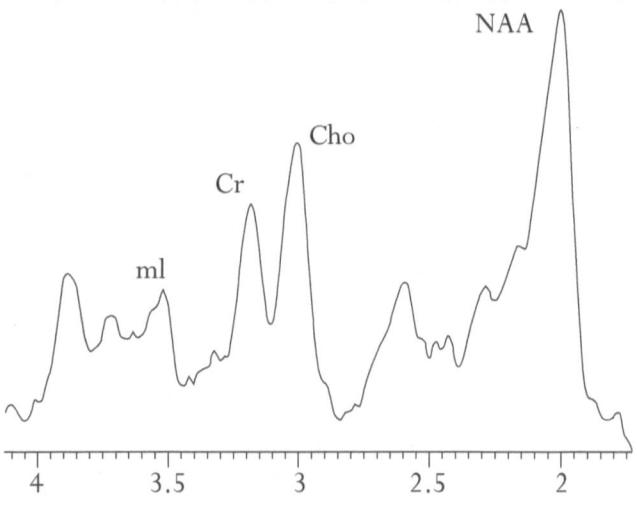

Figure 2.3 *¹H magnetic resonance spectrum (MRS) from the orbitofrontal cortex and a representative ¹H MRS from a 15-year-old healthy control subject. (Reprinted from Steingard et al.[106]) Cho, Choline compounds; Cr, creatine/phosphocreatine; mI, myoinositol; NAA, N-acetylaspartate.*

based on the viewing of fearful and neutral faces.[112] Amygdala response to fearful faces was heightened in anxious children (generalized anxiety disorder or panic disorder) and blunted in depressed children compared with healthy children. The amygdala signal difference between neutral and fearful face conditions was associated with severity of everyday anxiety symptoms. This study illustrates the power of fMRI studies to investigate the functional integrity of unique structures hypothesized to be involved in specific disorders.

Conclusions

The goal of this chapter was to review the most recent advances in pediatric functional neuroimaging in child psychiatry. This review is notable for the very limited number of published pediatric studies relative to the adult literature, despite the advent of the non-invasive fMRI and MRS techniques. Several factors may contribute to this observation, including the difficulties in acquiring quality data from children (e.g. not hampered by motion artifacts or weak unreliable signal), in recruiting ill children with clear diagnoses into research protocols, and in setting up ethical and feasible well-controlled experiments.

The studies reviewed herein are informative in showing how commonalities in abnormalities of brain function shared by adults and children for a given disorder coexist with differences, and how these relationships can change over time. Although providing more questions than answers at the present time, such knowledge can permit the research community to develop focused hypotheses to be tested at all levels of scientific inquiry, across molecular, neuroanatomical, neurofunctional, neurochemical and behavioral domains of investigation.

The lack of pediatric functional neuroimaging studies in psychiatric disorders such as substance-use disorders, eating disorders and anxiety (except for OCD) is disconcerting, particularly in the context of their relatively high prevalence in youth. The reasons for this situation are unclear. Research in substance abuse requires additional stringent ethical guidelines because of legal issues. Children with anxiety disorders, characterized by withdrawal from unfamiliar situations, may be more difficult to enroll in imaging protocols. As the field expands, strategies will be developed to incorporate these disorders into research agendas.

A fundamental message brought to light in this review is the critical need for normative developmental data as a basis for interpreting findings in diseased states. Methods need to be developed to expand normative studies while meeting ethical requirements. The ultimate goal of neuroscience is to understand, prevent, and treat illnesses. In this context, research in children is best suited to inform the major questions of vulnerability and protective factors, as well as of causality, which tend to be elusive in adult research.

References

1. Ernst M, Rumsey JM. *Functional Neuroimaging in Child Psychiatry*. (Cambridge University Press: Cambridge, 2000.)
2. Anderson AW, Marois R, Colson ER et al. Neonatal auditory activation detected by functional magnetic resonance imaging. *Magn Reson Imaging* 2001; **19**: 1–5.
3. Yamada H, Sadato N, Konishi Y et al. A milestone for normal development of the infantile brain detected by functional MRI. *Neurology* 2000; **55**: 218–23.
4. Gaillard WD, Grandin CB, Xu B. Developmental aspects of pediatric fMRI: considerations for image acquisition, analysis, and interpretation. *Neuroimage* 2001; **13**: 239–49.
5. Chung MK, Worsley KJ, Paus T et al. A unified statistical approach to deformation-based morphometry. *Neuroimage* 2001; **14**: 595–606.
6. Talairach J, Tournoux P. *Co-Planar Stereotaxic Atlas of the Human Brain: 3-Dimensional Proportional System: An Approach to Cerebral Imaging*. (Thieme Medical Publishers, Stuttgart, 1988.)
7. Durston S, Hulshoff Pol HE, Casey BJ, Giedd JN, Buitelaar JK, van Engeland H. Anatomical MRI of the developing human brain: what have we learned? *J Am Acad Child Adolesc Psychiatry* 2001; **40**: 1012–20.
8. Paus T, Zijdenbos A, Worsley K et al. Structural maturation of neural pathways in children and adolescents: in vivo study. *Science* 1999; **283**: 1908–11.
9. Hoagwood K, Jensen PS, Petti T, Burns BJ. Outcomes of mental health care for children and adolescents: I. A comprehensive conceptual model. *J Am Acad Child Adolesc Psychiatry* 1996; **35**: 1055–63.
10. Ernst M. PET in child psychiatry: the risks and benefits of studying normal healthy children. *Prog Neuropsychopharmacol Biol Psychiatry* 1999; **23**: 561–70.
11. Ernst M, Freed ME, Zametkin AJ. Health hazards of radiation exposure in the context of brain imaging research: special consideration for children. *J Nucl Med* 1998; **39**: 689–98.
12. Corina DP, Richards TL, Serafini S et al. fMRI auditory language differences between dyslexic and able reading children. *Neuroreport* 2001; **12**: 1195–201.
13. Georgiewa P, Rzanny R, Hopf JM et al. fMRI during word processing in dyslexic and normal reading children. *Neuroreport* 1999; **10**: 3459–65.

14. Richards TL, Corina D, Serafini S et al. Effects of a phonologically driven treatment for dyslexia on lactate levels measured by proton MR spectroscopic imaging. *Am J Neuroradiol* 2000; **21:** 916–22.

15. Richards TL, Dager SR, Corina D et al. Dyslexic children have abnormal brain lactate response to reading-related language tasks. *Am J Neuroradiol* 1999; **20:** 1393–8.

16. Simos PG, Breier JI, Fletcher JM, Bergman E, Papanicolaou AC. Cerebral mechanisms involved in word reading in dyslexic children: a magnetic source imaging approach. *Cereb Cortex* 2000; **10:** 809–16.

17. Simos PG, Breier JI, Fletcher JM et al. Brain activation profiles in dyslexic children during non-word reading: a magnetic source imaging study. *Neurosci Lett* 2000; **290:** 61–5.

18. Temple E, Poldrack RA, Salidis J et al. Disrupted neural responses to phonological and orthographic processing in dyslexic children: an fMRI study. *Neuroreport* 2001; **12:** 299–307.

19. American Psychiatric Association. *Diagnostic and Statistical Manual of Mental Disorders*, 4th edn [DSM-IV, 4 ed.]. (American Psychiatric Association: Washington, DC, 1994.)

20. Zametkin AJ, Ernst M. Problems in the management of attention-deficit-hyperactivity disorder. *N Engl J Med* 1999; **340:** 40–6.

21. Ernst M, Tata S. Review of functional neuroimaging research in attention deficit hyperactivity disorder. *Econom Neurosci* 2001; **3:** 58–66.

22. Ernst M, Zametkin AJ, Matochik JA, Jons PH, Cohen RM. DOPA decarboxylase activity in attention deficit hyperactivity disorder adults. A [fluorine-18]fluorodopa positron emission tomographic study. *J Neurosci* 1998; **18:** 5901–7.

23. Ernst M, Zametkin AJ, Matochik JA, Pascualvaca D, Jons PH, Cohen RM. High mid-brain [18F]DOPA accumulation in children with attention deficit hyperactivity disorder. *Am J Psychiatry* 1999; **156:** 1209–15.

24. Dougherty DD, Bonab AA, Spencer TJ, Rauch SL, Madras BK, Fischman AJ. Dopamine transporter density in patients with attention deficit hyperactivity disorder. *Lancet* 1999; **354:** 2132–3.

25. Dresel S, Krause J, Krause KH et al. Attention deficit hyperactivity disorder: binding of [99 m Tc]TRODAT-1 to the dopamine transporter before and after methylphenidate treatment. *Eur J Nucl Med* 2000; **27:** 1518–24.

26. Krause KH, Dresel SH, Krause J, Kung HF, Tatsch K. Increased striatal dopamine transporter in adult patients with attention deficit hyperactivity disorder: effects of methylphenidate as measured by single photon emission computed tomography. *Neurosci Lett* 2000; **285:** 107–10.

27. Teicher MH, Andersen SL, Hostetter JC. Evidence for dopamine receptor pruning between adolescence and adulthood in striatum but not nucleus accumbens. *Brain Res Dev Brain Res* 1995; **89:** 167–72.

28. Bush G, Frazier JA, Rauch SL et al. Anterior cingulate cortex dysfunction in attention-deficit/hyperactivity disorder revealed by fMRI and the Counting Stroop. *Biol Psychiatry* 1999; **45:** 1542–52.

29. Rubia K, Overmeyer S, Taylor E et al. Hypofrontality in attention deficit hyperactivity disorder during higher-order motor control: a study with functional MRI. *Am J Psychiatry* 1999; **156:** 891–6.

30. Schweitzer JB, Faber TL, Grafton ST, Tune LE, Hoffman JM, Kilts CD. Alterations in the functional anatomy of working memory in adult attention deficit hyperactivity disorder. *Am J Psychiatry* 2000; **157:** 278–80.

31. Langleben D, Austin G, Krikorian G, Ridlehuber H, Goris M, Strauss H. Interhemispheric asymmetry of regional cerebral blood flow in prepubescent boys with attention deficit hyperactivity disorder. *Nucl Med Commun* 2001; **22:** 1333–40.

32. Kim BN, Lee JS, Cho SC, Lee DS. Methylphenidate increased regional cerebral blood flow in subjects with attention deficit/hyperactivity disorder. *Yonsei Med J* 2001; **42:** 19–29.

33. Ernst M, Zametkin AJ, Matochik JA et al. Intravenous dextroamphetamine and brain glucose metabolism. *Neuropsychopharmacology* 1997; **17:** 391–401.

34. Matochik JA, Liebenauer LL, King C, Szymanski HV, Cohen RM, Zametkin AJ. Cerebral glucose metabolism in adults with attention deficit hyperactivity disorder after chronic stimulant treatment. *Am J Psychiatry* 1994; **151:** 658–64.

35. Matochik JA, Nordahl TE, Gross M et al. Effects of acute stimulant medication on cerebral metabolism in adults with hyperactivity. *Neuropsychopharmacology* 1993; **8:** 377–86.

36. Berquin PC, Giedd JN, Jacobsen LK et al. Cerebellum in attention-deficit hyperactivity disorder: a morphometric MRI study. *Neurology* 1998; **50:** 1087–93.

37. Mostofsky SH, Reiss AL, Lockhart P, Denckla MB. Evaluation of cerebellar size in attention-deficit hyperactivity disorder. *J Child Neurol* 1998; **13:** 434–9.

38. Teicher MH, Anderson CM, Polcari A, Glod CA, Maas LC, Renshaw PF. Functional deficits in basal ganglia of children with attention-deficit/hyperactivity disorder shown with functional magnetic resonance imaging relaxometry. *Nat Med* 2000; **6:** 470–3.

39. Vaidya CJ, Austin G, Kirkorian G et al. Selective effects of methylphenidate in attention deficit hyperactivity disorder: a functional magnetic resonance study. *Proc Natl Acad Sci USA* 1998; **95:** 14,494–9.

40. Volkow ND, Wang GJ, Fowler JS et al. Effects of methylphenidate on regional brain glucose metabolism in humans: relationship to dopamine D2 receptors. *Am J Psychiatry* 1997; **154:** 50–5.

41. Ilgin N, Senol S, Gucuyener K, Gokcora N, Sener S. Is increased D2 receptor availability associated with response to stimulant medication in ADHD. *Dev Med Child Neurol* 2001; **43:** 755–60.

42. Jin Z, Zang Y, Zeng Y, Zhang L, Wang Y. Striatal neuronal loss or dysfunction and choline rise in children with attention-deficit hyperactivity disorder: a 1H-magnetic resonance spectroscopy study. *Neurosci Lett* 2001; **315:** 45–8.

43. Flament MF, Whitaker A, Rapoport JL et al. Obsessive compulsive disorder in adolescence: an epidemiological study. *J Am Acad Child Adolesc Psychiatry* 1988; **27:** 764–71.

44. Valleni-Basile LA, Garrison CZ, Waller JL et al. Incidence of obsessive–compulsive disorder in a community sample of young adolescents. *J Am Acad Child Adolesc Psychiatry* 1996; **35:** 898–906.

45. Pauls DL, Alsobrook JP, Goodman W, Rasmussen S, Leckman JF. A family study of obsessive–compulsive disorder. *Am J Psychiatry* 1995; **152:** 76–84.

46. Riddle MA, Scahill L, King R et al. Obsessive compulsive disorder in children and adolescents: phenomenology and family history. *J Am Acad Child Adolesc Psychiatry* 1990; **29:** 766–72.

47. Last CG, Strauss CC. Obsessive–compulsive disorder in childhood. *J Anxiety Disord* 1989; **3:** 295–302.

48. Baxter Jr LR, Schwartz JM, Bergman KS et al. Caudate glucose metabolic rate changes with both drug and behavior therapy for obsessive–compulsive disorder. *Arch Gen Psychiatry* 1992; **49:** 681–9.

49. Benkelfat C, Nordahl TE, Semple WE, King C, Murphy DL, Cohen RM. Local cerebral glucose metabolic rates in obsessive–compulsive disorder: patients treated with clomipramine. *Arch Gen Psychiatry* 1990; **47:** 840–8.

50. Breiter HC, Rauch SL. Functional MRI and the study of OCD: from symptom provocation to cognitive-behavioral probes of cortico-striatal systems and the amygdala. *Neuroimage* 1996; **4:** S127–S138.

51. Hoehn-Saric R, Pearlson GD, Harris GJ, Machlin SR, Camargo EE. Effects of fluoxetine on regional cerebral blood flow in obsessive–compulsive patients. *Am J Psychiatry* 1991; **148:** 1243–5.

52. Rauch SL, Jenike MA, Alpert NM et al. Regional cerebral blood flow measured during symptom provocation in obsessive–compulsive disorder using oxygen 15-labeled carbon dioxide and positron emission tomography. *Arch Gen Psychiatry* 1994; **51:** 62–70.

53. Schwartz JM, Stoessel PW, Baxter Jr. LR, Martin KM, Phelps ME. Systematic changes in cerebral glucose metabolic rate after successful behavior modification treatment of obsessive–compulsive disorder. *Arch Gen Psychiatry* 1996; **53:** 109–13.

54. Swedo SE, Pietrini P, Leonard HL et al. Cerebral glucose metabolism in childhood-onset obsessive–compulsive disorder. Revisualization during pharmacotherapy. *Arch Gen Psychiatry* 1992; **49:** 690–4.

55. Rosenberg DR, MacMaster FP, Keshavan MS, Fitzgerald KD, Stewart CM, Moore GJ. Decrease in caudate glutamatergic concentrations in pediatric obsessive–compulsive disorder patients taking paroxetine. *J Am Acad Child Adolesc Psychiatry* 2000; **39:** 1096–103.

56. Gilbert AR, Moore GJ, Keshavan MS et al. Decrease in thalamic volumes of pediatric patients with obsessive–compulsive disorder who are taking paroxetine. *Arch Gen Psychiatry* 2000; **57:** 449–56.

57. Alexander GE, Crutcher MD. Functional architecture of basal ganglia circuits: neural substrates of parallel processing. *Trends Neurosci* 1990; **13:** 266–71.

58. Modell JG, Mountz JM, Curtis GC, Greden JF. Neurophysiologic dysfunction in basal ganglia/limbic striatal and thalamocortical circuits as a pathogenetic mechanism of obsessive–compulsive disorder. *J Neuropsychiatry Clin Neurosci* 1989; **1:** 27–36.

59. Fitzgerald KD, Moore GJ, Paulson LA, Stewart CM, Rosenberg DR. Proton spectroscopic imaging of the thalamus in treatment-naive pediatric obsessive–compulsive disorder. *Biol Psychiatry* 2000; **47:** 174–82.

60. Rosenberg DR, Amponsah A, Sullivan A, MacMillan S, Moore GJ. Increased medial thalamic choline in pediatric obsessive–compulsive disorder as detected by quantitative in vivo spectroscopic imaging. *J Child Neurol* 2001; **16:** 636–41.

61. Barker PB, Breiter SN, Soher BJ et al. Quantitative proton spectroscopy of canine brain: in vivo and in vitro correlations. *Magn Reson Med* 1994; **32:** 157–63.

62. Miller BL, Chang L, Booth R et al. In vivo 1H MRS choline: correlation with in vitro chemistry/histology. *Life Sci* 1996; **58:** 1929–35.

63. Apter A, Pauls DL, Bleich A et al. An epidemiologic study of Gilles de la Tourette's syndrome in Israel. *Arch Gen Psychiatry* 1993; **50:** 734–8.

64. Burd L, Kerbeshian J, Wikenheiser M, Fisher W. A prevalence study of Gilles de la Tourette syndrome in North Dakota school-age children. *J Am Acad Child Psychiatry* 1986; **25:** 552–3.

65. Comings DE, Himes JA, Comings BG. An epidemiologic study of Tourette's syndrome in a single school district. *J Clin Psychiatry* 1990; **51:** 463–9.

66. Nomoto F, Machiyama Y. An epidemiological study of tics. *Jpn J Psychiatry Neurol* 1990; **44:** 649–55.

67. Peterson BS, Thomas P. Tourette's syndrome: what are we really imaging? In: (Ernst M, Rumsey JM, eds) *Functional Neuroimaging in Child Psychiatry.* (Cambridge University Press: Cambridge, 2000.)

68. Peterson BS, Skudlarski P, Anderson AW et al. A functional magnetic resonance imaging study of tic suppression in Tourette syndrome. *Arch Gen Psychiatry* 1998; **55:** 326–33.

69. Brooks DJ, Turjanski N, Sawle GV, Playford ED, Lees AJ. PET studies on the integrity of the pre and postsynaptic dopaminergic system in Tourette syndrome. *Adv Neurol* 1992; **58:** 227–31.

70. Turjanski N, Sawle GV, Playford ED et al. PET studies of the presynaptic and post-synaptic dopaminergic system in Tourette's syndrome. *J Neurol Neurosurg Psychiatry* 1994; **57:** 688–92.

71. Malison RT, McDougle CJ, van Dyck CH et al. [123I]beta-CIT SPECT imaging of striatal dopamine transporter binding in Tourette's disorder. *Am J Psychiatry* 1995; **152:** 1359–61.

72. Wolf SS, Jones DW, Knable MB et al. Tourette syndrome: prediction of phenotypic variation in monozygotic twins by caudate nucleus D2 receptor binding. *Science* 1996; **273:** 1225–7.

73. Ernst M, Zametkin AJ, Jons PH, Matochik JA, Pascualvaca D, Cohen RM. High presynaptic dopaminergic activity in children with Tourette's disorder. *J Am Acad Child Adolesc Psychiatry* 1999; **38:** 86–94.

74. Ciaranello AL, Ciaranello RD. The neurobiology of infantile autism. *Annu Rev Neurosci* 1995; **18:** 101–28.

75. Courchesne E, Karns CM, Davis HR et al. Unusual brain growth patterns in early life in patients with autistic disorders. *Neurology* 2001; **57:** 245–54.

76. Eliez S, Reiss A. Neuroimaging of childhood psychiatric disorders: a selective review. *Child Psychol Psychiatry* 2000; **41:** 679–94.

77. Rumsey JM, Ernst M. Functional neuroimaging of autistic disorders. *Ment Retard Dev Disabil Res Rev* 2000; **6:** 171–9.

78. Baron-Cohen S, Ring HA, Wheelwright S et al. Social intelligence in the normal and autistic brain: an fMRI study. *Eur J Neurosci* 1999; **11:** 1891–8.

79. Muller RA, Behen ME, Rothermel RD et al. Brain mapping of language and auditory perception in high-functioning autistic adults: a PET study. *J Autism Dev Disord* 1999; **29:** 19–31.

80. Ring HA, Baron-Cohen S, Wheelwright S et al. Cerebral correlates of preserved cognitive skills in autism: a functional MRI study of embedded figures task performance. *Brain* 1999; **122:** 1305–15.

81. Chugani DC, Muzik O, Behen M et al. Developmental changes in brain serotonin synthesis capacity in autistic and nonautistic children. *Ann Neurol* 1999; **45:** 287–95.

82. Chugani DC, Muzik O, Rothermel R et al. Altered serotonin synthesis in the dentatothalamocortical pathway in autistic boys. *Ann Neurol* 1997; **42:** 666–9.

83. Ernst M, Zametkin AJ, Matochik JA, Pascualvaca D, Cohen RM. Low medial prefrontal dopaminergic activity in autistic children. *Lancet* 1997; **350:** 638.

84. Chugani DC, Sundram BS, Behen M, Lee ML, Moore GJ. Evidence of altered energy metabolism in autistic children. *Prog Neuropsychopharmacol Biol Psychiatry* 1999; **23:** 635–41.

85. Hashimoto T, Kawano N, Fukuda K et al. Proton magnetic resonance spectroscopy of the brain in three cases of Rett syndrome: comparison with autism and normal controls. *Acta Neurol Scand* 1998; **98:** 8–14.

86. Hashimoto T, Tayama M, Miyazaki M et al. Differences in brain metabolites between patients with autism and mental retardation as detected by in vivo localized proton magnetic resonance spectroscopy. *J Child Neurol* 1997; **12:** 91–6.

87. Minshew NJ, Goldstein G, Dombrowski SM, Panchalingam K, Pettegrew JW. A preliminary 31P MRS study of autism: evidence for undersynthesis and increased degradation of brain membranes. *Biol Psychiatry* 1993; **33:** 762–73.

88. Oktem F, Diren B, Karaagaoglu E, Anlar B. Functional magnetic resonance imaging in children with Asperger's syndrome. *J Child Neurol* 2001; **16:** 253–6.

89. Zilbovicius M, Boddaert N, Belin P et al. Temporal lobe dysfunction in childhood autism: a PET study. Positron emission tomography. *Am J Psychiatry* 2000; **157:** 1988–93.

90. Asano E, Chugani DC, Muzik O et al. Autism in tuberous sclerosis complex is related to both cortical and subcortical dysfunction. *Neurology* 2001; **57:** 1269–77.

91. Bolton PF, Griffiths PD. Association of tuberous sclerosis of temporal lobes with autism and atypical autism. *Lancet* 1997; **349:** 392–5.

92. Chugani HT, Da Silva E, Chugani DC. Infantile spasms: III. Prognostic implications of bitemporal hypometabolism on positron emission tomography. *Ann Neurol* 1996; **39:** 643–9.

93. Bachevalier J, Merjanian PM. The contribution of medial temporal lobe structures in infantile autism: a neurobehavioral study in primates. In: (Bauman ML, Kemper TL, eds) *The Neurobiology of Autism.* (Johns Hopkins University Press: Baltimore, 1994.)

94. Ohnishi T, Matsuda H, Hashimoto T et al. Abnormal regional cerebral blood flow in childhood autism. *Brain* 2000; **123:** 1838–44.

95. Kaya M, Karasalihoglu S, Ustun F et al. The relationship between 99mTc-HMPAO brain SPECT and the scores of real life rating scale in autistic children. *Brain Dev* 2002; **24:** 77–81.

96. Starkstein SE, Vazquez S, Vrancic D et al. SPECT findings in mentally retarded autistic individuals. *J Neuropsychiatry Clin Neurosci* 2000; **12:** 370–5.

97. Chugani DC, Muzik O, Chakraborty PK, Mangner TJ, Chugani HT. Brain serotonin synthesis measured with [11C]-methyl-tryptophan positron emission tomography in normal and autistic adults. *Soc Nuerosci* 1996; **22:** 22 (abstract).

98. Kemper TL, Bauman M. Neuropathology of infantile autism. *J Neuropathol Exp Neurol* 1998; **57:** 645–52.

99. Courchesne E, Yeung-Courchesne R, Press GA, Hesselink JR, Jernigan TL. Hypoplasia of cerebellar vermal lobules VI and VII in autism. *N Engl J Med* 1988; **318:** 1349–54.

100. Gordon CT, State RC, Nelson JE, Hamburger SD, Rapoport JL. A double-blind comparison of clomipramine, desipramine, and placebo in the treatment of autistic disorder. *Arch Gen Psychiatry* 1993; **50:** 441–7.

101. Sanchez LE, Campbell M, Small AM, Cueva JE, Armenteros JL, Adams PB. A pilot study of clomipramine in young autistic children. *J Am Acad Child Adolesc Psychiatry* 1996; **35:** 537–44.

102. Manji HK, Drevets WC, Charney DS. The cellular neurobiology of depression. *Nat Med* 2001; **7:** 541–7.

103. Dahlstrom M, Ahonen A, Ebeling H, Torniainen P, Heikkila J, Moilanen I. Elevated hypothalamic/midbrain serotonin (monoamine) transporter availability in depressive drug-naive children and adolescents. *Molec Psychiatry* 2000; **5:** 514–22.

104. Malison RT, Price LH, Berman R et al. Reduced brain serotonin transporter availability in major depression as measured by [123I]-2 beta-carbomethoxy-3 beta-(4-iodophenyl)tropane and single photon emission computed tomography. *Biol Psychiatry* 1998; **44:** 1090–8.

105. Kowatch RA, Devous Sr MD, Harvey DC et al. A SPECT HMPAO study of regional cerebral blood flow in depressed adolescents and normal controls. *Prog Neuropsychopharmacol Biol Psychiatry* 1999; **23:** 643–56.

106. Steingard RJ, Yurgelun-Todd DA, Hennen J et al. Increased orbitofrontal cortex levels of choline in depressed adolescents as detected by in vivo proton magnetic resonance spectroscopy. *Biol Psychiatry* 2000; **48:** 1053–61.

107. Charles HC, Lazeyras F, Krishnan KR, Boyko OB, Payne M, Moore D. Brain choline in depression: in vivo detection of potential pharmacodynamic effects of antidepressant therapy using hydrogen localized spectroscopy. *Prog Neuropsychopharmacol Biol Psychiatry* 1994; **18:** 1121–7.

108. Dilsaver SC. Cholinergic mechanisms in affective disorders. Future directions for investigation. *Acta Psychiatr Scand* 1986; **74:** 312–34.

109. Fritze J. The adrenergic–cholinergic imbalance hypothesis of depression: a review and a perspective. *Rev Neurosci* 1993; **4:** 63–93.

110. Mesulam MM. Frontal cortex and behavior. *Ann Neurol* 1986; **19:** 320–5.

111. Sackeim HA, Prohovnik I, Moeller JR et al. Regional cerebral blood flow in mood disorders. I. Comparison of major depressives and normal controls at rest. *Arch Gen Psychiatry* 1990; **47:** 60–70.

112. Thomas KM, Drevets WC, Dahl RE et al. Amygdala response to fearful faces in anxious and depressed children. *Arch Gen Psychiatry* 2001; **58:** 1057–63.

113. Gustafsson P, Thernlund G, Ryding E, Rosen I, Cederblad M. Associations between cerebral blood-flow measured by single photon emission computed tomography (SPECT), electroencephalogram (EEG), behaviour symptoms, cognition and neurological soft signs in children with attention-deficit hyperactivity disorder (ADHD). *Acta Paediatr* 2000; **89**: 830–5.

3. NEUROIMAGING AND AGING

Domonick J Wegesin, Yaakov Stern

Introduction

As the percentage of the population that is over the age of 65 continues to increase, the need to understand the brain–behavior relationships that differentiate successful and unsuccessful aging is clear. Advances in structural and functional brain imaging technologies continue to enhance our abilities to probe the normal and pathological changes that occur in the aging brain. This chapter provides a brief review of imaging studies that explore the aging brain, including computed tomography (CT), single photon emission computed tomography (SPECT), positron emission tomography (PET), and magnetic resonance imaging (MRI). Findings in healthy elders are initially described, followed by reports of dementing geriatric patients, e.g. those with Alzheimer's disease (AD), vascular dementia, Huntington's disease (HD), and Parkinson's disease (PD). Due to the limited scope of the review, electroencephalographic (EEG) studies and event-related brain potential (ERP) studies will not be covered (for a review of ERP studies in aging see Friedman and Johnson[1]). We begin with an overview of specific brain regions that are most vulnerable to age- and disease-related decline, and then examine the functional changes that are hypothesized to underlie cognitive aging.

Structural changes in the aging brain

After the second decade of life, a gradual decline in brain size ensues that slowly accelerates with each passing year. Brain atrophy (up to 15% of adult brain weight) is evidenced by a progressive increase in the size of the ventricles and cortical sulci in CT imaging and by a progressive decrease in brain volume in MRI. The decrease in total brain size is thought to primarily reflect atrophic processes within gray matter, as the volume of white matter is relatively more resilient to atrophy across the lifespan.

Within gray matter, cortical atrophy is clearly not global, as some regions are more vulnerable than others to the effects of aging. The pattern of loss appears to follow a 'last in, first out' rule, whereby structures that developed last (phylogenetically and ontogenetically) are the first to deteriorate with age. The hippocampus is an exception. Though it develops early in ontogeny, it commonly shows an early age-related decline, especially in cases of dementia. Consequently, it has been proposed that the 'last in, first out' rule applies to normal aging, whereas changes in medial temporal lobe structures, including the hippocampus, may represent pathological processes.[2] The areas showing the greatest age-related atrophy, including the frontal–temporal cortex, hippocampus, and subcortical gray areas are highlighted below.

Prefrontal gray matter volume shows the strongest negative correlation with age ($r = -0.55$).[3] Reductions in temporal lobe volume with age nearly parallel losses to frontal lobe volume,[4,5] and in some cases have been reported to exceed the reductions in the frontal cortex.[6] The pattern of age-related cortical loss has been shown to vary with sex: men experience greater loss in the frontal and temporal lobes, whereas women have greater losses in the hippocampus and parietal lobes.[7] Thus, the gender composition of group data may affect study outcomes and should be considered when comparing research reports.

Post-mortem studies have shown clear decreases in hippocampal volume with age (for a review see Geinisman et al[8]). Imaging studies of the hippocampus have been less consistent, with several recent anatomical studies reporting no change with aging in hippocampal cell size or volume,[9] and others reporting clear reductions in volume in older adults.[3,10,11] Longitudinal studies with multiple scans have reported minimal changes in hippocampal formation in normal elderly.[12] Overall, reviews of the literature demonstrate a mild age-related decrease in hippocampal volume ($r = -0.30$).[2] Within the hippocampal formation, subregions appear to atrophy differentially, with posterior regions being more vulnerable to age-related decline. This variability within the hippocampus may help account for inconsistent findings between studies, since those that do not include that anterior portion of the hippocampus are less likely to show age-related differences.[13] Within the striatum, both the caudate and putamen show moderate to strong negative associations between age and volume[14,15] (but see Backman et al[16] for null findings). These two subcortical structures constitute part of an important frontal–striatal circuit that is thought to be relevant to higher cognitive function, which may be particularly sensitive to age-related decline.[17]

Though gray matter undergoes the greatest amount of atrophy across the lifespan, the majority of age-related abnormalities detected with brain imaging are hyperintensities located in the deep subcortical white matter. Leukoaraiosis on CT scans are seen as bilateral patchy or diffuse areas of hypodensity. On MRI scans, which is a superior technique compared to CT in detecting these white matter changes, they appear as white matter hyperintensities (WMHI). White matter changes are reported with increasing frequency in adults over the age of 60. In one community sample, 11% of those aged 65–69 and 59% of those aged 80–84 showed WMHI.[18]

WMHI are thought to represent structural changes affecting the small intraparenchymal cerebral arteries and arterioles. These microvascular changes are most likely caused by repeated transient events involving reductions in blood flow that produce an incomplete form of infarction, e.g. transient cerebral ischemia.[19] Epidemiological studies have reported an association between WMHI and certain cerebrovascular diseases.[20,21] In addition, MR blood flow data have shown decreased cerebral blood flow (CBF) in areas with WMHI compared with normal white matter areas.[22] WMHI also appear more frequently in demented groups compared to control groups,[23] and WMHI scores are higher in patients with vascular dementia compared to those with dementia with Lewy bodies or AD. Together, these findings suggest that ischemia makes an instrumental contribution to the development of WMHI.

The relationship between WMHI and cognitive function remains unclear. In the Austrian Stroke Prevention Study, MR measures of WMHI were evaluated in 273 participants (mean age of 60) over 3 years.[24] Lesion progression was reported in 49 (17.9%) cases. Changes in WMHI had no impact on the course of cognitive test performance over the 3-year period. Cross-sectional studies provide limited evidence for a negative relationship between the extent of WMHI and performance on tests of executive function, e.g. digit span, Wisconsin Card Sorting Test (WCST)[25] and the Trails tests.[26] However, the relationship between WMHI and these frontal/subcortical functions has been shown to diminish or disappear when the variance related to age and education are controlled.[27]

In sum, WMHI constitute a common finding in healthy geriatric patients and are more extensive in patients with dementia. More data are required to delineate the relationship between WMHI and cognition in the elderly. In addition, data informing the relationship between WMHI and late-life depression are also needed, as these lesions have been shown to be common in old adults suffering from depression.[28] Given the hypothesis that WMHI result from transient ischemic events, geriatric patients showing subclinical levels of WMHI should be encouraged to reduce risks associated with vascular disease.

Functional changes in the aging brain

The most encouraging developments in geriatric brain imaging are reflected in studies of age-related changes in brain function, both at rest and during cognitive activation tasks. Initially, it is critical to determine if age is associated with alterations in the function of neural and cerebrovascular systems at rest. To date, it remains controversial whether global changes in cerebral metabolic rate for oxygen or CBF occur with aging in healthy individuals (for a review see Grossman et al[29]). Several studies have shown significant CBF decreases with age,[30–33] whereas others have not found age-related declines (e.g. de Leon et al[34]). Many studies have implemented corrections for estimated cerebral atrophy associated with aging and reported that these corrections account for the correlation between CBF and age.[35] Despite the inconsistencies reported on global changes in CBF, evidence for age-related reductions in regional CBF has been more consistent. Specifically, reductions have been reported for frontal, temporal, and parietal areas.[30,33,36] The age-related hypometabolism in the frontal lobes reported during rest [30,37] is significant in the light of the frontal lobe hypothesis of cognitive aging highlighted below.

Brain imaging and memory

One of the most frequent complaints of the elderly involves self-perceived age-related changes in cognitive abilities, particularly those associated with memory. Though memory decline is not an inevitable part of the aging process, neuropsychological studies have shown memory loss to be pervasive in adults over the age of 65.[38] Two patterns have emerged in the brain imaging literature that may account for age-related memory decline. First, old adults have shown diminished activation in brain networks activated by younger individuals. This pattern of results reflects a functional deficit in the old adults. Second, old adults have shown activation of additional brain areas that are not active in young adults during performance of the same task. This pattern has been described as a compensatory mechanism in the old adults.

Traditionally, investigators examining age-associated memory impairment have acknowledged the similarities in the pattern of memory loss seen in the elderly and that seen in amnesic patients, and therefore have focused their attention on structures commonly associated with amnesia, specifically those within the medial temporal lobe (MTL). However, many of these studies have shown that MTL activity is typically preserved in healthy old adults.[39–41] These findings are consistent with the structural imaging data reported above that showed that in healthy elderly MTL regions undergo relatively little age-related structural decline.[3]

A second neuropsychological hypothesis of cognitive aging proposes that selective frontal lobe decline underlies age-related cognitive decline.[42,43] In support of this claim, studies have reported severe memory impairment in patients with frontal lobe lesions.[44,45] Meta-analysis revealed that frontal lobe patients are impaired not only on tests of free recall, which is known to rely on greater executive processes subserved by the frontal lobes, but also on tests of cued recall and simple item recognition.[46] Studies of healthy elderly using neuroimaging techniques have also drawn focus to the importance of the frontal lobes in accounting for age-related memory loss.

Imaging studies have revealed a pattern in which old adults show diminished left prefrontal activity during encoding compared to young adults.[47–49] The decreases in activation during encoding are thought to reflect less efficient use of the neural network involved in encoding.[49] Grady et al[48] examined the left frontal activity in young and old adults under different encoding conditions: shallow encoding, semantic encoding and a memorization condition. In the two elaborative conditions (semantic encoding and memorization), young adults showed greater left prefrontal activation compared to the old, suggesting that the decreased activation during encoding in the old may reflect deficient use of elaborative strategies during encoding.

For retrieval, more extensive (bilateral) prefrontal activity has been reported in old compared to young adults.[39,47,50,51] For example, in a paired-associate memory task, young adults showed right prefrontal activation during cued recall (the first word of the pair was presented, and the subjects were asked to recall the second word of the pair), but older adults showed bilateral prefrontal activation. The increase in activation in old adults was proposed to reflect functional compensation.[47] This compensatory mechanism has also been shown in tests of working memory. Grady[52] reported that in young adults, the right prefrontal activation increased with longer working memory delays. In the old, no increases in the right prefrontal activation were seen with increasing delays, though the elderly showed more activity in left prefrontal areas. In another study, old adults who exhibited a bilateral pattern of prefrontal activity performed better on a verbal working memory task than those who did not,[53] as would be predicted if the additional left prefrontal activity is, in fact, compensatory.

Though the frontal cortex remains a focus in the cognitive aging literature, its role in age-associated cognitive decline has been challenged. Rubin[54] suggested that deficits attributed exclusively to frontal lobe changes might better be described by changes within the striatum. (Structural changes within the caudate and putamen are described above.) Additional evidence on the role of the striatum in cognitive aging derives from recent PET studies that have allowed an inspection of age-associated changes within particular neurotransmitter systems. Such studies are dependent on the availability of ligands for specific neurotransmitters that can be labeled with short-lived radionuclides. The radioligands are injected intravenously, and radioactivity in the brain is measured continuously over a short period (typically < 1 hour). For example, aging studies have examined alterations in the dopaminergic (DA) system using these techniques.

Age-related changes in the DA biochemistry and neurotransmission in the striatum are considerably larger than reported structural changes within this region.[55] Backman et al[16] examined striatal DA binding associated with two age-sensitive functional domains, episodic memory and perceptual speed, in healthy controls between the ages of 21 and 68. The authors observed age-related reduction of DA binding in the putamen and caudate in subjects as young as the age of 30. While age was not reliably related to either caudate or putamen volume in their study, it was found to relate significantly to DA binding on the cognitive tasks. Importantly, DA binding predicted cognitive performance better than age, confirming other reports showing a strong correlation between DA binding and cognitive function.[56,57] Others have demonstrated a strong relationship between DA binding and frontal metabolism.[58] Therefore, it seems that cognitive aging may reflect changes in both striatal and frontal function, and in the striatal–frontal circuitry connecting these two systems.

Indeed, it is clear that enhancing our understanding of age-related cognitive decline will depend upon improvements in understanding not just the changes in isolated brain structures but also in understanding the highly interconnected networks that constitute the thinking brain. A recent study reported differences in interactions of the hippocampus with other brain areas as a function of aging.[59] While hippocampal activation during task performance was comparable across groups, it was associated in the young subjects with activation of Brodmann's area 10, and the fusiform gyrus and posterior cingulate gyrus. In contrast, in the older subjects hippocampal activation was associated with activation of the dorsolateral prefrontal cortex, middle cingulate gyrus and caudate nucleus. Anatomic studies support the idea that the functional connectivity of the hippocampus is altered in aging. For example, hippocampal physiology is affected in aging by receptor number changes and changes in dendritic arborization.[60,61] This change in functional connectivity may, in part, result in age-related memory changes. Mathematical modeling of such circuitry based on functional imaging data (e.g. Moeller et al[62]) promises to become a more consequential player as the technology for brain imaging continues to evolve.

Imaging and dementia

As imaging technologies become more widely available and more capable of detecting small changes in brain structure and function, clinicians rely more on imaging data in the diagnosis of geriatric patients. At present it remains difficult to differentiate changes in the brain associated with normal aging and changes associated with pathological processes, like dementia, especially early in the course of a disease. A brief review of studies reflecting the current understanding of brain-related changes in AD-type dementia, as well as other dementias, is provided below.

AD

At least 50% of dementia cases are due to AD, and a large body of data is available detailing the neuropathology of AD (e.g. neurofibrillary tangles, senile plaques, granulovacuolar degeneration). However, using brain imaging to differentiate changes associated with normal aging and changes associated with AD remains difficult, in part because the differences between AD and normal aging are quantitative, not qualitative. Imaging studies have detailed the regional specificity of volume reductions associated with AD pathology, with the greatest loss in cortical volume seen in the medial temporal structures. One study reported hippocampal volumes of AD patients were 14% less than those of similar age controls.[63] Perihippocampal areas, specifically the entorhinal cortex, have been shown to be affected earliest in AD.[64] Reductions in AD are also larger in gray matter compared to white matter, though changes in white matter have also been reported. For example, decreases in the volume of the corpus callosum have been shown to relate to dementia severity.[65] The callosal changes appear to be focused more on the genu of the corpus callosum, whereas more global changes in callosal volume has been reported in normal aging.[66]

Cross-sectional studies of brain atrophy or brain metabolism have thus far not been promising in diagnosing AD (for a review see Cutler et al[67]). In fact, MR and CT imaging usually do not exceed an 80% correct classification rate of patients and healthy controls.[68] However, longitudinal studies of changes in brain function are more promising (for a review, see de Leon et al[69]). For example, one MR study[12] mapped the rate of change over a 12-month period and found that AD patients showed a significantly faster rate of atrophy compared to age-matched controls. In addition, the authors reported that non-demented individuals at risk of AD (based on family history) showed greater rates of volume loss than the controls – and subsequently developed symptoms of AD. Another longitudinal study using CT performed over a 4-year follow-up period reported that hippocampal atrophy is predictive of dementia status.[70]

Functional imaging studies indicate that the medial temporal lobe and temporoparietal association areas discriminate best between controls and patients at risk for AD.[71] SPECT studies have reported sensitivity rates of 90–100% in discriminating AD patients and healthy controls.[72,73] The distinct pattern of changes associated with AD pathology are illustrated in Figure 3.1, which compares SPECT images of an AD patient to those of a healthy elderly control. However, the differentiation of AD from other dementias, e.g. vascular dementia, is much less clear.

High-resolution scanning provides an ever-increasing sensitivity to monitor and record detailed functional neuroanatomical changes important in detecting the early onset of AD. The relevance of early detection will increase as potential treatments for AD become available. Small et al[74] used anatomical landmarks to identify subregions of the hippocampus with sub-millimeter resolution. During a recognition memory task, AD patients showed a diminished signal compared to controls. Changes were most notable in the entorhinal cortex.[64]

Functional studies have also begun to delineate how the brain may attempt to compensate for AD pathology by implementing different brain networks to process cognitive tasks. For example, Stern and Small[75] recently showed that healthy elders engaged a specific brain network when performing a continuous verbal recognition task, and that differential expression of this network was strongly related to memory performance

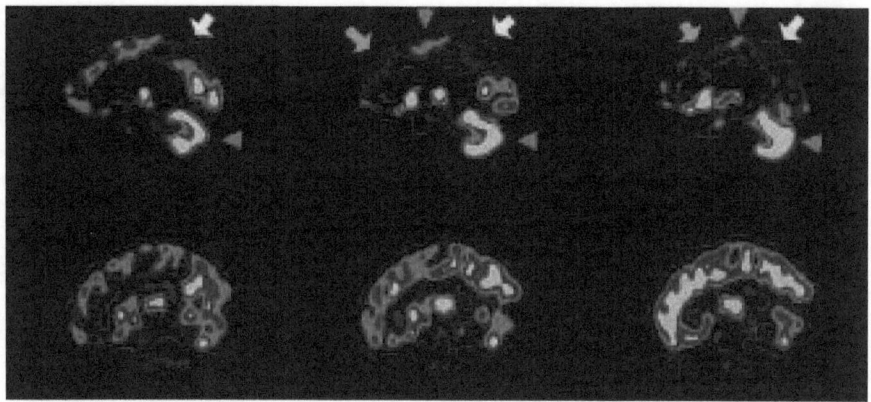

Figure 3.1 *These single photon emission computed tomography (SPECT) scan images show the brain blood flow (perfusion) in three sagittal brain slices each of a patient with Alzheimer's disease (top row of three images) and a person without dementia (bottom row of three images). These images are color coded so that higher perfusion to lower perfusion is coded as white (highest)–gray–orange–red–brown–green–blue (lowest). In the Alzheimer's brain, there is relatively less perfusion of overlying brain cortex, compared to deeper, lower structures such as basal ganglia, thalamus, and cerebellum. Particular deficits are noted in the parietal regions (white arrows), and less so in the frontal regions (green arrows). Red arrowheads show relative preservation of perfusion to sensorimotor cortex (areas directly controlling movement and sensation; arrowheads pointing downwards), and the cerebellum (controlling coordination of movements; arrowheads pointing to the right). These areas are less affected than other areas in the patient with Alzheimer's disease.*

(Figure 3.2). AD patients failed to express the topography seen in the controls, but instead activated a different network that was associated with their performance. Such findings provide a framework for further investigation of compensation in response to brain pathology, and highlight the importance of studying the interconnected pathways of the brain rather than studying changes in neuroanatomical structures in isolation.

Other dementias

Vascular dementia accounts for approximately 20–30% of all dementia cases,[76] though many patients diagnosed as having vascular dementia have been shown to exhibit coexistent pathologic changes related to AD at autopsy. Diagnosis of vascular dementia is dependent upon laboratory evidence of significant cerebrovascular disease. MRI is more sensitive than CT in detecting ischemic changes underlying vascular dementia. However, as

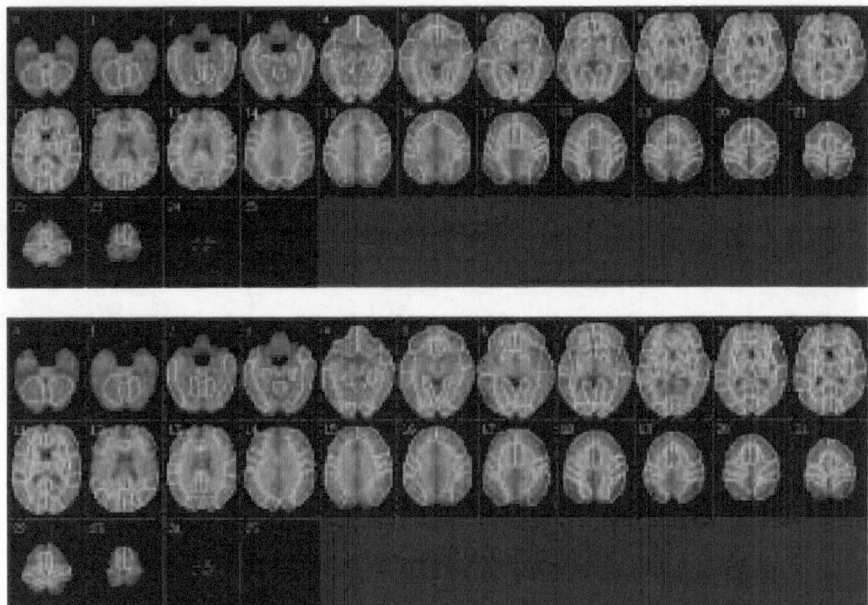

Figure 3.2 *Within each group of healthy elderly and Alzheimer's disease subjects, differential expression of these networks correlated with size of the study list on the activation task. Weights for each region's participation in the topography have been overlaid on standard, Tailarach-transformed axial magnetic resonance imaging (MRI) sections, with positive weights indicated in red and negative weights indicated in blue. (a) The healthy elders' network. Higher study list size was associated with increased activation in left anterior cingulate and anterior insula, and decreased activation of the left basal ganglia. (b) Alzheimer's disease network. Higher study list size was associated with the increased activation of the left posterior temporal cortex, calcarine cortex, posterior cingulate, and the vermis.*

noted earlier, a significant percentage of psychometrically normal people over the age of 60 will have some white matter changes on MRI. Therefore, the distinction between normal age-related change and change indicative of vascular dementia is difficult to discern. Diagnosis of vascular dementia is dependent upon the extent of cerebral infarction. For instance, one study comparing patients with vascular dementia, patients with strokes without dementia, and healthy controls, found that the total area of white matter lesions was the strongest factor differentiating the three groups.[77]

SPECT has not proven effective at differentiating patients with AD and patients with vascular dementia. The differentiation is complicated by the heterogeneity in the topography of the ischemic lesions, though some studies have shown that the temporoparietal focus seen in AD is not typical of vascular dementia, and thus provides a means to assist in a differential diagnosis.[78] Algorithms based on neural networks have provided further enhanced discrimination – up to 83% – of AD patients from those with vascular dementia.[79]

Neuropathology associated with Huntington's disease (HD) is noted by a loss of spiny neurons in the striatum, which has a high number of postsynaptic DA receptors.[80] Structural imaging using both CT[81] and MRI[82] show age-related reductions in striatum that are related to cognitive decline associated with HD. MRI shows greater accuracy than CT in the volumetric measure of the caudate heads, and is thus preferred in examining structural changes associated with HD. Functional changes in the brains of HD patients can be detected prior to detection of structural brain changes. For example, PET studies show glucose hypometabolism in the striatum early in HD, even in asymptomatic carriers.[83] Also, focal hypoperfusion in the striatum shown in SPECT studies precedes tissue atrophy measures revealed with CT or MRI.[84] As such, functional imaging has proven effective in assisting in the early diagnosis of patients at risk for HD.

Parkinson's disease (PD) involves a decline in the striato–nigral DA system. Brain imaging of PD patients is characterized by an abnormal signal hypointensity in the putamen, thought to reflect the accumulation of iron deposit in this region. However, specificity for detecting PD can be low since iron deposits are common in normal aging.[85] Signal hypointensity can also be detected in the substantia nigra and may reflect iron deposits in the pars compacta of this region,[86] or be a manifestation of the atrophy of the pars compacta.[87]

Overall, emerging imaging techniques have already improved our understanding of the brain changes associated with these and other dementing illnesses. Particularly promising are findings of changes in neural function that precede changes in brain structure that can be detected in individuals at risk for developing a disease. The availability of earlier detection, and consequently earlier treatment, create hope for eventually reducing the burden these diseases place on society.

Issues in brain imaging and aging

One central concern in the field of imaging and aging relates to what the imaging signal represents. In both functional MRI (fMRI) and PET studies, blood flow is measured and is presumed to reflect neural activity. The close coupling between CBF and neuronal function was first suggested by Roy and Sherrington.[88] However, the assumption that neural activity in aged brains will create a similar hemodynamic response to an equivalent amount of neural activity in young brains remains an unsettled issue. Recent data suggests that this basic tenet underlying imaging and aging research is most likely not true. D'Esposito et al[89] examined the spatial and temporal characteristics of the blood oxygenation-level dependent (BOLD) fMRI hemodynamic response in primary sensorimotor cortex during a simple reaction time task, thought to be behaviorally invariant, in young and elderly subjects. Differences in hemodynamic coupling between neural activity and the BOLD fMRI signal were reported, with young adults showing a greater signal:noise ratio compared to the old adults (elders showed greater noise per voxel). Since old adults have been previously shown to produce more artifacts due to head movement during scanning, the authors ruled out the possibility that the increased noise they reported was due to differences in head motion. Instead, they suggested that age-related vascular changes (arteriolar change such as narrowing due to endothelial proliferation, fibrinoid necrosis, and atherosclerosis and stiffening) might account for the reported aging effect. The fact that 25% of the elderly participants in the study failed to show a detectable BOLD response is of particular concern, given that they presumably produced the neural activity related to button pressing that would induce the changes in the local deoxyhemoglobin concentrations that underlie the fMRI signal.

Greater variability in the fMRI hemodynamic responses of old versus young adults have been reported elsewhere (e.g. Aguirre et al[90]). Increases in the temporal lag and spatial extent of BOLD signal in elders, which have been attributed to vascular changes associated with age, are important because they translate into differences in signal intensity after spatial smoothing of the imaged data.[89]

A related confound in interpreting signal differences between young and old subjects involves the cerebral atrophy associated with aging. Loss of gray matter may produce lower values of perfusion through partial volume effects in older adults. Thus, differences in signal intensity may not reflect differences in neural activation between young and old subjects, but instead reflect differences in brain volume. Studies benefit by incorporating structural variation into the analysis of their functional effects and by including co-registration of functional imaging data with structural imaging data.[91] One recent study failed to find age-related declines in CBF in normal elders once age-related volume changes were accounted for.[92]

The still limited literature on brain imaging and aging is notable for the amount of conflicting data emanating from different laboratories. One issue that contributes to the conflicting findings involves the criteria that are used for the inclusion of 'healthy normal elderly'. Including subjects with cerebrovascular risk factors, and consequently those with potentially more ischemic damage and/or vascular changes that affect CBF, will likely affect the study outcomes. Similarly, including participants who are taking medications that may affect CBF measures will impact upon the findings. On the other hand, limiting participation to those 'super-healthy' elders may not provide an accurate assessment of the changes that occur in the more typical aging brain. These inclusion/exclusion criteria should be considered when evaluating the aging and imaging literature.

Another confounding issue relates to the quantification and interpretation of imaging findings. For example, measurement of WMHI varies between studies since many sites still rely on the naked eye assessment of an expert rater. Volumetric techniques are preferable, as they are less susceptible to variation associated with the subjective judgments of individual raters and are more sensitive than visual inspection (e.g. Breteler et al[18]).

Overall, it is clear that we do not yet command a full understanding of what is reflected in brain imaging signals of PET and fMRI studies. In regards to aging, preliminary studies indicate that the neural activity in aged brains may not create a similar hemodynamic response to an equivalent amount of neural activity in young brains. Despite these data, most neuroimaging studies of aging use a cross-sectional design that assumes equivalence in young and old brains in the coupling of neural activity to the hemodynamic signal. In these cases, it appears that we may have put the cart before the horse. An understanding of the neurophysiological basis of PET and fMRI signals and an understanding of how these signals change across the age span ideally should precede studies examining age-related differences in cognitive activation. Since these areas of study are progressing in tandem, it is important to keep in mind the limitations of our knowledge of basic brain imaging when evaluating more complex imaging studies of aging.

Conclusions

The role of neuroimaging in the diagnosis of various conditions commonly seen by geriatric psychiatrists continues to evolve. Technological advances are driving progress in this field. For example, improvements in the spatial resolution of imaging methodologies is providing a clearer picture of the neurophysiological changes that occur across the age span. Already studies report submillimeter resolution in T2*-weighted fMRI,[74] allowing the anatomical dissection of brain function *in vivo* that was even recently considered inconceivable. Higher spatial resolution in brain imaging may parlay into earlier detection of diseases of aging, and thereby provide a means of earlier treatment and prevention. However, despite the promise brain imaging represents, it is clear that our understanding of what the changes in brain signaling with age reflect remains unclear. Therefore, a cautious evaluation of the literature is warranted as we continue to enhance our understanding of the neuropharmacology and pathophysiology of the aging brain.

Acknowledgment

The authors gratefully acknowledge Dr Larry Honig for assistance with the figures.

References

1. Friedman D, Johnson R. Event-related potential (ERP) studies of memory encoding and retrieval: a selective review. *Microsc Res Tech* 2000; **51:** 6–28.
2. Raz N. Aging of the brain and its impact on cognitive performance: integration of structural and functional findings. In: (Craik FIM, Salthouse TA, eds) *Handbook of Aging and Cognition.* (Erlbaum: Mahwah, NJ, 2000) 1–90.
3. Raz N, Gunning FM, Head D et al. Selective aging of the human cerebral cortex observed in vivo: differential vulnerability of the prefrontal gray matter. *Cereb Cortex* 1997; **7:** 268–82.
4. Jernigan TL, Archibald SL, Berhow MT et al. Cerebral structure on MRI. Part I: localization of age-related changes. *Biol Psychiatry* 1991; **29:** 55–67.
5. Sullivan EV, Marsh L, Mathalon DH et al. Age-related decline in MRI volumes of temporal lobe gray matter but not hippocampus. *Neurobiol Aging* 1995; **18:** 609–15.
6. Pfefferbaum A, Lim KO, Zipursky RB et al. Brain gray and white matter volume loss accelerates with aging in chronic alcoholics: a quantitative MRI study. *Alcohol Clin Exp Res* 1992; **16:** 1078–89.
7. Murphy DG, DeCarli C, McIntosh AR et al. Sex differences in human brain morphometry and metabolism: an in vivo quantitative magnetic resonance imaging and positron emission tomography study on the effect of aging. *Arch Gen Psychiatry* 1996; **53:** 585–94.

8. Geinisman Y, Detoledo-Morrell L, Morrell F, Heller RE. Hippocampal markers of age-related memory dysfunction: behavioral, electrophysiological and morphological perspectives. *Prog Neurobiol* 1995; **45**: 223–52.

9. Rapp PR, Gallagher M. Preserved neuron number in the hippocampus of aged rats with spatial learning deficits. *Proc Natl Acad Sci USA* 1996; **93**: 9926–30.

10. Mu Q, Xie J, Wen Z et al. A quantitative MR study of the hippocampal formation, the amygdala, and the temporal horn of the lateral ventricle in healthy subjects 40 to 90 years of age. *Am J Neuroradiol* 1999; **20**: 207–11.

11. Morrison JH, Hof PR. Life and death of neurons in the aging brain. *Science* 1997; **278**: 412–19.

12. Fox NC, Freeborough PA, Rossor MN. Visualisation and quantification of rates of atrophy in Alzheimer's disease. *Lancet* 1996; **348**: 94–7.

13. Petersen RC, Jack CR, Smith GE et al. MRI in the diagnosis of mild cognitive impairment and Alzheimer's disease. *J Int Neuropsychol Soc* 1998; **4**: 22.

14. Krishnan KRR, Husain MM, McDonald WM et al. In vivo stereological assessment of caudate volume in man: effect of normal aging. *Life Sci* 1990; **47**: 1325–9.

15. Raz N, Torres IJ, Acker JD. Age, gender, and hemispheric differences in human striatum: a quantitative review and new data from in vivo MRI morphometry. *Neurobiol Learn Mem* 1995; **63**: 133–42.

16. Backman L, Ginovart N, Dixon RA et al. Age-related cognitive deficits mediated by changes in the striatal dopamine system. *Am J Psychiatry* 2000; **157**: 635–7.

17. Parent A, Hazrati LN. Functional anatomy of the basal ganglia I: the cortico–basal ganglia–thalamo–cortical loop. *Brain Res Rev* 1995; **20**: 91–127.

18. Breteler MM, van Swieten JC, Bots ML et al. Cerebral white matter lesions, vascular risk factors, and cognitive function in a population-based study: the Rotterdam Study. *Neurology* 1994; **44**: 1246–52.

19. Pantoni L, Garcia JH. Pathogenesis of leukoaraiosis: a review. *Stroke* 1997; **28**: 652–9.

20. Awad IA, Spetzler RF, Hodak JA et al. Incidental subcortical lesions identified on magnetic resonance imaging in the elderly, I: correlation with age and cerebrovascular risk. *Stroke* 1986; **17**: 1084–9.

21. Longstreth Jr WT, Manolio TA, Arnold A et al. Clinical correlates of white matter finding on cranial magnetic resonance imaging of 3301 elderly people: the Cardiovascular Health Study. *Stroke* 1996; **27**: 1274–82.

22. Meguro K, Hatazawa J, Yamaguchi T et al. Cerebral circulation and oxygen metabolism associated with subclinical periventricular hyperintensity as shown by magnetic resonance imaging. *Ann Neurol* 1990; **28**: 378–83.

23. Barber R, Scheltens P, Gholkar A et al. White matter lesions on magnetic resonance imaging in dementia with Lewy bodies, Alzheimer's disease, vascular dementia, and normal aging. *J Neurol Neurosurg Psychiatry* 1999; **67**: 66–72.

24. Schmidt SL, Oliveira RM, Krahe TE, Filgueiras CC. The effects of hand preference and gender on finger tapping performance asymmetry by the use of an infra-red light measurement device. *Neuropsychologia* 2000; **38**: 529–34.

25. Boone KB, Ghaffarian S, Lesser IM et al. Wisconsin Card Sorting Test performance in healthy, older adults: relationship to age, sex, education, and IQ. *J Clin Psychol* 1993; **49**: 54–60.

26. Schmidt R, Fazekas F, Offenbacher H et al. Neuropsychologic correlates of MRI white matter hyperintensities: a study of 150 normal volunteers. *Neurology* 1993; **43**: 2490–4.

27. Tupler LA, Coffey CE, Logue PE et al. Neuropsychological importance of subcortical white matter hyperintensity. *Arch Neurol* 1992; **49**: 1248–52.

28. Campbell JJ, Coffey CE. Neuropsychiatric significance of subcortical hyperintensity. *J Neuropsychiatry Clin Neurosci* 2001; **13**: 261–88.

29. Grossman H, Harris G, Jacobson S, Folstein M. The normal elderly. In: (Ames D, Chiu E, eds) *Neuroimaging and the Psychiatry of Late Life*. (Cambridge University Press: Cambridge, 1997) 77–99.

30. Kuhl DE, Metter EJ, Riege WH, Phelps ME. Effects of human aging on patterns of local cerebral glucose utilization determined by the fluorodeoxyglucose method. *J Cereb Blood Flow Metab* 1982; **2**: 163–71.

31. Levine RL, Hanson JM, Nickles RJ. Cerebral vasocapacitance in human aging. *J Neuroimaging* 1994; **4**: 130–6.

32. Takada H, Nagata K, Hirata Y et al. Age-related decline of cerebral oxygen metabolism in normal population detected with positron emission tomography. *Neurol Res* 1992; **14**: 128–31.

33. Waldemar G, Hasselbalch SG, Andersen AR et al. 99mTc-d,l-HMPAO and SPECT of the brain in normal aging. *J Cereb Blood Flow Metab* 1991; **11**: 508–21.

34. de Leon MJ, George AE, Tomanelli J. Positron emission tomography studies of normal aging: a replication of PET III and 18-FDG using PET VI and 11-CDG. *Neurobiol Aging* 1987; **8**: 319–23.

35. Yoshii F, Barker WW, Chang JY et al. Sensitivity of cerebral glucose metabolism to age, gender, brain volume, brain atrophy, and cerebrovascular risk factors. *J Cereb Blood Flow Metab* 1988; **8**: 654–61.

36. Gur RC, Gur RE, Resnick SM et al. The effect of anxiety on cortical cerebral blood flow and metabolism. *J Cereb Blood Flow Metab* 1987; **7**: 173–7.

37. Meyer JS, Kawamura J, Terayama Y. Cerebral blood flow and metabolism with normal and abnormal aging, In: (Albert ML, Knoefel, JE, eds) *Clinical Neurology of Aging*, 2nd edn. (Oxford University Press: New York, 1994.)

38. Spencer W, Raz N. Differential effects of aging on memory for content and context: a meta-analysis. *Psychol Aging* 1995; **10**: 527–39.

39. Backman L, Almkvist O, Andersson J et al. Brain activation in young and older adults during implicit and explicit retrieval. *J Cogn Neurosci* 1997; **9**: 378–91.

40. Cabeza R, Anderson ND, Houle S et al. Age-related differences in neural activity during item and temporal-order memory retrieval: a positron emission tomography study. *J Cogn Neurosci* 2000; **12**: 197–206.

41. Schacter DL, Savage CR, Alpert NM et al. The role of hippocampus and frontal cortex in age-related memory changes: a PET study. *Neuroreport* 1996; **7**: 1165–9.

42. Dempster FN. The rise and fall of the inhibitory mechanism: toward a unified theory of cognitive development and aging. *Devel Rev* 1992; **12**: 45–75.

43. West R. An application of prefrontal cortex function theory to cognitive aging. *Psychol Bull* 1996; **120**: 272–92.

44. Gershberg F, Shimamura AP. Impaired use of organizational strategies in free recall following frontal lobe damage. *Neuropsychologia* 1995; **33**: 1305–33.

45. Shimamura AP. The role of prefrontal cortex in controlling and monitoring memory processes. In: (Reder L, ed) *Implicit Memory and Metacognition*. (Erlbaum: Mahwah, 1996.)

46. Wheeler MA, Stuss DT, Tulving E. Frontal lobe damage produces episodic memory impairment. *Int Neuropsychol Soc* 1995; **1:** 525–36.

47. Cabeza R, Grady CL, Nyberg L et al. Age-related differences in neural activity during memory encoding and retrieval: a positron-emission tomography study. *J Neurosci* 1997; **17:** 391–400.

48. Grady CL, McIntosh AR, Horwitz B et al. Age-related reductions in human recognition memory due to impaired encoding. *Science* 1995; **269:** 218–21.

49. Anderson ND, Iidaka T, Cabeza R et al. The effects of divided attention on encoding- and retrieval-related brain activity: a PET study of younger and older adults. *J Cogn Neurosci* 2000; **12:** 775–92.

50. Madden DJ, Turkington TG, Provezale JM et al. Adult age difference in the functional neuroanatomy of verbal recognition memory. *Hum Brain Mapping* 1999; **7:** 115–35.

51. McIntosh AR, Sekuler AB, Penpeci C et al. Recruitment of unique neural systems to support visual memory in normal aging. *Curr Biol* 1999; **9:** 1275–8.

52. Grady CL. Brain imaging and age-related changes in cognition. *Exp Gerontol* 1998; **33:** 661–73.

53. Reuter-Lorenz PA, Jonides J, Smith EE et al. Age differences in the frontal lateralization of verbal and spatial working memory revealed by PET. *J Cogn Neurosci* 2000; **12:** 174–87.

54. Rubin DC. Frontal–striatal circuits in cognitive aging: evidence for caudate involvement. *Aging Neuropsychol Cogn* 1999; **6:** 241–59.

55. Backman L, Farde L. Dopamine and cognitive functioning: brain imaging findings in Huntington's disease and normal aging. *Scand J Psychol* 2001; **42:** 287–96.

56. Wang Y, Chan GL, Holden JE et al. Age-dependent decline of dopamine D1 receptors in human brain: a PET study. *Synapse* 1998; **30:** 56–61.

57. Volkow ND, Wang GJ, Fowler JS et al. Parallel loss of presynaptic and post-synaptic dopamine markers in normal aging. *Ann Neurol* 1998; **44:** 143–7.

58. Volkow ND, Logan J, Fowler JS et al. Association between age-related decline in brain dopamine activity and impairment in frontal and cingulate metabolism. *Am J Psychiatry* 2000; **157:** 75–80.

59. Della-Maggiore V, Sekuler AB, Grady CL et al. Corticolimbic interactions associated with performance on a short-term memory task are modified by age. *J Neurosci* 2000; **20:** 8410–16.

60. Barnes CA, McNaughton BL. Neurophysiological comparison of dendritic cable properties in adolescent, middle-aged, and senescent rats. *Exp Aging Res* 1979; **5:** 195–206.

61. Barnes CA, McNaughton BL. Physiological compensation for loss of afferent synapses in rat hippocampal granule cells during senescence. *J Physiol* 1980; **309:** 473–85.

62. Moeller JR, Ghez C, Antonini A et al. Brain networks of motor behavior assessed by principal component analysis. In: (Carson R, ed) *Quantitative Functional Brain Imaging with Positron Emission Tomography*. (Academic Press: San Diego, 1998) 247–52.

63. Smith CD. Quantitative computed tomography and magnetic resonance imaging in aging and Alzheimer's Disease. *J Neuroimaging* 1995; **6:** 44–53.

64. Braak H, Braak E. Neuropathological staging of Alzheimer-related changes. *Acta Neuropathol* 1991; **82:** 239–59.

65. Yamauchi H, Fukayama H, Harada K et al. Callosal atrophy parallels decreased cortical oxygen metabolism and neuropsychological impairment in Alzheimer's disease. *Arch Neurol* 1993; **50:** 1070–4.

66. Biegon A, Eberling JL, Richardson BC et al. Human corpus callosum in aging and Alzheimer's disease: a magnetic resonance imaging study. *Neurobiol Aging* 1994; **15:** 393–7.

67. Cutler NR, Duara R, Creasey H. Brain imaging: aging and dementia. *Ann Intern Med* 1984; **101:** 355–69.

68. Sandor T, Jolesz F, Tieman J et al. Comparative analysis of computed tomographic and magnetic resonance imaging scans in Alzheimer patients and controls. *Arch Neurol* 1992; **49:** 381–4.

69. de Leon MJ, George AE, Reisberg B. Alzheimer's disease: longitudinal CT studies of ventricular change. *Am J Roentgenol* 1989; **152:** 1527–62.

70. de Leon MJ, Golomb J, George AE et al. Radiologic prediciton of Alzheimer's disease: the atrophic hippocampus. *Am J Neuroradiol* 1993; **14:** 897–906.

71. de Leon MJ, Convit A, DeSanti S et al. Hippocampus in aging and Alzheimer's disease. *Neuroimaging Clin N Am* 1995; **5:** 1–17.

72. Johnson KA, Kijewski MR, Becker A. Quantitative brain SPECT in Alzheimer's disease and normal aging. *J Nucl Med* 1993; **34:** 2044–8.

73. Waldemar G, Bruhn P, Kristensen M et al. Heterogeneity of neocortical cerebral blood flow deficits in dementia of the Alzheimer type: a [99mTc]-d,l-HMPAO SPECT study. *J Neurol Neurosurg Psychiatry* 1994; **57:** 285–95.

74. Small SA, Nava AS, Perera GM et al. Evaluating the function of hippocampal sub-regions with high-resolution MRI in Alzheimer's disease and aging. *Microsci Res Tech* 2000; **51:** 101–8.

75. Stern Y, Small SA. Imaging the consequences of Alzheimer's disease pathology. In: (Iqbal K, Swaab DF, Winblad B, Wisniewski HM, eds) *Alzheimer's Disease: Advances in Etiology, Pathogenesis and Therapeutics.* (Chichester: John Wiley & Sons Ltd: 2001) 181–92.

76. Khujneri R, De Sousa JA. Magnetic resonance imaging of the ageing brain. *East Afr Med J* 1997; **74:** 656–9.

77. Liu CK, Miller BL, Cummings JL et al. A quantitative MRI study of vascular dementia. *Neurology* 1992; **42:** 138–43.

78. Gemmell HG, Sharp PF, Smith FW et al. Cerebral blood flow measured by SPECT as a diagnostic tool in the study of dementia. *Psychiatry Res* 1989; **29:** 327–9.

79. de Figueiredo RJ, Shankle WR, Maccato A et al. Neural-network-based classification of cognitively normal, demented, Alzheimer disease and vascular dementia from single photon emission with computed tomography image data from brain. *Proc Natl Acad Sci USA* 1995; **92:** 5530–4.

80. Filloux F, Wagster MV, Folstein M et al. Nigral dopamine type-1 receptors are reduced in Huntington's disease striatum. *Exp Neurol* 1990; **110:** 219–27.

81. Bamford KA, Caine ED, Kido DK et al. Clinical–pathologic correlation in Huntington's disease: a neuropsychological and computed tomography study. *Neurology* 1989; **39:** 796–801.

82. Brandt J, Bylsma FW, Aylward EH et al. Impaired source memory in Huntington's disease and its relation to basal ganglia atrophy. *J Clin Exp Neuropsychol* 1995; **17:** 877.

83. Berent S, Giordani B, Lehtinen S et al. Positron emission tomographic scan investigations of Huntington's disease. *Ann Neurol* 1988; **23:** 541–6.

84. Bruyn RPM, Hageman G, Geelan JAG et al. SPECT, CT, and MRI in a Turkish family with Huntington's disease. *Neuroradiology* 1993; **35:** 525–8.

85. Drayer B, Burger P, Darwin R et al. Magnetic resonance imaging of brain iron. *Am J Roentgenol* 1986; **147:** 373–80.

86. Drayer BP, Olanow W, Burger P et al. Parkinson plus syndrome: diagnosis using high field MR imaging of brain iron. *Radiology* 1986; **159:** 493–8.

87. Duguid JR, de la Paz R, de Groot JC. Magnetic resonance imaging of the midbrain in Parkinson's disease. *Ann Neurol* 1986; **20:** 744–7.

88. Roy CS, Sherrington CS. On the regulation of the blood supply of the brain. *J Physiol* 1890; **11:** 85–108.

89. D'Esposito M, Zarahn E, Aguirre GK, Rypma B. The effect of normal aging on the coupling of neural activity to the bold hemodynamic response. *Neuroimage* 1999; **10:** 6–14.

90. Aguirre GK, Zarahn E, D'Esposito M. The variability of human, BOLD hemodynamic responses. *Neuroimage* 1998; **8:** 360–9.

91. Nobler MS, Mann JJ, Sackeim HA. Serotonin, cerebral blood flow, and cerebral metabolic rate in geriatric major depression and normal aging. *Brain Res Rev* 1999; **30:** 250–63.

92. Cidis Meltzer C, Cantwell MN, Greer PJ et al. Does cerebral blood flow decline in healthy aging? A PET study with partial-volume correction. *J Nucl Med* 2000; **41:** 1842–50.

4. NEUROIMAGING STUDIES OF HUMAN DRUG ADDICTION

Natalia S Lawrence, Elliot A Stein

Introduction

Modern, non-invasive neuroimaging provides, for the first time, a vehicle to address questions about the acute effects of drugs of abuse on the human brain, the consequences of their chronic use and ultimately the mechanisms leading to the development of drug dependence and addiction. Contrary to popular belief, addiction is not defined by physical dependence on a drug but by the lack of control over drug intake, i.e. the compulsive use of a drug against one's will and at the expense of other behaviors.[1] Hence, addicts often report continued drug self-administration despite the absence of its ability to produce an acute pleasurable feeling and, instead, having considerable adverse physical, personal and financial consequences.[1] Recent theories argue that drug addiction involves neuroadaptive, plastic brain mechanisms driving the transition from casual, recreational drug taking to a regular, compulsive habit.[2,3] While it has been argued that certain individuals may have an innate predisposition to developing a drug addiction,[3,4] it has been difficult to isolate specific differences in brain neurochemistry [e.g. numbers of dopamine (DA) receptors or transporters] responsible for this predisposition, since comparison of drug addicts to healthy, non-drug users is confounded by the effects of chronic drug use on the brain. This problem of trait (innate) versus state (induced) causes of differences in brain structure and function also plagues many other areas of brain imaging research in psychiatry. However, these alternatives can potentially be disentangled by examining the time course of drug effects on the brain in experiments employing both drug-naïve and experienced animals, and by studying healthy control subjects showing certain addictive tendencies.

The changes in regional brain structure and function that mediate the initial rewarding effects of drugs, the triggers that lead to compulsive drug use, and the long-term consequences of drug use on these regions and mechanisms are among the subjects of current neuroimaging studies of drug addiction. This chapter reviews these studies by arranging them into categories based on the stage of the addictive process, combining across different classes of drug. A basic theoretical overview of each stage in the addictive process is first presented, followed by a review of recent findings from neuroimaging research. Although most human imaging research has focused on cocaine use, a discussion of those common brain mechanisms involved in the abuse of different drugs is given, since these are the likely targets for therapeutic intervention and are of broadest interest. The review focuses on imaging studies using positron emission tomography (PET), single photon emission computed tomography (SPECT) and functional magnetic resonance imaging (fMRI) studies; electroencephalographic (EEG) and event-related potentials (ERP) studies have not been included. The interested reader is referred to Alper,[5] Little[6], and Bauer.[7]

PET and SPECT studies have concentrated on where drugs bind in the brain, and how drugs change blood flow, metabolic rate and the number of neurotransmitter (particularly DA) receptors and transporters in the brains of addicts and healthy controls. In addition, a number of studies have examined changes in brain resting activity and/or chemistry in drug addicts over varying periods of withdrawal in an attempt to determine potential normalization of function.[8–10] Visualization of regional drug binding can be achieved by injecting a ^{11}C-radiolabelled form of the drug of interest. Drug-induced changes in the regional cerebral blood flow (rCBF) can be measured using radiotracers such as [15]O water in PET and technetium-99m (Tc-99m)-d,l-hexamethylpropyleneamineoxime (HMPAO) in SPECT studies; the regional cerebral metabolic rate (rCMR) is generally measured with PET imaging using a form of labelled glucose ([^{18}F]fluorodeoxyglucose (FDG)). Both rCBF and rCMR methods are based on the principle of coupling local changes in metabolism (and the blood flow necessary to provide the oxygen and glucose substrates for energy production) with neuronal activity.[11] Since the principal energy driver in the brain is nerve terminal synaptic activity,[12] metabolic markers provide a good, albeit delayed, index of how drugs (or other sensory, motor or cognitive stimuli) alter neurotransmission.[13,14] Perhaps the most prevalent means of determining the effects of abused drugs on DA transmission is to determine alterations in the specific binding of tracer amounts of 'reversible' D2 receptor radioligands, such as [^{11}C]raclopride. This method is based on the theory that the more DA release induced by a drug (or other treatment), the greater the displacement of, and decrease in, radioligand binding.[15,16]

fMRI has the ability to measure changes in rCBF [using arterial spin-labelling (ASL) techniques], cerebral blood volume (CBV) or, most often used, changes in blood oxygenation [the blood oxygenation-level dependent (BOLD) signal. Although some fMRI studies have investigated direct drug effects on the resting BOLD signal,[17,18] most have focused on the activation differences between healthy controls and drug addicts during performance of cognitive tasks, or in response to drug-related cues (i.e. studies of drug craving). fMRI studies offer a number of technical advantages over PET and SPECT methods, including superior temporal (seconds compared to minutes) and spatial (a few millimetres compared to about 1 cm) resolution, which is crucial when investigating rapid activation changes in small structures implicated in drug effects, such as the nucleus accumbens and amygdala.[19] In addition, since fMRI, unlike PET or SPECT, does not involve administering ionizing radiation, subjects can be scanned on repeated occasions, enabling within-subject design experiments examining responses to several doses of a drug or monitoring extended periods of time during withdrawal or treatment.

Neuroimaging studies are increasingly examining the interaction between drugs of abuse and various cognitive processes, since recent theories of drug addiction posit that changes in brain circuitry related to learning and memory[3,20] and impulsivity[9] may underlie the development and maintenance of the addicted state. Understanding drug effects on cognitive processes is therefore important, since these effects not only reinforce drug-taking behaviour but cognitive deficits in chronic drug users may impede the success of cognitive–behavioural therapies during rehabilitation.[21]

Stages of drug addiction

The initiation stage of drug abuse is characterized by a desire to obtain the drug and successful experience of a drug's pleasurable effects, i.e. drug-induced activation of the brain's reward pathway which, for many abused drugs, involves activation (via enhanced nucleus accumbens DA release[22]) of the ventral striatal–thalamic–frontal circuitry.[3,23,24] As mentioned above, an individual's initial response to drugs may be largely determined by innate factors. The first two sections of this review are therefore concerned with innate predispositions to drug addiction and the effects of acute administration of drugs of abuse on brain activation. Results to date support the hypothesis that most drugs of abuse increase DA release and activate limbic striato–thalamic–frontal regions associated with the perception of salient, rewarding stimuli. Drug-induced activation of this circuitry, and of related limbic structures such as the amygdala and hippocampus, are thought to result, at least in part, in the formation of conditioned associations between internal and external stimuli (such as dysphoric mood, money, drug-using friends), and the rewarding effects of the drug. Subsequent exposure to these drug-associated stimuli cues expectation of the associated drug (consciously perceived as craving) by activating implicit and/or explicit memories, leading to further drug-seeking and drug-taking behaviour.[25] The third section of this review therefore examines research into cue- and drug-induced drug craving, which currently constitutes the most extensive area of fMRI research within the field of drug addiction. The findings from these studies strongly implicate activation of limbic brain regions associated with emotional learning and memory (the dorsolateral prefrontal cortex, anterior cingulate, amygdala and hippocampus) in drug addicts in response to drug-related cues. A recent comprehensive review of neurobiological mechanisms underlying the development of drug addiction is provided in Robinson and Berridge.[3]

Chronic drug use also disrupts functioning of the striato–thalamo–orbitofrontal circuit, which regulates, among others, behavioural drive[26] and is associated with learning the positive/aversive significance of stimuli, as well as reversing this learning when contingencies change.[9,27,28] During drug craving, drug-seeking behaviour and ultimately drug self-administration, an addict is likely to experience a degree of conflict about certain behavioural options, especially if s/he no longer finds the drug pleasurable and has started to suffer adverse consequences. Despite this conflict, addicts maintain their drug-taking behaviour, suggesting that drug addiction involves deficits in reversing previously learnt contingencies (i.e. extinguishing stimulus–response associations), as well as impairments in the ability to control, or inhibit, prepotent behaviour, i.e. enhanced behavioural impulsivity (see Jentsch and Taylor[29] for a review). The fourth section of this review therefore summarizes the potential deficits in drug addicts in the circuitry involved in decision-making and the inhibitory control of behaviour. In this context, abnormalities in orbitofrontal cortex and anterior cingulate function in drug addicts may be especially important. Studies into the long-term consequences of chronic drug use on the brain are discussed, and whether these recover during abstinence. Understanding the brain mechanisms underlying drug addiction is important since the potential exists for therapeutic intervention at all stages of addiction. Finally, this chapter describes some of the concerns and limitations related to utilizing and interpreting data from neuroimaging studies of drug effects.

Evidence for innate predispositions to drug use and abuse

Volkow et al[30] observed that cocaine, methamphetamine, heroin and alcohol abusers tend to show decreased levels of striatal DA D2 receptors when compared to healthy controls (see Figure 4.1a). In addition, decreased D2 receptor expression in cocaine and methamphetamine addicts was associated with a decreased 'resting' metabolism in frontal (orbitofrontal and anterior cingulate) regions (Figure 4.1b). In order to clarify whether this characteristic was drug induced or an innate difference predisposing one to drug use, Volkow et al[4,31] examined D2-receptor levels and metabolic and subjective responses in healthy controls to acute administration of methylphenidate, a drug that, like cocaine, enhances synaptic DA but has considerably lower abuse liability. Their results showed that the 'high' induced by methylphenidate was only experienced in those non-drug using subjects with low levels of D2 receptors, and these same individuals showed less of an increase in frontal metabolism following acute drug administration, similar to that seen in drug addicts. These findings were followed by pioneering investigations into the effects of increasing D2-receptor expression in rats trained to self-administer alcohol.[32] Intriguingly, this manipulation decreased the rats' liking and intake of alcohol, suggesting that increased D2-receptor expression might protect individuals from experiencing a drug's pleasurable effects, possibly because excessive dopaminergic stimulation is aversive.

Another PET study compared individuals with a family history of alcoholism to those with no such family history, and found a reduction in baseline cerebellar metabolism in people with alcoholism in their families.[33] In addition, those with a family history of alcoholism showed a blunted metabolic response to the benzodiazepine lorazepam, which facilitates gamma-aminobutyric acid (GABA) transmission. Together, these studies suggest the existence of innate differences in drug liking correlated with D2-receptor density and, possibly, GABAergic transmission, and illustrate how neuroimaging coupled with selective drug administration and behavioural

(a)

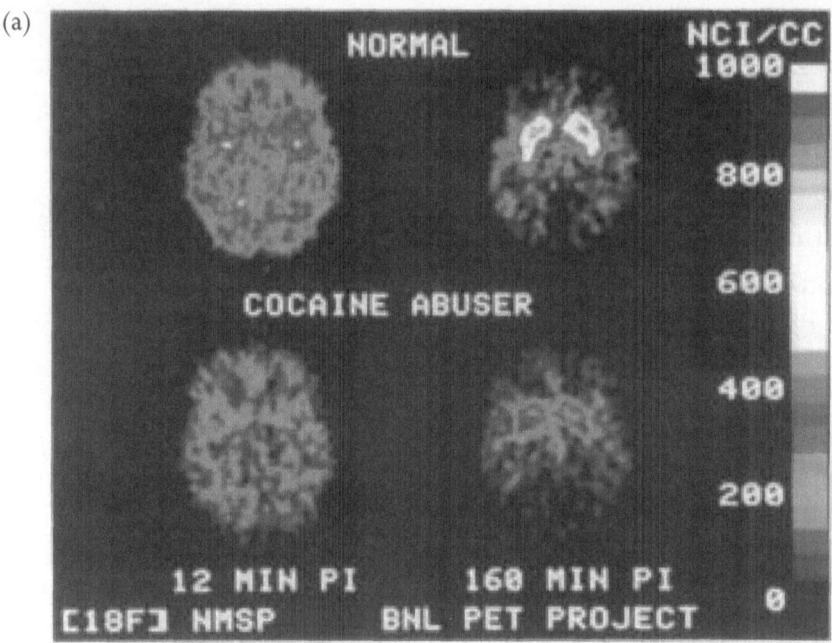

(b)

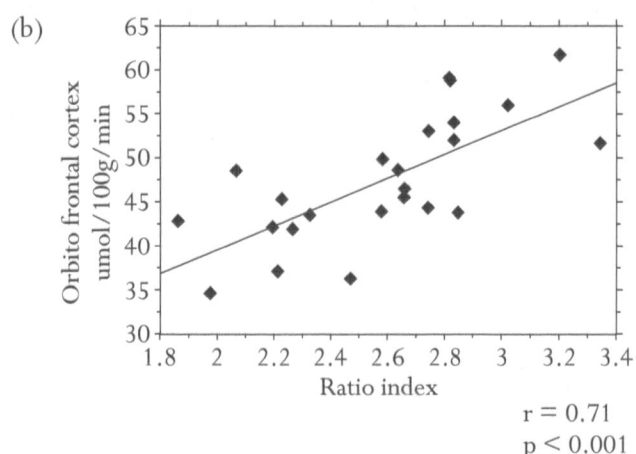

r = 0.71
p < 0.001

Figure 4.1 *Decreased D2 receptors in a cocaine abuser (a) and association of reduced orbitofrontal cortex metabolism with lower D2 receptor levels (b). (a) Dopamine (DA) D2 receptors in a normal subject (top) and in a cocaine abuser undergoing detoxification (bottom). Images were taken at 12 and 160 min after injection of [^{18}F]N-methylspiroperidol to assess D2-receptor availability. There is a marked reduction in [^{18}F]N-methylspiroperidol binding in the cocaine abuser at 160 min, revealing the decrease in D2 receptors. (Scale is to the right.) (b) A strong association between low levels of D2 receptors (ratio index) and low metabolism in the orbitofrontal cortex is shown. (Reproduced with kind permission from Volkow et al.[31])*

monitoring has begun to address questions related to the initiation of drug-taking behaviour.

Initial rewarding effects of drugs of abuse ('Ah that feels good')

As mentioned above, animal studies demonstrate that many abused drugs share the ability to elicit DA release in the nucleus accumbens; to date, this has been demonstrated following the administration of alcohol, amphetamine, cocaine, 3,4-methylenedioxymethamphetamine (MDMA; Ecstasy), nicotine, opiates, phencyclidine and tetrahydrocannabinol, the active ingredient in marijuana.[24,34–37] Brain imaging studies discussed below have shown that similar dopaminergic mechanisms underpin drug-induced reward in humans. For example, the 'high' induced by cocaine is linked to the drug's ability to block the striatal dopamine transporter (DAT), thereby increasing synaptic DA in the striatum.[8,14] The extent and time course of cocaine binding to striatal DAT (peak binding to 50–77% of DAT sites within 4–6 min) paralleled the 'high' induced by the drug. Similarly, another DAT-blocker, methylphenidate (Ritalin), induced a 'high' after rapid binding to striatal DAT (within 4–8 min). The euphoria induced by these drugs appears dependent on their rapid uptake into the brain since methylphenidate induces euphoria after intravenous (IV) (Administration blocking DAT-binding sites within 4–10 min) but not after oral administration (blocking DAT-binding sites within 60 min).[38] The ability of methylphenidate to induce euphoric feelings in healthy controls also correlated with its ability to increase striatal DA release as assessed by [^{11}C]raclopride displacement.[39] Interestingly, cocaine addicts showed a blunted increase in DA response and experience of 'high' in response to methylphenidate compared to non-drug-using control subjects.[40] These PET studies demonstrate important associations between drug-induced euphoria and striatal DA transmission in humans, and support the observation that, in chronic cocaine users, there is a decreased rather than increased experience of a drug's pleasurable effects. A similar adaptation is seen with DA and GABA transmission in alcoholics.[14] Although alcohol's rewarding effects have been linked to increased GABA transmission, alcoholics show decreased GABA neurotransmission when compared to healthy controls. Hence, alcoholics show a blunted metabolic decrease in response to benzodiazepines (which facilitate GABA transmission) in the striato–thalamic–orbitofrontal circuit[9] as well as reduced levels of benzodiazepine receptors in the orbitofrontal cortex.[41]

Together these studies suggest that chronic drug users show a decreased capacity to activate brain reward mechanisms in response to administered abused drugs. However, as tolerance to a drug's acute effects occurs in at least some brain areas following chronic drug use, other regions such as the orbitofrontal cortex may develop a sensitized (hyperactivation) response to drugs. For example, administration of procaine, a drug pharmacologically similar to cocaine, activates the orbitofrontal cortex more in cocaine addicts than in healthy controls.[42] Conversely, non-drug users show a much greater activation of striatal and anterior cingulate limbic regions than cocaine addicts following procaine administration. It is possible that this shift in the brain's response to drugs – with tolerance to activation of reward mechanisms and sensitization of regions involved in compulsive behaviours – mediates the transition from casual to compulsive use that underlies the development of addiction.[3]

Pharmacokinetic studies of drugs such as cocaine and methylphenidate have also led to suggestions for therapeutic intervention. The rapid clearance of cocaine from the striatum enhances the probability of frequent repeated administration of the drug, which is believed to underlie its highly addictive qualities. In contrast, methylphenidate is rewarding when administered IV but is not very addictive, possibly because of it's much longer half-life (> 90 min). This has led to the proposal that substances that bind to striatal DAT with very long half-lives will prevent cocaine binding and thus drug-induced euphoria, and may therefore help reduce cocaine abuse.[8,43] Studies investigating selective DAT blockers, such as RTI–55, PTT and GBR-12909, are now underway in animal models of addiction.[43] In sum, PET and SPECT studies of drug pharmacokinetics are enhancing the understanding of the neural basis of drugs' rewarding properties, potentially leading towards the development of novel therapeutic agents.

PET and fMRI studies have traced changes in brain metabolism and regional blood oxygenation following drug challenge. Acute administration of cocaine, amphetamine, morphine, benzodiazepines and alcohol to addicts and (in some cases) healthy controls often results in a decrease in global CBF and CMR,[14,44] leading to the hypothesis that a general inhibition of cognitive activity, especially in the cortex (e.g. reduction in anxiety), is related to a drug's pleasurable effects.[45] Why this common response exists following administration of agents from different pharmacological classes with different mechanisms of action remains uncertain, and is difficult to reconcile with other studies that demonstrate that many drugs cause regional increases in brain activity, notably in reward regions receiving dopaminergic input from the midbrain ventral tegmentum. For example, alcohol increases rCMR in the left basal ganglia and temporal cortex,[46] Δ^9-tetrahydrocannabinol (THC) increases rCMR and frontal, insula, cingulate and subcortical rCBF,[14] nicotine increases activity in, among other areas, the nucleus accumbens, amygdala, cingulate and frontal lobes,[18] and euphorigenic doses of amphetamine induce a manic-like state that correlates with increased metabolism in the anterior cingulate, basal ganglia and thalamus.[47] Various methodological differences across imaging techniques and/or differences in individual drug-use patterns and histories of subjects may help explain these discrepancies.

fMRI studies also indicate increased regional brain activation following acute IV administration of cocaine. The superior temporal and spatial resolution of fMRI has enabled the elucidation of finer time-related changes in activation in distinct brain regions in response to drugs. Unfortunately, many small subcortical structures mediating drug effects are located near air–tissue interfaces, and magnet susceptibility artefacts often lead to MR signal dropout, making these regions difficult to visualize. Nevertheless, recent studies have revealed drug-induced changes in several subcortical structures. For example, Breiter et al[17] reported that IV cocaine increased activation in multiple brain regions including the nucleus accumbens, basal forebrain, basal ganglia, insula, ventral tegmentum, and various frontal and other cortical regions when compared to pre-drug activity levels. Signal decreases were observed in three regions, including the amygdala, but the significance of decreases in the BOLD signal, whilst possibly reflecting inhibition of or reduction in neuronal activity, are still unclear.[48] Subjects' reported feelings of 'rush' over time correlated with transient activation in the ventral tegmentum, basal forebrain, thalamus, caudate, and lateral prefrontal and cingulate cortices, whereas their more delayed feelings of 'craving' were correlated with sustained activation in the nucleus accumbens and parahippocampal gyrus, and deactivation in the amygdala. This study highlights the importance of mesocorticolimbic DA system regions, traditionally associated with reward in animals, in mediating the acute effects of cocaine in humans. In addition, it illustrates how fMRI time-course data can help dissociate brain mechanisms associated with temporally discrete affective responses to drugs, such as the initial 'rush' versus delayed 'craving' responses.

Another method that takes advantage of the fine temporal resolution of fMRI to study drug-induced changes in brain activation employs a template-matching technique to isolate voxels whose time course of activation matches the pharmacokinetics of the drug under investigation (e.g. the time to reach peak plasma, and presumably brain, concentration, the magnitude of the peak and the time to fall back to baseline).[49] Using this method, Stein et al,[18] observed that acute IV nicotine, given in a cumulative dosing procedure, activated cortical (frontal, parietal, occipital, insula, temporal, cingulate cortex) and subcortical limbic regions (nucleus accumbens, amygdala, thalamus) in non-abstinent cigarette smokers. Further analysis of these data revealed specific dose-dependent activations in the anterior cingulate, right orbitofrontal and left dorsolateral frontal cortices, insula and right caudate/nucleus accumbens.[50] Preliminary findings using similar pharmacokinetic analysis methods point to IV cocaine injections activating many of the same regions as nicotine,[50] which may explain why many cocaine addicts fail to discriminate between IV nicotine and IV cocaine.[51] Finally, also using the pharmacokinetic template-matching method, IV THC was found to decrease the BOLD signal in the cerebellum, including the region of the dentate nucleus, and specific frontal and parietal regions, and to increase activation in some visual, temporal and parietal cortical areas in experienced marijuana smokers.[52]

In summary, PET and fMRI studies have revealed that acute administration of several abused drugs increases DA transmission and activates regions associated with the mesocorticolimbic DA system. Furthermore, the changes in DA transmission and neuronal activity, particularly in the striatum, are correlated with the experience of a drug-induced 'high'.[8,17,53] Whilst these findings constitute important advances in our understanding of how abused drugs affect brain activity in humans, and reveal a high degree of similarity with drug effects in animal models, an important challenge that faces neuroimaging is to explore the differences between passive (i.e. experimenter delivered) and self-administration of drugs. To date, all published human studies have concentrated on the effects of passively administered drugs, but evidence from animal studies suggests that self-administration of drugs (which is obviously more germane to real-life drug abuse) is associated with different activation of the mesolimbic DA system from that discussed above.[54]

In this regard, using fMRI and real-time behavioural ratings during human cocaine self-administration, Salmeron et al[55] reported that drug-induced 'high' ratings correlated inversely with activity in a number of limbic, paralimbic and mesocortical regions, including the nucleus accumbens, inferior frontal/orbitofrontal gyrus and anterior cingulate, while 'craving' correlated positively with activity in the anterior cingulate, nucleus accumbens, and inferior frontal and orbitofrontal cortices. A dissociation between the behavioural ratings and neuronal activity also occurred, in that as 'high' continued to increase with successive injections during a 1 h self-administration session, phasic activity in the nucleus accumbens/orbitofrontal cortex was seen only during the initial two cocaine self-injections. Finally, consistent with preclinical electrophysiological data, a decrease in orbitofrontal cortex and ventral striatal activity was seen prior to the first two injections of the session, possibly reflecting rapid learning of the expectation of reward. These data provide evidence that complex plastic, time-dependent patterns of neural activity in limbic reward regions are associated with the behavioural planning for, and consequences of, cocaine self-administration in human drug abusers, and that motivation, expectation and active planning for drug administration have large effects on the brain's response to an acute drug injection compared to that seen after an experimenter-administered drug.

Craving ('I want more')

Considerable neuroimaging research in the past few years has focused on brain activity underlying craving – operationally defined as the intense desire or powerful motivational state that often precedes drug seeking and taking. The rationale for this area of research is that a better understanding of the neurobiological, anatomical and cognitive mechanisms underlying craving may help minimize, or even eliminate this state, thereby preventing or reducing drug seeking and taking, and minimize relapse in individuals trying to quit.[56] A preliminary model of the brain circuitry involved in craving suggested dysfunction in the ventral striatal–thalamic– orbitofrontal loop.[57] This proposal followed observations that this circuitry shows abnormalities in obsessive–compulsive disorder patients[58] and is activated during symptom provocation,[59,60] which, like craving, is associated with intrusive thoughts and intense urges to carry out ritualized behaviours in response to certain internal or external cues.

Craving for drugs has been induced using a number of methods – videotapes of simulated drug-taking/drug-related paraphernalia, directed recall of past experiences/mental imagery and low doses of pharmacological stimulants (i.e. drug-induced drug craving). In addition, since craving putatively directs the subject into a certain affective/motivational state, studies have examined differences in more general affective processing in drug addicts. One principal goal of these studies is to determine if affective responses to drug cues are exaggerations of normal emotions or new pathological brain responses. To this end, studies have typically compared the brain activation response to drug-related cues and other affectively charged stimuli with that to neutral cues in both drug addicts and non-drug using controls in order to isolate brain regions specifically involved in drug craving in addicts. In general, evidence largely supports increased activation of the ventral striatum, caudate nucleus, thalamus and orbitofrontal cortex as the principal brain circuitry underlying craving (as proposed by Modell et al[57]). In addition, a number of regions associated with learning, memory and emotional arousal, such as the amygdala, parahippocampal gyrus and dorsolateral prefrontal cortex, have also been generally activated in response to visually presented drug-related cues.

Numerous studies have examined the response to cocaine-related visual cues in cocaine addicts undergoing treatment and in withdrawal,[61–63] or cocaine-free but not withdrawn,[20,64,65] compared to control subjects. Brain areas demonstrating increased metabolism, rCBF or BOLD responses in cocaine addicts viewing cocaine videotapes include the orbitofrontal, dorsolateral prefrontal, anterior cingulate, parietal and medial temporal cortices, amygdala, insula and cerebellum.[20,61,62,64,65] Reports of craving in addicts correlated with dorsolateral, medial temporal cortex and cerebellar metabolism,[20] and anterior cingulate[62,64] and left dorsolateral prefrontal cortex BOLD signal increases.[64] Except for Garavan et al,[65] none of these studies showed increases in basal ganglia or thalamic metabolism during craving, although Childress et al[61] reported a decrease in basal ganglia rCBF. Interestingly, Garavan et al[65] showed that many of the cortical activations evoked by a cocaine film in cocaine addicts were also induced by a erotic film in both addicts and healthy controls (see Figure 4.2), implying that cocaine craving may be subserved by the same brain regions and mechanisms that respond to naturally rewarding/evocative stimuli. In addition, the cocaine users showed a blunted activation response to the sexual film when compared with healthy controls (Figure 4.2), suggesting a diminished capacity to crave and possibly appreciate natural rewards in favour of a stronger desire for drugs.

Similarly, Wexler et al[62] observed that cocaine addicts show different temporal dynamics of brain activation in response to tapes inducing happy and sad moods when compared to controls, suggesting general affective

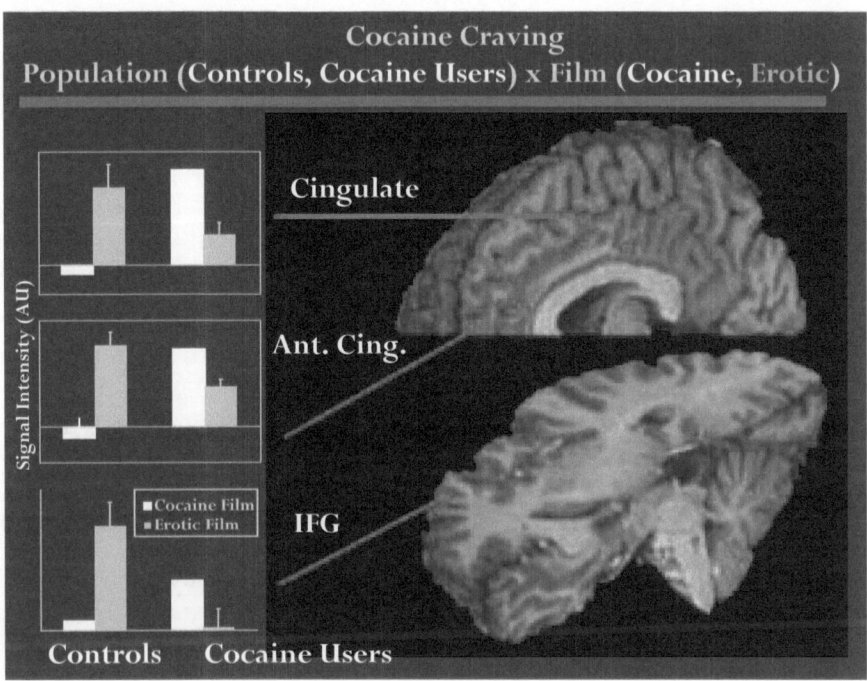

Figure 4.2 *Brain activation in cocaine users and healthy volunteers during viewing of cocaine-related and erotic videotapes. Regions activated by viewing the two videotapes are shown in red on a rendered brain. Graphs show the mean blood oxygenation-level dependent (BOLD) signal intensity in healthy controls and cocaine users in response to the cocaine-related (black) and erotic (orange) videotapes. Note that in all three regions illustrated, the volunteers responded with greater activity while viewing the erotic video, while the cocaine users showed both greater activation while viewing the cocaine-related scenes versus the erotic scenes and less activation to the erotic scenes compared with the volunteers viewing the erotic film. (Ant. Cing., anterior cingulate; IFG, inferior frontal gyrus.)*

dysregulation in chronic cocaine users. Of particular interest were findings of increased activation in 'sad mood' areas in cocaine users following the onset of sad feelings, and in response to the cocaine film, pointing to an association between cocaine use and dysphoric mood, which is borne out by the high incidence of depression in cocaine users.[66]

In addition to a limited number of cortical regions, studies investigating drug-induced drug craving have revealed activation in more subcortical sites than those outlined above, activated in response to visual drug cues. Hence, small doses of alcohol elicited craving in alcoholics, which correlated with increased rCBF in the right caudate nucleus.[67] A more recent fMRI study of

113

craving in 1-week-abstinent alcoholics found increased craving along with right amygdala and cerebellar activation in response to ethanol odour, which normalized following a 3-week recovery programme.[68] As mentioned in the preceding section, Breiter et al[17] suggested that nucleus accumbens and parahippocampal gyrus activation correlated with cocaine-induced cocaine craving, whilst craving induced by methylphenidate administration to cocaine addicts was associated with increased metabolism in the right orbitofrontal cortex and right caudate nucleus,[69] and increased DA release in the thalamus.[8] Therefore, it seems that the compulsive desire to take drugs in addicted individuals can be triggered by at least two distinct mechanisms: activation of cortical areas associated with forms of explicit and implicit memory (episodic, working and emotional) are triggered by presentation of visual cues related to drug use, suggesting that craving occurs due to the activation of autobiographical memories of previous drug-taking experiences,[20] leading to heightened attention towards drug-related stimuli and thoughts.[65] In fact, increased metabolism in the insula, orbitofrontal cortex and cerebellum,[70] and increased rCBF in the amygdala, insula, anterior cingulate, nucleus accumbens and subcallosal cortex,[63] have been observed during script-guided recall of previous drug-taking experiences in cocaine users. Similarly, heroin addicts listening to audiotapes of personalized craving scripts showed increased rCBF in the anterior cingulate, basal ganglia, insula, cerebellum and parahippocampal gyrus.[71] In contrast, pharmacological stimulation of craving appears to act via a more striatal/basal ganglia/thalamic mechanism, possibly by generating the expectation of further reinforcement.[72] Both mechanisms of craving appear to involve the activation of a learnt association or memory, prompting the suggestion that possible pharmacotherapeutic interventions in drug addiction may involve the development of agents that selectively block the formation of, or reduce already-formed memories of, associations between drug cues and reward.[3] However, it is difficult to envisage pharmacotherapies that could selectively alter drug-related associations and memories, as drugs appear to activate mechanisms also involved in learning about natural reinforcers.

The neuronal sites activated during drug craving outlined above seemingly converge in the anterior cingulate and orbitofrontal regions. Anterior cingulate activation may arise from the powerful motivational states elicited by drug-related cues or, alternatively, as a consequence of individuals' attempts to inhibit drug craving and drug taking, since the anterior cingulate is activated by conflicting responses.[73,74] In addition, the anterior cingulate seems to be involved in the inhibition of externally triggered automatic behaviour.[74]

Orbitofrontal cortex activation could generate the anticipation of reward and result in compulsive seeking and taking of a drug. The functional significance of changes in the orbitofrontal cortex and anterior cingulate function in chronic drug users are explored in the following section.

Cognitive effects of drug use ('I can't control my behaviour')

Chronic use of cocaine, amphetamine and alcohol has been associated with cognitive deficits similar to those seen in patients with orbitofrontal lobe lesions, i.e. problems in decision-making and lack of concern for the long-term consequences of one's actions. It is easy to see how such deficits could perpetuate compulsive drug use. Hence, drug-free stimulant and alcohol abusers perform similarly poorly (although not as severely) compared to frontal lobe patients on gambling tasks that depend on, and activate, the orbitofrontal cortex and amygdala.[75–78] Both drug addicts and frontal lobe patients show slowed decision-making and chose the riskier, ultimately less advantageous, option. This behavioural profile can also be induced in non-drug users by reducing serotonergic transmission, which putatively causes hypoactivity in the orbitofrontal cortex.[75] These findings are consistent with the reported reductions in orbitofrontal cortex serotonergic transmission in methamphetamine users,[79] and abnormal orbitofrontal cortex function in cocaine and alcohol abusers.[9] Animal studies suggest that these effects are the direct result of prolonged cocaine and alcohol administration.[80,81] If increased risk-taking and compulsive behaviour is associated with decreased orbitofrontal serotonergic function in alcoholism and stimulant abusers,[9,75] pharmacotherapy with selective serotonin reuptake inhibitors (SSRI) may be effective in maintaining abstinence in some recovering addicts.[82]

The loss of control that often accompanies human drug addiction suggests that disrupted executive functioning, including impaired behavioural inhibition arising from altered frontal cortical (including anterior cingulate and orbitofrontal cortex) function may be one component of addiction. Successful behavioural inhibitions in healthy controls performing a go/no-go paradigm, where subjects must press whenever they see an 'X' or 'Y' except on the odd occasions that it is preceded by the same target letter, are associated with right-hemispheric activations in ventromedial and dorsolateral frontal, anterior insula and inferior parietal cortical regions.[83]

More recently, event-related fMRI was used to examine potential cognitive deficits in otherwise healthy active cocaine users. Active cocaine users and non-users completed a go/no-go task based on Garavan et al,[83] but now in which they were presented with a serial stream of alternating Xs and Ys, all of which required a button-press response. Periodic lures (no-go stimuli), where the stimuli did not alternate required inhibition of the pre-potent button response. Despite attempts to equilibrate task difficulty across subjects by changing the amount of time to make or not make the response, cocaine users made significantly more commission and omission errors than non-users, suggesting that they did not maintain the task set throughout the entire session. Cocaine users also showed significantly less activation than non-users for inhibitions in the right superior temporal gyrus and the anterior cingulate, regions implicated in error detection.[84,85] For errors, users showed hypoactivity relative to non-users in the cingulate, left insula, left inferior frontal gyrus and right medial frontal gyrus. Notably, no between-group differences were found for regions previously suggested to be important for inhibitory control.[86] These findings may represent a unique executive function profile for cocaine users in an inhibitory task and suggests a dysexecutive sequelae of cocaine abuse such that while cocaine users are able to perform inhibitory control tasks, task maintenance and error detection may be impaired.

Another task involving behavioural conflict and requiring inhibition of prepotent responses is the Stroop task, which although not impaired in cocaine and alcohol users, is associated with altered brain activation when compared to healthy controls.[87] Hence, higher relative activation of the orbitofrontal gyrus at baseline predicts better Stroop performance in drug addicts but worse performance in controls, suggesting a reversal of the role of the orbitofrontal gyrus as a function of addiction. Goldstein et al[87] suggested that the orbitofrontal cortex develops a role in bottom-up conflict-monitoring processes in drug addicts, which replaces its more top-down evaluative role in controls and may, ultimately, lead to impaired behavioural inhibition in cases where resources are more limited.

Finally, not all abused drugs are necessarily associated with cognitive deficits. Nicotine, which stimulates (among others) DA and cholinergic neurotransmission, has been shown to enhance cognitive performance in humans and animals,[88,89] particularly in tests of sustained and visuospatial attention. Such cognitive improvements could contribute to the maintenance of smoking behaviour in addicted individuals. Indeed, smokers often report that a cigarette helps them concentrate.[90] In an attempt to elucidate the neural substrates of nicotine's cognitive effects, Ghatan et al[45] observed that acute IV nicotine administered to abstinent smokers and non-smokers enhanced rCBF in parieto-occipital regions during performance of a complex spatial attention maze test. Similarly, nicotine gum enhanced pre-frontal and parietal cortex rCBF in non-smokers performing a two-back working memory task,[91] although no behavioural improvement was reported in either study. In contrast, Lawrence et al[92] found a significant improvement in performance on a test of visual sustained attention in mildly abstinent smokers wearing a nicotine, but not a placebo, patch, which was accompanied by enhanced activation in several task-related (parietal, thalamic, caudate and occipital) areas. When compared to non-smokers performing the same attention task, smokers with a placebo patch showed regional hypoactivity in the parietal cortex and caudate, along with mild behavioural impairment in mood and performance. These findings support observations of cognitive impairment and decreased brain activation in smokers compared to non-smokers during performance of a concept-formation task.[93] In the Lawrence et al[92] study, nicotine replacement in smokers led to identical task-induced brain activation and behavioural responding compared to non-smokers, supporting earlier suggestions that nicotine brings smokers up from a hypoactive to a normal baseline level of mood and cognition.[94]

Changes in brain function in chronic drug users

As the previous sections have illustrated, long-term, chronic drug use is associated with changes in brain function, notably decreases in baseline frontal cortical activity and blunted responses to acute administration of drugs. Some of these alterations show normalization during detoxification but others persist, suggesting that drug use can permanently alter the brain.

During abstinence (1 week to 4 months), frontal cortical rCBF is reduced in the orbitofrontal cortex and cingulate gyrus of cocaine abusers, and this decrease correlates with persistent reductions in D2-receptor availability.[8,95] In addition, decreased metabolism in the dorsomedial and dorsolateral pre-frontal cortices has been reported in cocaine users who were up to 4 months abstinent.[96] Evidence also points to persistent reductions in D2 receptors in the brains of alcoholic individuals,[97] although the deficits in rCMR seen in alcoholics, particularly in frontal regions, show some recovery during abstinence.[98]

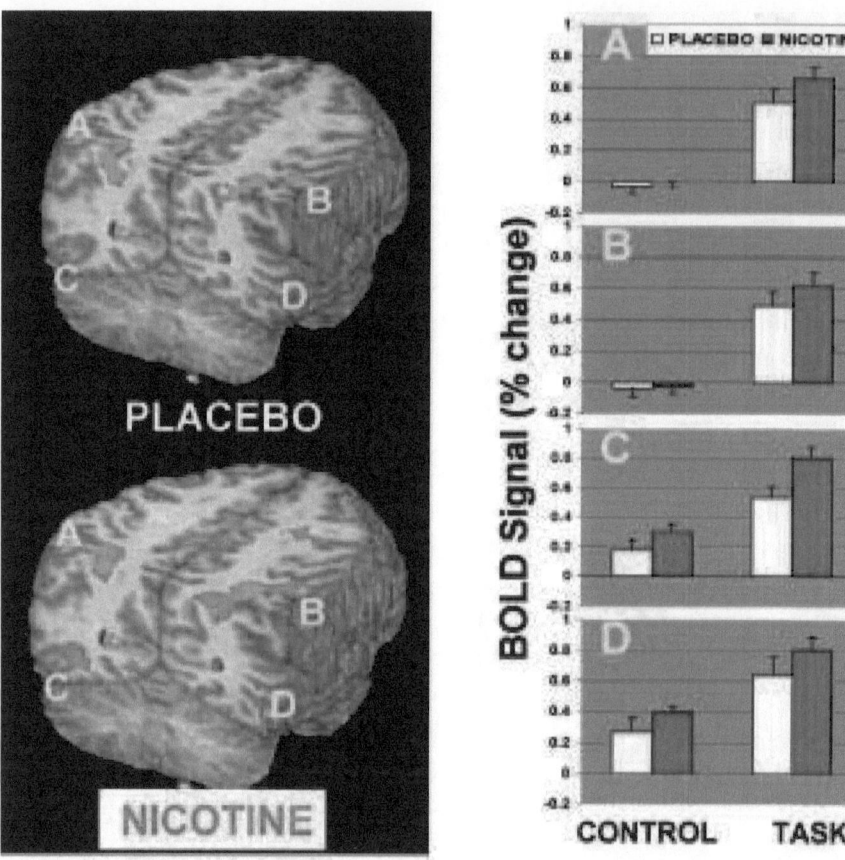

Figure 4.3 Nicotine enhances activation in parietal and occipital cortex. Activated clusters are shown on a representative rendered brain and reflect the activation difference between the attention task and a control task in smokers with placebo and with nicotine patch (cuts made at 60 mm anterior and 43 mm superior to the anterior commissure). The graphs show the change in activation (from baseline) during performance of each task in smokers with placebo and with nicotine. A = left parietal cortex, B = right parietal cortex, C = left occipital cortex, D = right occipital cortex. (Reproduced from Lawrence et al. Neuron 2002; **36:** 539–548.[92])

Use of cocaine has been associated with cerebral strokes and haemorrhages (see Kosten[99] for a review), which likely contribute to the deficits in cerebral perfusion observed in cocaine users and may contribute to their cognitive impairment.[100] Deficits in cerebral perfusion following chronic cocaine use can be reversed when abstinence is combined with buprenorphine, a mixed opioid agonist/antagonist,[101] or aspirin treatment,[99] which may help alleviate cognitive deficits associated with hypofrontality in recovering addicts.

Prolonged cocaine use may also induce a reduction in endogenous opioid transmission, resulting in an upregulation of mu opioid receptors in the frontal and temporal cortices, anterior cingulate and amygdala that persists for at least 4 weeks of abstinence.[102] Administration of buprenorphine, an agonist at the mu opioid receptor, may therefore normalize opioid neurotransmission and help reduce cocaine intake.[103]

Proton magnetic resonance spectroscopy (^{1}H MRS) is an MRI technique that allows for the *in vivo* measurement of brain chemistry and has recently been employed in several drug-abuse studies. Li et al[104] found N-acetyl aspartate (NAA, a marker of neuronal viability) decreases in the left thalamus in active cocaine users compared to normal controls, but no changes in the basal ganglia. In abstinent cocaine users, Chang et al[105] found increases in creatine (Cr, a metabolic marker) and myoinositol (MI) in temporoparietal white matter and a trend toward increased Cr in mid-occipital grey matter, again compared to non-drug-using controls. A similar increase in MI was seen in abstinent users of MDMA (Ecstasy) in white matter.[106]

Recently, Ross et al[107] used ^{1}H MRS to measure metabolite level changes in the anterior cingulate gyrus in experienced cigarette smokers after an acute nicotine challenge both in the presence and absence of previously applied nicotine patches. These were administered to determine alterations in any effect in the face of increased chronic levels of nicotine. A 23% decrease in MI levels was seen 30 min after an acute nicotine injection (0.75 mg) compared to that seen at the pre-drug baseline. Pretreatment with two 21 mg nicotine patches prevented this acute response. In contrast, acute nicotine has no effect on Cr levels no matter what the pretreatment, although patch application was sufficient to increase Cr by about 10% independent of acute nicotine administration.

Since MI is generally thought to be a marker of glial cell activity,[108] and since astrocytes possess nicotinic and muscarinic binding sites,[109] acute nicotine administration may have altered glial cell membrane potential and/or other cellular biochemical processes. As neuronal nicotinic receptors are known to undergo profound desensitization and upregulation, leading to the well-known pharmacodynamic tolerance to nicotine,[110,111] no change in MI levels after patch administration suggests that these glial cell binding sites were desensitized after chronic drug administration. The increase in Cr may represent a new equilibrium state of an upregulated metabolic rate due to chronic drug administration. Since nicotine can acutely induce cingulate neuronal activity[18] and as the cingulate is implicated in attention[112] – an effect often reported after nicotine – cingulate Cr levels may reflect drug-induced changes in vigilance and arousal. It is important to note that these studies demonstrate long-term changes in neurochemistry due to substance abuse but do not address possible reversible changes mediated by acute pharmacological challenge.

The effects of MDMA have not been extensively studied in humans but animal research indicates neurotoxic effects in serotonergic neurons.[113] A PET study in abstinent human MDMA users corroborates the animal findings by revealing decreased serotonin (5-hydroxytryptamine; 5-HT) transporter binding that correlated with previous MDMA use.[114]

Structural studies using computerized tomography (CT) scans suggest that chronic use of alcohol is associated with enlarged ventricles,[115] although this may normalize with prolonged abstinence.[116] In cocaine addicts, cocaine-induced euphoria is lower in individuals with larger ventricles, suggesting that tolerance may develop following reduced periventricular grey matter.[117] A structural MRI study also pointed to reduced prefrontal grey matter in cocaine abusers, with larger reductions in addicts reporting more years of use.[103]

Limitations of neuroimaging studies of drug effects on brain function

This chapter concludes with several disclaimers related to employing neuroimaging to study acute drug effects on the brain, as well as subject safety concerns, drug-induced motion and the effects of drugs on the physiological variables underlying the BOLD signal. More detailed discussions of these issues have recently been reviewed.[19,93]

First, as it is generally agreed that it is unethical to administer highly addictive or toxic substances to non-drug-using individuals, direct comparisons of drug-induced activations in healthy controls and chronic users are limited to a few substances. This makes isolating causation from consequence of drug use difficult if not impossible. Some also find it questionable on ethical grounds or safety concerns to administer abused drugs to any individual, even those with long histories of choosing to self-administer the drug. The former concern may be addressable with analogy to a disease-state model, i.e. it is impossible to study a disease in its absence. As to the latter, it clearly seems possible to utilize rigorous safety measures in order to preclude using individuals of questionable health to ensure minimal complications and/or side effects.

These include in-depth medical screening, including 12-lead electrocardio-gram (ECG), full blood and urine chemistries, complete medical histories and urine testing to confirm prior drug use. Once a decision is made to use an individual in an experimental study, sufficient safety precautions must be adopted, including limiting the drug dose and frequency of administration, and performing initial drug administration in a hospital bed with appropriate monitoring, emergency personnel and equipment available in the event of an untoward response. The latter is considered absolutely necessary as medical interventions in a PET or MRI environment are challenging due to, among other considerations, the presence of radioisotopes in the former and the metal-free environment requirements of the latter. Drug administrations should always be performed in the presence of continuous monitoring of heart rate, ECG, blood pressure and, in some instances, $ETCO_2$ (end tidal CO_2) and respiration rate.

Secondly, head movement in fMRI studies is always a critical issue, as spatial resolutions of just a few millimetres are generally employed. Rapid administration of stimulant drugs such as cocaine, nicotine and ampheta-mine are likely to exacerbate head movement, even in the most compliant of subjects. In addition, experience of the 'high' induced by, for example, IV cocaine is often accompanied by relaxation of the neck muscles, resulting in the head falling backwards out of the imaging plane. In an event-related study, in which the drug-induced 'high' is the only 'event' of interest, this is a considerable problem. Some excessive head movement may be alleviated by applying effective motion-correction algorithms during acquisition and by improving head restraints inside the scanner during analysis. Nevertheless, it is probably fair to assume that successful scan sessions will be less frequent than in non-drug experiments.

Finally, many abused drugs, e.g. nicotine, induce profound cardiovas-cular effects and psychostimulants increase heart rate and blood pressure, which may in itself lead to direct cerebrovascular effects[118,119] that may be sufficient to alter CBF and the BOLD signal. In addition, drugs may alter the coupling of neural activity with rCBF and/or the extraction of oxygen from the blood, causing further changes in the BOLD signal that are unrelated to neural activity. For these reasons, it is critical to ensure simi-larities between rCBF/BOLD changes and changes in metabolic rate (which are not as vulnerable to such confounding variables) and/or to perform control experiments to delineate any non-specific drug effects on CBF and BOLD. These control procedures include use of alternative fMRI pulse sequences in addition to the echo-planar BOLD signal, such as

ASL, or the injection of contrast agents such as gadolinium to measure CBF or CBV. Control experiments have shown that although cocaine causes small (approximately 10%) decreases in the BOLD signal and CBF, there are no changes in task-induced BOLD activation during finger-tapping or visual stimulation, suggesting that neuronal–vascular coupling mechanisms are intact.[50,120] THC and nicotine administration also fail to alter CBF and/or BOLD activation during finger tapping.[52,93] These and other control procedures suggest that in spite of some non-neuronal effects of abused drugs, neuroimaging techniques can be successfully employed to follow the acute effects of drug administration in the human brain.

Conclusions

Neuroimaging enables the visualization of changes in brain activity, as indexed by blood flow, brain metabolism and blood oxygenation, following acute and chronic administration of abused drugs. In contrast to animal experiments, these studies in humans allow one to correlate these changes with subjective experience and alterations in specific cognitive abilities. Findings to date suggest significant overlap in basic drug effects in animals and humans, and point to distinct mechanisms underlying the acute rein-forcing effects of drugs and the development and maintenance of the addicted state. Results strongly suggest that with repeated use, tolerance develops to drugs' reinforcing effects mediated by activation of striatal–thalamic–orbitofrontal circuitry, whilst sensitized responses develop to drug-associated cues and produce powerful urges to maintain drug-taking behaviour. Deficits in frontal cortical perfusion and activity may impair drug users' abilities to inhibit prepotent or ritualized behaviours, or to alter responses with adverse future consequences. Continued methodological and technological improvements in brain imaging are likely to overcome present limitations associated with susceptibility and motion artefacts, and promise to enhance the spatial and temporal resolution of measurement of the brain's response to drugs and its neurobiological consequences. The developing understanding of the neural basis of addiction is expected to advance the development and evaluation of cognitive and pharmacological therapies for drug addiction, which will hopefully help people regain and maintain control over their lives.

Acknowledgements

This review and the studies from the authors' laboratory were supported by funds from the US National Institute on Drug Abuse (DA09465) and National Centre for Research Resources General Clinical Research Centre (M01 RR00058) while they were on the faculty at the Medical College of Wisconsin Department of Psychiatry. We gratefully acknowledge our colleagues Drs Alan Bloom, Hugh Garavan, Robert Risinger, Thomas Ross and Betty Jo Salmeron, without whom much of the data from our laboratory would not exist.

References

1. American Psychiatric Association. *Diagnostic and Statistical Manual for Mental Disorders.* (American Psychiatric Association: Washington, DC, 1994.)
2. Berke JD, Hyman SE. Addiction, dopamine and the molecular mechanisms of memory. *Neuron* 2000; **25:** 515–32.
3. Robinson TE, Berridge KC. The psychology and neurobiology of addiction: an incentive-sensitization view. *Addiction* 2000; **95:** 91–117.
4. Volkow ND, Wang G-J, Fowler JS et al. Prediction of reinforcing responses to psychostimulants in humans by brain dopamine D2 receptor levels. *Am J Psychiatry* 1999; **156:** 1440–3.
5. Alper KR. The EEG and cocaine sensitization: a hypothesis. *J Neuropsychiatry Clin Neurosci* 1999; **11:** 209–21.
6. Little HJ. The contribution of electrophysiology to knowledge of the acute and chronic effects of ethanol. *Pharmacol Therapeut* 1999; **84:** 333–53.
7. Bauer LO. Psychomotor and electroencephalographic sequelae of cocaine dependence. *NIDA Res Mono* 1996; **163:** 66–93.
8. Volkow ND, Wang G-J, Fowler JS. Imaging studies of cocaine in the human brain and studies of the cocaine addict. *Ann NY Acad Sci* 1997; **820:** 41–55.
9. Volkow ND, Fowler JS. Addiction, a disease of compulsion and drive: involvement of the orbitofrontal cortex. *Cerebral Cortex* 2000; **10:** 318–25.
10. Volkow ND, Chang L, Wang GJ et al. Higher cortical and lower subcortical metabolism in detoxified methamphetamine abusers. *Am J Psychiatry* 2001; **158:** 383–9.
11. Sokoloff L. Relationships among local functional activity, energy metabolism and blood flow in the central nervous system. *Fed Proc* 1981; **40:** 2311–16.
12. Mata M, Fink DJ, Gainer H et al. Activity-dependent energy metabolism in rat posterior pituitary primarily reflects sodium pump activity. *J Neurochemistry* 1980; **34:** 213–15.
13. Kuschinsky W, Wahl M. Local chemical and neurogenic regulation of cerebral vascular resistance. *Physiol Rev* 1978; **58:** 656–89.

14. Gatley SJ, Volkow ND. Addiction and imaging of the living human brain. *Drug Alcohol Depend* 1998; **51:** 97–108.

15. Volkow ND, Wang G-J, Fowler JS et al. Imaging endogenous dopamine competition with [^{11}C]raclopride in the human brain. *Synapse* 1994; **16:** 255–62.

16. Laruelle M, D'Souza D, Baldwin RM et al. Imaging D2 receptor occupancy by endogenous dopamine in humans. *Neuropsychopharmacology* 1997; **17:** 162–74.

17. Breiter HC, Gollub RL, Weisskoff RM et al. Acute effects of cocaine on human brain activity and emotion. *Neuron* 1997; **19:** 591–611.

18. Stein EA, Pankiewicz J, Harsch HH et al. Nicotine-induced limbic cortical activation in the human brain: a functional MRI study. *Am J Psychiatry* 1998; **155:** 1009–15.

19. Salmeron BJ, Stein EA. Pharmacological applications of magnetic resonance imaging. *Psychopharmacol Bull* 2002; **36:** 102–29.

20. Grant S, London ED, Newlin DB et al. Activation of memory circuits during cue-elicited cocaine craving. *Proc Natl Acad Sci USA* 1996; **93:** 12040–5.

21. Rogers RD, Robbins TW. Investigating the neurocognitive deficits associated with chronic drug misuse. *Curr Opin Neurobiol* 2001; **11:** 250–7.

22. Di Chiara G. A motivational learning hypothesis of the role of dopamine in compulsive drug use. *J Psychopharmacol* 1998; **12:** 54–67.

23. Koob GF, Bloom FE. Cellular and molecular mechanisms of drug dependence. *Science* 1988; **242:** 715–23.

24. Pontieri FE, Tanda G, Orzi, Di Chiara G. Effects of nicotine on the nucleus accumbens and similarity to those of addictive drugs. *Nature* 1996; **382:** 255–7.

25. White, NM. Addictive drugs as reinforcers: multiple partial actions on memory systems. *Addiction* 1996; **91:** 921–49.

26. Stuss DT, Benson DF. *The Frontal Lobes*. (Raven Press: New York, 1986.)

27. Tremblay L, Schultz W. Relative reward preference in primate orbitofrontal cortex. *Nature* 1999; **398:** 704–8.

28. Rolls ET. The orbitofrontal cortex and reward. *Cerebral Cortex* 2000; **10:** 284–94.

29. Jentsch JD, Taylor JR. Impulsivity resulting from frontostriatal dysfunction in drug abuse: implications for the control of behavior by reward-related stimuli. *Psychopharmacology* 1999; **146:** 373–90.

30. Volkow ND, Chang MD, Wang GJ et al. Low level of brain dopamine D$_2$ receptors in methamphetamine abusers: association with metabolism in the orbitofrontal cortex. *Am J Psychiatry* 2001; **158:** 2015–21.

31. Volkow ND, Wang G-J, Fowler JS et al. Effects of methylphenidate on regional brain glucose metabolism in humans: relationship to dopamine D2 receptors. *Am J Psychiatry* 1997; **154:** 50–5.

32. Thanos PK, Volkow ND, Freimuth P et al. Overexpression of dopamine D2 receptors reduces alcohol self-administration. *J Neurochem* 2001; **78:** 1094–103.

33. Volkow ND, Wang G-J, Begleiter H et al. Regional brain metabolic response to lorazepam in subjects at risk for alcoholism. *Alcohol Clin Exp Res* 1995; **19:** 510–16.

34. Di Chiara G, Imperato A. Drugs abused by humans preferentially increase synaptic dopamine concentrations in the mesolimbic system of freely moving rats. *Proc Natl Acad Sci USA* 1988; **85:** 5274–8.

35. Carboni E, Imperato A, Perezzani L, Di Chiara G. Amphetamine, cocaine, phencyclidine and nomifensine increase extracellular dopamine in the nucleus accumbens of freely-moving rats. *Neuroscience* 1989; **28:** 653–61.

36. Chen JP, Paredes W, Li J et al. Delta 9-tetrahydrocannabinol produces naloxone-blockable enhancement of presynaptic basal dopamine efflux in nucleus accumbens of conscious, freely-moving rats as measured by intracerebral microdialysis. *Psychopharmacology* 1990; **102:** 156–62.

37. Kankaanpaa A, Meririnne E, Lillsunde P, Seppala T. The acute effects of amphetamine derivatives on extracellular serotonin and dopamine levels in rat nucleus accumbens. *Pharmac Biochem Behav* 1998; **59:** 1003–9.

38. Volkow ND, Fowler JS, Wang G-J. Imaging studies on the role of dopamine in cocaine reinforcement and addiction in humans. *J Psychopharmacology* 1999; **13:** 337–45.

39. Volkow ND, Wang G-J, Fowler JS et al. Reinforcing effects of psychostimulants are associated with increases in brain dopamine and occupancy of D(2) receptors. *J Pharmac Exp Ther* 1999; **291:** 409–15.

40. Volkow ND, Wang G-J, Fowler JS et al. Decreased striatal responsiveness in detoxified cocaine-dependent subjects. *Nature* 1997; **386:** 830–3.

41. Lingford-Hughes AR, Acton PD, Gacinovic S et al. Reduced levels of GABA-benzodiazepine receptor in alcohol dependency in the absence of grey matter atrophy. *Br J Psychiatry* 1998; **173:** 116–22.

42. Adinoff B, Devous Sr MD, Best SM et al. Limbic responsiveness to procaine in cocaine-addicted subjects. *Am J Psychiatry* 2001; **158:** 390–8.

43. Howell LL, Wilcox KM. The dopamine transporter and cocaine medication development: drug self-administration in nonhuman primates. *J Pharmac Exp Ther* 2001; **289:** 1–6.

44. London ED, Cascella NG, Wong DF et al. Cocaine-induced reduction of glucose utilization in human brain. A study using positron emission tomography and [fluorine 18]-fluorodeoxyglucose. *Arch Gen Psychiatry* 1990; **47:** 567–74.

45. Ghatan PH, Ingvar M, Eriksson L et al. Cerebral effects of nicotine during cognition in smokers and non-smokers. *Psychopharmacology* 1998; **136:** 179–89.

46. Wang GJ, Volkow ND, Franceschi D et al. Regional brain metabolism during alcohol intoxication. *Alcohol Clin Exp Res* 2000; **24:** 822–9.

47. Vollenweider FX, Maguire RP, Leenders KL et al. Effects of high amphetamine dose on mood and cerebral glucose metabolism in normal volunteers using positron emission tomography (PET). *Psychiatry Res* 1998; **83:** 149–62.

48. Gusnard DA, Raichle ME. Searching for a baseline: functional imaging and the resting human brain. *Nat Neurosci Rev* 2001; **2:** 685–94.

49. Bloom AS, Hoffmann RG, Fuller SA et al. Determination of drug-induced changes in functional MRI signal using a pharmacokinetic model. *Hum Brain Mapping* 1999; **8:** 235–44.

50. Stein EA. fMRI: A new tool for the in vivo localization of drug actions in the brain. *J Anal Toxicol* 2001; **25:** 419–24.

51. Henningfield JE, Miyasato K, Jasinski DR. Cigarette smokers self-administer intravenous nicotine. *Pharmac Biochem Behav* 1983; **19:** 887–90.

52. Bloom AS, Risinger RC, Ross TJ et al. Dose-dependent effects of tetrahydrocannabinol (THC) on brain activity in humans: a functional magnetic resonance imaging (fmri) study. *Neurosci Abs* 2001; **27**: 668–9.

53. Pearlson GD, Jeffrey PJ, Harris GJ et al. Correlation of acute cocaine-induced changes in local cerebral blood flow with subjective effects. *Am J Psychiatry* 1993; **150**: 495–7.

54. Hemby SE, Co C, Koves TR et al. Differences in extracellular dopamine concentrations in the nucleus accumbens during response-dependent and response-independent cocaine administration in the rat. *Psychopharmacology* 1997; **133**: 7–16.

55. Salmeron BJ, Risinger RC, Ross TJ et al. Neural correlates of high and craving during human cocaine self-administration. *NIDA Monograph 182, 2001.*

56. Wallace BC. Psychological and environmental determinants of relapse in crack cocaine smokers. *J Subst Abuse Treat* 1989; **6**: 95–106.

57. Modell JG, Mountz JM, Beresford TP. Basal ganglia/limbic striatal and thalamocortical involvement in craving and loss of control in alcoholism. *J Neuropsychol Clin Neurosci* 1990; **2**: 123–44.

58. Insel TR. Toward a neuroanatomy of obsessive–compulsive disorder. *Arch Gen Psychiatry* 1992; **49**: 739–44.

59. Breiter HC, Rauch SL, Kwong KK et al. Functional magnetic resonance imaging of symptom provocation in obsessive–compulsive disorder. *Arch Gen Psychiatry* 1996; **49**: 595–606.

60. Rauch SL, Jenike MA, Alpert NM et al. Regional cerebral blood flow measured during symptom provocation in obsessive–compulsive disorder using oxygen 15-labeled carbon dioxide and positron emission tomography. *Arch Gen Psychiatry* 1994; **51**: 62–70.

61. Childress AR, Mozley PD, McElgin W et al. Limbic activation during cue-induced cocaine craving. *Am J Psychiatry* 1999; **156**: 11–18.

62. Wexler BE, Gottschalk CH, Fulbright RK et al. Functional magnetic resonance imaging of cocaine craving. *Am J Psychiatry* 2001; **158**: 86–95.

63. Kilts CD, Schweitzer JB, Quinn CK et al. Neural activity related to drug craving in cocaine addiction. *Arch Gen Psychiatry* 2001; **58**: 334–41.

64. Maas LC, Lukas SE, Kaufman MJ et al. Functional magnetic resonance imaging of human brain activation during cue-induced cocaine craving. *Am J Psychiatry* 1998; **155**: 124–6.

65. Garavan H, Pankiewicz J, Bloom A et al. Cue-induced cocaine craving: neuro-anatomical specificity for drug users and drug stimuli. *Am J Psychiatry* 2000; **157**: 1789–98.

66. Withers NW, Pulvirenti L, Koob GF, Gillin JC. Cocaine abuse and dependence. *J Clin Psychopharmac* 1995; **15**: 63–78.

67. Modell JG, Mountz JM. Focal cerebral blood flow change during craving for alcohol measured by SPECT. *J Neuropsychiatry Clin Neurosci* 1995; **7**: 15–22.

68. Schneider F, Habel U, Wagner M et al. Subcortical correlates of craving in recently abstinent alcoholic patients. *Am J Psychiatry* 2001; **158**: 1075–83.

69. Volkow ND, Wang G-J, Fowler JS et al. Association of methylphenidate-induced craving with changes in right striato-orbitofrontal metabolism in cocaine abusers: implications in addiction. *Am J Psychiatry* 1999; **156**: 19–26.

70. Wang GJ, Volkow ND, Fowler JS et al. Regional brain metabolic activation during craving elicited by recall of previous drug experiences. *Life Sci* 1999; **64:** 775–84.

71. Weinstein A, Feldtkeller B, Malizia A et al. Integrating the cognitive and psychological aspects of craving. *J Psychopharmac* 1998; **12:** 31–8.

72. Knutson B, Adams CM, Fong GW, Hommer D. Anticipation of increasing monetary reward selectively recruits nucleus accumbens. *J Neurosci* 2001; **21:** 1–5.

73. Carter CS, Macdonald AM, Botvinick M et al. Parsing executive processes: strategic vs. evaluative functions of the anterior cingulate cortex. *Proc Natl Acad Sci USA* 2000; **97:** 1944–8.

74. Paus T. Primate anterior cingulate cortex: where motor control, drive and cognition interface. *Nature Neurosci* 2001; **2:** 417–24.

75. Rogers RD, Everitt BJ, Baldacchino A et al. Dissociable deficits in the decision-making cognition of chronic amphetamine abusers, opiate abusers, patients with focal damage to prefrontal cortex, and tryptophan-depleted normal volunteers: evidence for monoaminergic mechanisms. *Neuropsychopharmacology* 1999; **20:** 322–39.

76. Rogers RD, Owen AM, Middleton HC et al. Choosing between small, likely rewards and large, unlikely rewards activates inferior and orbital prefrontal cortex. *J Neurosci* 1999; **20:** 9029–38.

77. Grant S, Contoreggi C, London ED. Drug abusers show impaired performance in a laboratory test of decision-making. *Neuropsychologia* 2000; **38:** 1180–7.

78. London ED, Ernst M, Grant S et al. Orbitofrontal cortex and human drug abuse: functional imaging. *Cerebral Cortex* 2000; **10:** 334–42.

79. Wilson JM, Kalasinsky KS, Levey AI et al. Striatal dopamine nerve terminal markers in human, chronic methamphetamine users. *Nat Med* 1996; **2:** 699–703.

80. Corso TD, Mostafa HM, Collins MA, Neafsey EJ. Brain neuronal degeneration caused by episodic alcohol intoxication in rats: effects of nimodipine, 6,7-dinitro-quinoxaline-2,3-dione, and MK-801. *Alcohol Clin Exp Res* 1998; **22:** 217–24.

81. Porrino LJ, Lyons D. Orbital and medial prefrontal cortex and psychostimulant abuse: studies in animal models. *Cerebral Cortex* 2000; **10:** 326–33.

82. Balldin J, Berggren U, Bokstrom K et al. Six-month open trial with Zimelidine in alcohol-dependent patients: reduction in days of alcohol intake. *Drug Alcohol Depend* 1994; **35:** 245–8.

83. Garavan H, Ross TJ, Stein E. Right hemispheric dominance of inhibitory control: an event-related functional MRI study. *Proc Natl Acad Sci USA* 1999; **96:** 8301–6.

84. Dehaene S, Posner MI, Tucker DM. Localization of a neural system for error detection and compensation. *Psychol Sci* 1994; **5:** 303–5.

85. Kiehl KA, Liddle PF, Hopfinger JB. Error processing and the rostral anterior cingulate: an event-related fMRI study. *Psychophysiology* 2000; **37:** 216–23.

86. Kaufman JN, Ross TJ, Stein EA, Garavan H. Cingulate hypoactivity in cocaine users during a GO/NOGO task as revealed by event-related fMRI. *J Neurosci* (in press).

87. Goldstein RZ, Volkow ND, Wang GJ. et al. Addiction changes orbitofrontal gyrus function: involvement in response inhibition. *Neuroreport* 2001; **12:** 2595–9.

88. Sherwood N. Effects of nicotine on human psychomotor performance. *Hum Psychopharmac* 1993; **8:** 155–84.

89. Stolerman IP, Mirza NR, Shoaib M. Nicotine psychopharmacology: addiction, cognition and neuroadaptation. *Med Res Rev* 1995; **15**: 47–72.

90. Russell MA, Peto J, Patel UA. The classification of smoking by factorial structure of motives. *J Roy Stat Soc* 1974; **137**: 313–33.

91. Ernst M, Matochik JA, Heishman SJ et al. Effect of nicotine on brain activation during performance of a working memory task. *Proc Natl Acad Sci USA* 2000; **98**: 4728–33.

92. Lawrence NS, Ross TJ, Stein EA. Cognitive mechanisms of nicotine on visual attention. *Neuron* 2002; **36**: 539–48.

93. Stein EA, Risinger R, Bloom AS. Functional MRI in pharmacology. In: (Moonen C, Bandettini PA, eds) *Medical Radiology. Diagnostic Imaging.* (Berlin: Springer-Verlag: 1999) 525–38.

94. Parrott AC. Nesbitt's Paradox resolved? Stress and arousal modulation during cigarette smoking. *Addiction* 1998; **93**: 27–39.

95. Volkow ND, Fowler JS, Wang GJ et al. Decreased D2 receptor availability is associated with reduced frontal metabolism in cocaine abusers. *Synapse* 1993; **14**: 169–77.

96. Volkow ND, Hitzemann R, Wang G-J et al. Long-term frontal brain metabolic changes in cocaine abusers. *Synapse* 1992; **11**: 184–90.

97. Volkow ND, Wang G-J, Overall JE et al. Regional brain metabolic response to lorazepam in alcoholics during early and late alcohol detoxification. *Alcohol Clin Exp Res* 1997; **21**: 1278–84.

98. Volkow ND, Wang G-J, Hitzemann R et al. Decreased cerebral response to inhibitory neurotransmission in alcoholics. *Am J Psychiatry* 1993; **150**: 417–22.

99. Kosten TR. Pharmacotherapy of cerebral ischaemia in cocaine dependence. *Drug Alcohol Depend* 1998; **49**: 133–44.

100. Volkow ND, Mullani N, Gould KL et al. Cerebral blood flow in chronic cocaine users: a study with positron emission tomography. *Br J Psychiatry* 1988; **152**: 641–8.

101. Levin JM, Mendelson JH, Holman BL et al. Improved regional cerebral blood flow in chronic cocaine polydrug users treated with buprenorphine. *J Nucl Med* 1995; **36**: 1211–15.

102. Zubieta JK, Gorelick DA, Stauffer R et al. Increased mu opioid receptor binding detected by PET in cocaine-dependent men is associated with cocaine craving. *Nat Med* 1996; **2**: 1225–9.

103. London ED, Bonson KR, Ernst M, Grant S. Brain imaging studies of cocaine abuse: implications for medication development. *Crit Rev Neurobiol* 1999; **13**: 227–42.

104. Li SJ, Wang Y, Pankiewicz J et al. Neurochemical adaptation to cocaine abuse: reduction of N-acetyl aspartate in thalamus of human cocaine abusers. *Biol Psychiatry* 1999; **45**: 1481–7.

105. Chang L, Mehringer CM, Ernst T et al. Neurochemical alterations in asymptomatic abstinent cocaine users: a proton magnetic resonance spectroscopy study. *Biol Psychiatry* 1997; **42**: 1105–14.

106. Chang L, Ernst T, Grob CS et al. Cerebral (1)H MRS alterations in recreational 3, 4-methylenedioxymethamphetamine (MDMA, 'ecstasy') users. *J Magn Reson Imaging* 1999; **10**: 521–6.

107. Ross TJ, Schneider E, Prost R et al. Effects of acute and chronic nicotine on ^{1}H MRS in the anterior cingulate. *Int Soc Magn Reson Med* 2000; **8:** 1079.

108. Shonk T, Ross BD. Role of increased cerebral myo-inositol in the dementia of Down syndrome. *Magn Reson Med* 1995; **33:** 858–61.

109. Hosli E, Hosli L. Autoradiographic localization of binding sites for muscarinic and nicotinic agonists and antagonists on cultured astrocytes. *Exp Brain Res* 1988; **71:** 450–4.

110. Henningfield JE, Schuh LM, Jarvik ME. Pathophysiology of tobacco dependence. In: (Bloom FE, Kupfer DJ, eds) *Psychopharmacology: The Fourth Generation of Progress.* (Raven Press: New York, 1995) 1715–29.

111. Dani JA, Heinemann S. Molecular and cellular aspects of nicotine abuse. *Neuron* 1996; **16:** 905–8.

112. Warburton D. Psychopharmacological aspects of nicotine. In: (Wonnacott S, Russell M, Stolerman I, eds) *Nicotine Psychopharmacology: Molecular, Cellular and Behavioral Aspects.* (Oxford University Press: New York, 1990) 77–111.

113. Ricaurte GA, Yuan J, McCann UD. (+/−)3,4-Methylenedioxymethamphetamine ('Ecstasy')-induced serotonin neurotoxicity: studies in animals. *Neuropsychobiology* 2000; **42:** 5–10.

114. McCann UD, Szabo Z, Scheffel U et al. Positron emission tomographic evidence of toxic effects of MDMA ('Ecstasy') on brain serotonin neurons in human beings. *Lancet* 1998; **352:** 1433–7.

115. Cascella NG, Pearlson G, Wong DF et al. Effects of substance abuse on ventricular and sulcal measures assessed by computerised tomography. *Br J Psychiatry* 1991; **159:** 217–21.

116. Pfefferbaum A, Sullivan EV, Rosenbloom MJ et al. A controlled study of cortical gray matter and ventricular changes in alcoholic men over a 5-year interval. *Arch Gen Psychiatry* 1998; **55:** 905–12.

117. Morgan MJ, Cascella NG, Stapleton JM et al. Sensitivity to subjective effects of cocaine in drug abusers: relationship to cerebral ventricular size. *Am J Psychiatry* 1993; **150:** 1712–17.

118. Fischman MW, Schuster CR, Javaid J et al. Acute tolerance development to the cardiovascular and subjective effects of cocaine. *J Pharmac Exp Ther* 1985; **235:** 677–82.

119. Johanson CE, Fischman MW. The pharmacology of cocaine related to its abuse. *Pharmac Rev* 1989; **41:** 3–52.

120. Gollub RL, Breiter HC, Kantor H et al. Cocaine decreases cortical cerebral blood flow but does not obscure regional activation in functional magnetic resonance imaging in human subjects. *J Cereb Blood Flow Metab* 1998; **18:** 724–34.

5. NEUROIMAGING STUDIES OF MOOD DISORDERS

Cynthia HY Fu, Nicholas D Walsh, Wayne C Drevets

Introduction

Our understanding of mood disorders has progressed from a notion of black bile causing melancholia to a realization that they develop from a complex interaction of genetic, psychological and social factors. That these disorders of the mind derive from some form of dysfunction of the brain is supported by evidence from clinical, neurochemical, neuroendocrine and histological studies. A high prevalence of depression has been observed in patients with neurological disorders, such as Parkinson's and Huntington's diseases,[1,2] and in patients following a stroke.[3-5] This clinical evidence of secondary mood disorders (i.e. a mood disorder that is secondary to a medical/neurological disorder) indicates an underlying pathology within the brain and further suggests some regions where the dysfunction may be localized. Researchers have been examining the expression of similar abnormalities in primary mood disorders using structural and functional neuroimaging techniques.

Since the initial studies, it has been evident that mood disorders are associated with regional, functional neuroanatomical abnormalities. Subsequent research goals have involved elucidation of the neurobiological mechanisms underlying these findings and characterization of their clinical correlates. Ongoing research questions include identifying abnormalities that are specific to mood disorders and distinct from other psychiatric disorders such as schizophrenia or anxiety disorders, and determining whether abnormalities are specific to currently recognized mood disorder subtypes, such as unipolar as compared to bipolar disorder; or melancholic as compared to atypical subtypes. It also remains unclear whether abnormalities are specific to major depressive episodes or also extend to manic episodes, or whether they are associated with specific symptoms, such as anhedonia, psychomotor retardation and cognitive impairment. Such questions are, nevertheless, imminently tractable to neuroimaging studies, as a major advantage of this technology is that non-invasive, serial measures of brain function can be acquired both during an illness episode and upon recovery, allowing discrimination of state versus trait markers, and in depressed samples manifesting a particular psychopathological signs or symptom versus those without. Finally, the value of applying neuroimaging technology in clinical psychiatry to aid in optimizing treatment regimens for individuals and for identifying early markers of treatment responses that can predict clinical outcome, remains under investigation.

In this chapter, we review how structural and functional neuroimaging techniques have contributed to our understanding of the pathophysiology of mood disorders. The focus is on adult-onset mood disorders, specifically major depressive disorder [primary unipolar depression (UP)] and bipolar disorder (BP), as based on current diagnostic systems. From the early studies there has been a rapid evolution in the sophistication and complexity of experimental designs. At the same time, there have been significant improvements in instrumentation providing greater spatial and temporal resolution. This review emphasizes the most consistent findings while presenting contrasting data and possible reasons for the discrepancies. The chapter is divided into two sections: (1) structural neuroimaging, with computed tomography (CT) and magnetic resonance imaging (MRI) measurements of neuroanatomic abnormalities; and (2) functional neuroimaging, with findings from the xenon-133 (^{133}Xe) inhalation technique, single photon emission computed tomography (SPECT), positron emission tomography (PET) and functional magnetic resonance imaging (fMRI) studies.

Initial structural neuroimaging studies sought to identify general cerebral abnormalities by examining global cerebral and ventricular volumes. As technology improved, greater spatial resolution became available, allowing examination of regional cortical and subcortical structures, and more recent studies have been able to further discern individual gyri and regional structures, such as distinguishing the hippocampus and amygdala, which may have a particular relevance in mood disorders. The early functional neuroimaging studies measured global cerebral activity and the ratio of anterior to posterior regional activity, along with correlations of resting state cerebral activity with clinical symptoms and cognitive impairments. In order to directly examine dynamic cerebral function, several more recent studies have used particular cognitive activation or mood-induction tasks. Furthermore, researchers have been specifically examining those regions that are associated with, and predictive of, a successful response to therapy.

The major findings in mood disorders are reviewed below using this general outline as a guide, and their implications for current neuroanatomical models are discussed.

Structural neuroimaging studies

There have been several comprehensive reviews of the early literature on structural neuroimaging studies of mood disorders,[6–10] including a few meta-analyses.[11–13] We shall summarize pertinent findings and discuss some of the more recent and significant data on regions that were poorly examined in the early studies.

Global brain measurements have been in the form of global cerebral volume, ventricular volume, ventricular-to-brain (VBR) volume ratio and sulcal size. In a meta-analysis of 29 studies with a total of 912 patients and 932 controls, Elkis et al[11] found a moderate effect size for ventricular enlargement and sulcal widening in patients with mood disorders as compared to healthy controls. However, similar differences are also evident in schizophrenia,[14] albeit perhaps to a greater degree than in mood disorders,[12,15] indicating a lack of specificity of these abnormalities. Further correlations with outcome measures have revealed mixed results, with findings of larger ventricles being associated with a poorer outcome,[16–18] and of no relationship between ventricular size and outcome.[19,20] Measures of global cerebral volume have not indicated any differences between patients with mood disorders and healthy controls,[10,21,22] in contrast to schizophrenia in which smaller global cerebral volumes have been observed.[14] Most studies of total grey matter volumes have similarly found no difference between UP patients and controls,[23] nor between BP patients and controls,[24–29] with the exception of one study.[30]

One of the most consistent findings has been an increased number of signal hyperintensities (also known as white matter hyperintensities or white matter lesions), which are small discrete regions that appear brighter or hyperintense on T2-weighted MRI scans, reflecting a localized change in water content in that tissue. They are associated with cerebrovascular disease with greater rates found with increasing age.[31,32] From a meta-analysis of 10 studies of BP patients (296 patients, 516 controls) and seven studies of UP patients (254 patients, 511 controls), Videbech[13] reported significantly increased rates of signal hyperintensities in BP patients, irrespective of age, and in UP patients, particularly in late-onset depression. Further associations with a poorer outcome in BP disorder[33,34] and a history of suicide attempts in UP patients[35] have been reported. Their etiology in BP patients remains unclear,[10,13,36,37] although a neuropathology associated with atherosclerotic, cerebrovascular disease has been proposed for elderly UP patients who have a late age at depression onset.[6,31,38] Interestingly, increased rates of signal hyperintensities are not a common finding in schizophrenia, suggesting a more specific association with mood disorders.[13,39,40]

Measurements of the frontal lobes have revealed mixed findings.[10,41] However, as the frontal lobes comprise over half of the human brain, and are composed of several functionally distinct components, examination of individual regions becomes essential for elucidating conditions such as mood disorders which involve relatively specific cognitive/emotional domains. For example, Drevets et al[42] reported a reduced volume of the left subgenual anterior cingulate cortex (i.e. ventral to the genu of the corpus callosum) in UP and BP patients with a family history of mood disorders, and Hirayasu et al[43] similarly observed a decreased volume in the same region in patients with a first episode of affective psychosis and a family history of mood disorders. Recently, Bremner et al[21] additionally found reduced orbitofrontal cortical volumes in UP patients. In other cortical regions, there has been little evidence of abnormalities of the parietal lobes, and findings have been inconclusive for the temporal lobes.[10,44,45]

Initial studies of hippocampal volume were equivocal in their findings, possibly due to the poor resolution of the early neuroimaging techniques which did not allow separation of the hippocampus and the adjacent amygdala.[46,47] Some recent studies with high-resolution MRI have reported bilaterally decreased volumes of the hippocampus in UP patients,[41,48,49] ranging from 8 to 19%,[50] although others found no volumetric difference relative to healthy controls.[51–55] In BP disorder, the findings have been less consistent with reports of increased,[56] decreased[47,57] and no difference in hippocampal volume.[26,44,58] Measurements of the amygdala in UP patients have found reduced core nuclei volumes but no significant difference in total amygdalar volumes,[59] asymmetry with the right smaller than the left amygdala,[60] increased bilateral volumes[61] and no difference.[41] Similarly, in BP patients the amygdala volumes have been reported to be increased[20,44] as well as decreased[26] with respect to healthy controls. Precise and reliable identification and measurement of the amygdala has been difficult due to its small size and juxtaposition to multiple other grey matter structures,[62] and future MRI studies focusing on delineation of the amygdala from the hippocampal complex, basal forebrain, anteromedial temporal cortex, and parahippocampal cortex ought to provide more reliable data on this important region.

In subcortical regions, volumetric abnormalities of the thalamus and basal ganglia have been an inconsistent finding.[6,10,22] In UP patients, particularly older patients, decreased caudate and putamen volumes have been reported.[63–65] However, several groups have not found any differences,[66–69] with Lenze and Sheline[68] suggesting that a confounding factor in previous studies may have been cerebrovascular disease causing atrophy of these regions.

Impaired function in the hypothalamic–pituitary–adrenal axis has significant neuroendocrine and physiological implications in mood disorders. Initial studies found increased volume of the pituitary gland in UP patients[70,71] but a recent study, which had greater spatial resolution, did not report any differences between UP patients and healthy controls.[72] In the same study, Sassi et al[72] reported a decreased pituitary volume in BP patients.

A reduced cerebellar volume has been reported by a number of studies of both UP and BP patients.[10,73] Recent findings, including data from neuroimaging studies, have consistently implicated a role in affective and cognitive processes.[74–76] Neuroanatomical mapping of cerebellar projections have also revealed that they extend into the prefrontal cortex, which may provide the anatomical substrate for its cognitive and emotional functions.[77]

In summary, non-specific ventricular enlargement is evident in mood disorders, mostly in chronic UP. However, specific measurements in UP and BP disorders, and with chronicity, are particularly relevant. Specific cortical regions have been implicated, such as the subgenual anterior cingulate in familial depression, but further examinations of subdivisions of the prefrontal cortex and other regions are necessary. Decreased hippocampal volumes have been observed in UP patients, with reports of increased amygdalar volumes in BP patients and reduced cerebellar volumes in both UP and BP patients. One of the most replicated findings has been an increased number of signal hyperintensities in BP patients and elderly UP patients who have a late age at depression onset. Elucidation of the significance of these structural abnormalities awaits integration with findings from histological investigations, genetic studies and their functional correlates.

Box 5.1 Summary of structural abnormalities

Major depressive disorder [primary unipolar depression (UP)]

Increased signal hyperintensities in late-onset depression

Reports of decreased left subgenual anterior cingulate and orbitofrontal volumes

Some evidence of decreased bilateral hippocampal volume

Reports of decreased caudate and putamen volume, particularly in chronic UP

Bipolar disorder (BP)

Increased signal hyperintensities

Reports of abnormal amygdala volumes

Both UP and BP

Reports of ventricular enlargement, particularly in chronic BP

Sulcal widening

Reports of decreased cerebellar volume

Studies of neuroreceptor systems: neuroreceptors and neuroendocrine studies

Functional brain imaging has afforded a unique opportunity to study neuro-receptor systems *in vivo*. The key neurotransmitter systems implicated in the pathophysiology of mood disorders include serotonin, dopamine and norepinephrine. For each neurotransmitter (NT) system, the process of investigation is similar as impairments may be possible at each stage of NT metabolism: an insufficient supply of the NT precursor, defects in the uptake of the NT precursor, impaired release of NT, and dysfunction of NT receptors and transporters. Neuroimaging methods include neuroreceptor mapping and functional neuroimaging studies incorporating pharmacologi-cal challenge or neuroendocrine probes. Measurement and regional localiza-tion of neuroreceptors have been conducted with SPECT and PET studies, but a major limitation has been the limited availability of radiotracers that are selective for a particular receptor, which had restricted early investiga-tions to the serotonergic and dopaminergic systems. Ongoing research though is expanding the repertoire to include studies of excitatory amino acid function with mapping of N-methyl-D-aspartate (NMDA) receptors.[78] We shall review the findings in turn for each of the major neurotransmitter systems.

Serotonergic system

Forty years of research have established a fundamental role for the serotonergic system in the pathophysiology of mood disorders.[79,80] The serotonergic system derives from the dorsal and median raphe nuclei in the brain stem, which have extensive neural projections to all regions of the brain,[81] and more than 16 serotonin (5-hydroxytryptamine; 5-HT) receptor subtypes have been identified.[82] To date, neuroimaging studies of the 5-HT system have examined the presynaptic 5-HT transporter, pre- and postsynaptic 5-HT_{1A} receptor, postsynaptic 5-HT_{2A} receptor, and measures of serotonergic function by pharmacological manipulation with fenfluramine challenge and tryptophan modulation studies.

The most commonly studied receptor has been the 5-HT_{2A} subtype. In an early SPECT study with $[^{123}\text{I}]$ketanserin, D'haenen et al[83] found increased uptake of the radioligand in the parietal cortex in depressed subjects. However, this finding has not been replicated in PET studies with more selective radiotracers. Using the radioligand $[^{18}\text{F}]$altanserin, Biver et al[84] reported decreased uptake in the orbitofrontal and insular cortices, while Meltzer et al[85] found no differences between depressives and controls. In studies using the radioligand $[^{18}\text{F}]$setoperone, reduced binding was reported in the frontal cortex[86] in all cortical regions[87] in depressives versus controls, although Meyer et al[88] found no difference in medication-free UP patients as compared to healthy controls. The evidence from these studies of abnormalities in 5-HT_{2A} receptor density is inconclusive. Though following antidepressant treatment with selective serotonin reuptake inhibitor (SSRI) medications, increased binding potentials have been found, measured with $[^{18}\text{F}]$setoperone.[89] However, $[^{18}\text{F}]$setoperone measurements have also shown decreased binding potentials following clomipramine treatment,[86,90] and with paroxetine in younger patients but no change in patients > 30 years of age.[91] In these studies, changes in 5-HT_{2A} receptor binding potential were observed with antidepressant medication treatment,[86,89–91] but a specific association with clinical treatment response was less clear. Instead, Zanardi et al[92] have reported that UP patients who responded to treatment with paroxetine showed greater frontal cortical 5-HT_{2A} receptor binding potential than patients who remained depressed, as measured with

[^{18}F]fluoroethylspiperone and PET. These findings suggest that antidepressant drug treatment may be associated with a decreased 5-HT$_{2A}$ receptor binding potential, but a relationship with treatment response awaits further investigation (Figure 5.1).

Widespread cerebral reductions in 5-HT$_{1A}$ receptor density in depressed patients have been reported by PET studies with the [carbonyl-^{11}C]WAY-100635 compound in both UP and BP patients,[93–97] and these decreases appear to persist following antidepressant treatment in UP patients.[97] These findings may reflect a reduction in 5-HT innervation,[98] down-regulation of 5-HT$_{1A}$ receptor gene expression in the hippocampus due to elevated cortisol associated with depression,[93,96,98] or abnormal reductions in cellular elements (e.g. glial cells) on which 5-HT$_{1A}$ receptors are expressed (reviewed by Drevets et al[94]). Clinical studies have indicated that augmentation of SSRI medications with pindolol may reduce the time of onset of the antidepressant response.[99] This improved response is believed to be mediated through blockade of presynaptic, somatodendritic 5-HT$_{1A}$ autoreceptors,[99] with pindolol revealing a selectivity for 5-HT$_{1A}$ auto-

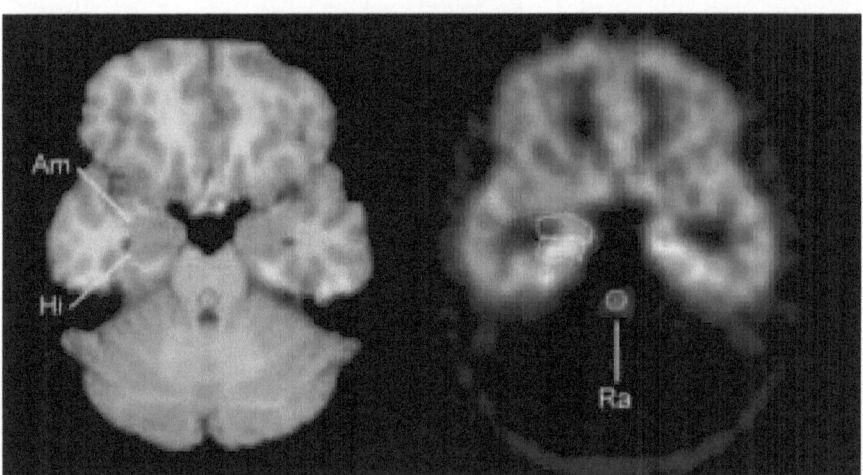

Figure 5.1 Co-registered PET and MRI sections through the mesiotemporal cortex and midbrain. This region included areas of high 5HT$_{1A}$ receptor density (hippocampus; Hi) along with areas of moderate density (amygdala (Am), periamygdaloid cortex). The hippocampal region of interest (ROI) assessed post hoc is delimited from amygdala by the alveus (thin white matter tract). The raphe (Ra) ROI was defined on the PET, but in the co-registered MRI it is evident that this circular ROI overlies the midbrain area where the dorsal raphe nucleus is known to be situated. (Modified from Drevets et al. PET imaging of serotonin 1A receptor binding in depression. Biol Psychiatry 1999; **46**: 1375–87.)

receptors in the dorsal raphe nucleus in the brainstem.[100–102] However, its clinical effectiveness has been variable, which appears to be related to the degree of pre- versus postsynaptic receptor occupancy.[101] A correlation between receptor occupancy levels and clinical response has been observed in treatment studied in schizophrenia,[103,104] and a similar approach in mood disorders would offer an exciting and heuristic application of receptor binding studies (Figure 5.2).[101]

Reductions in the density of 5-HT transporter binding sites in the brain stem have been found in medication-free UP patients[105] and following SSRI antidepressant treatment,[106] as measured with [^{123}I]B-CIT and SPECT. Using a more selective radiotracer, [^{11}C]DASB and PET, Meyer et al[107] did not find any differences in the striatum between medication-free UP patients and healthy controls, but did report decreased 5-HT transporter density following SSRI antidepressant treatment. With the ligand [^{11}C](+)McN5652 and PET, Ichimiya et al[108] found increased binding sites in the midbrain for medication-free UP patients and in the thalamus for both medication-free UP and BP patients, but acknowledged that these findings may have been an overestimate due to greater non-specific binding

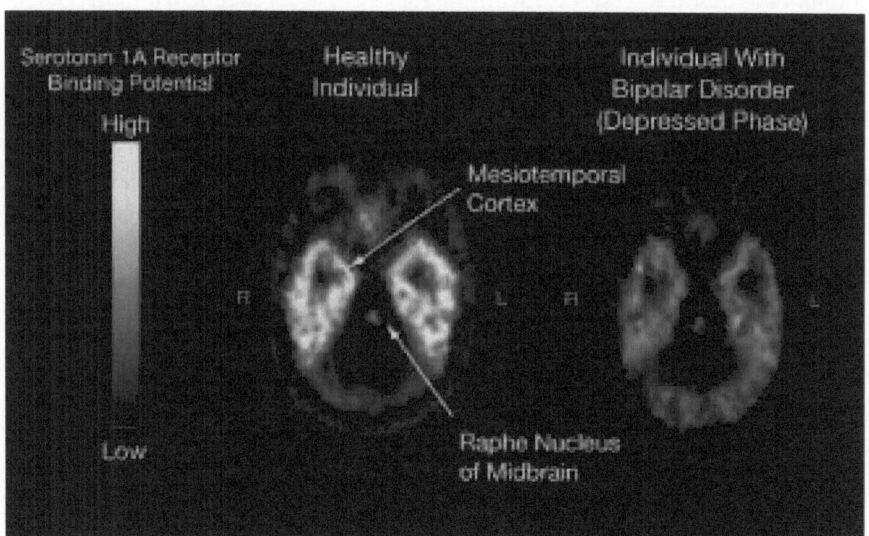

Figure 5.2 *Transverse PET scans showed marked deficiency of 5HT$_{1A}$ receptor activity in the mesiotemporal cortex (including the amygdala and hippocampus) and in the midbrain raphe nucleus in an individual during an acute depressive episode. (Reproduced from Vastag. Decade of work show depression is physical. JAMA 2002; 287: 1787–8.)*

associated with the ligand. Post-mortem brain studies have revealed decreased 5-HT transporter binding in both ventral and dorsal regions of the prefrontal cortex in patients with depression,[109–111] which may not be explained by substance abuse nor suicide.[110] The magnitude of these differences was small though, which may have contributed to the discrepant receptor neuroimaging data of Meyer et al[107] and Ichimiya et al.[108] However, decreased binding has been observed following SSRI antidepressant treatment and may be understood as occupancy (with inhibition) of the 5-HT transporter, which would reduce serotonin reuptake and clearance and, thus, elevate synaptic serotonin levels.[105,107]

Researchers have also sought to evaluate the neural correlates of neurotransmitter function by incorporating neuroendocrine function with functional neuroimaging measures. To investigate the serotonergic system, researchers have used fenfluramine, which produces a temporary release of serotonin from presynaptic neurons.[112,113] Using PET and [^{18}F]fluorodeoxyglucose (FDG), Mann et al[112] found that depressed patients failed to show the pattern of activation that was observed in the healthy subjects, in whom fenfluramine was associated with increased glucose metabolism in the left prefrontal and temporoparietal cortices, and decreases in the right prefrontal cortex. The finding of a 'blunted' response would putatively be consistent with purported impaired serotonin function in depression. However, in a [^{15}O] H$_2$O PET study, Meyer et al[113] did not find any significant differences between depressed and healthy subjects. These studies though had several methodological differences which may account for their discrepant findings: different isomers of fenfluramine and methods of administration; oral d,l-fenfluramine[112] versus intravenous d-fenfluramine,[113] which is more selective for serotonin,[114] different timings of the scans; an earlier scan time[113] in which depletion of presynaptic 5-HT stores may not have been fully observed in depressed patients as with a delayed scan time;[112] and the method of analysis in which measurements were restricted to regions that had shown the maximal differences in the healthy control sample, creating a bias towards finding a diminished response in the depressed sample[112] rather than a global cortical comparison between groups.[113]

Investigating the serotonin precursor tryptophan with PET and L-[^{11}C]hydroxytryptophan, Agren et al[115] found impaired uptake in the whole brain and prefrontal cortex in UP patients, suggesting impaired transport of tryptophan across the blood–brain barrier. Bremner et al[116] examined the effects of tryptophan depletion on regional cerebral metabolism in UP patients who were in remission. They found that those patients who developed a temporary worsening of depressive symptoms following tryptophan depletion had reduced metabolism in a number of regions, including the middle frontal and orbitofrontal cortices and thalamus, as compared to patients with no change in symptoms. As both groups of patients had comparable plasma levels of tryptophan, the differences in regional cerebral metabolism could not be merely attributed to differences in brain serotonin levels; rather, the finding suggests dysfunction in postsynaptic receptor bindings or other postsynaptic mechanisms.[116] Smith et al[117] combined tryptophan depletion with a cognitive task in remitted UP patients and observed comparable findings; that a worsening mood was associated with decreased cerebral blood flow in the anterior cingulate and orbitofrontal cortices, as well as in the parietal and occipital cortices and caudate. Furthermore, a mood–task interaction was found in the dorsal anterior cingulate cortex, which raises some intriguing queries on the interplay of specific neurotransmitter systems with cognitive function in depression.

Norepinephrine system

Several lines of evidence have implicated a primary role for the noradrenergic system in the pathophysiology of mood disorders. Norepinephrine originates from neuronal cell bodies in the brainstem, in particular the locus coeruleus, which have extensive projections throughout the brain.[118] One of the most consistent findings in depression has been an attenuation of the growth hormone response to clonidine, an α_2-adrenoceptor agonist, suggesting an underlying dysregulation in the noradrenergic system.[119] In a $[^{15}O]$ H_2O PET study, Fu et al[120] examined noradrenergic function in medication-free UP patients in combination with clonidine as a neuromodulatory probe. Although a significant difference in growth hormone response was not evident between UP patients and healthy controls, differential activity in the right prefrontal cortex was elicited, with the healthy controls showing decreased activity but the UP patient group revealing increased activity in this region. The authors suggested that this differential effect of clonidine in the prefrontal cortex may have arisen from impaired presynaptic α_2-adrenoceptors as well as regionally 'supersensitive' postsynaptic cortical α_2-adrenoceptors.[120] As subjects were engaged in a simple attentional task during the scans, the finding suggests a possible interaction in the right prefrontal cortex of depression, the noradrenergic neurotransmitter system, and the cognitive process of attention. Although further investigations with dynamic mapping of adrenoceptors and their function are needed

---

Box 5.2 Summary of neuroendocrine studies

Serotonergic system

Little evidence for abnormalities in presynaptic function with fenfluramine challenge in depressed patients

Decreased activation in middle and orbitofrontal cortices and thalamus associated with temporary worsening of depressive symptoms following tryptophan depletion; postsynaptic receptor abnormalities have been implicated

Combining tryptophan depletion with a cognitive task reveals a mood–task interaction in the dorsal anterior cingulate cortex

Norepinephrine system

Abnormal function in right prefrontal cortex has been observed in depressed UP patients following a clonidine challenge

---

to fully delineate the dysregulation of the noradrenergic system and its effect in mood disorders, PET or SPECT radioligands with sufficient selectivity for norepinephrine binding sites are not currently available.

Dopaminergic system

The dopaminergic system has also been postulated to have a role in the pathophysiology of mood disorders based upon evidence that concentrations of the dopamine metabolite homovanillic acid are decreased in the cerebral spinal fluid of depressed patients. In particular, in those with psychomotor retardation, the mesolimbic dopamine projections into the ventral striatum and medial prefrontal cortex play a critical role in reward processing. The prevalence of depression is increased in Parkinson's disease (relative to other similarly disabling conditions), and some medications with dopaminergic actions exert antidepressant effects.[121–123] Several studies have examined the dopamine D_2 receptor in patients with major depression using SPECT and the radiotracer [^{123}I]iodobenzamide (IBZM).[124–128] Three studies did not report a significant difference in striatal binding between patients and controls,[124,127,128] while two studies found higher binding rates in depressed patients.[125,126] Parsey et al[127] calculated the weighted effect size for these five studies to be a 4% increase in D_2 receptors in UP patients as compared to healthy controls, suggesting that there is little evidence for a mediating role of striatal D_2 receptors in UP depression.

Pearlson et al[129] showed that psychotic BP subjects have an increased striatal uptake of $[^{11}C]N$-methylspiperone binding to D2-like dopamine receptor sites relative to controls or to non-psychotic BP subjects. The striatal D2 binding in the psychotic BP subjects correlated positively with psychosis ratings in this study. As a measure of endogenous dopamine stores, an amphetamine challenge showed no significant change in D2 receptor binding, despite subjective reports of an improved mood in depressed UP[127] or euthymic BP patients.[130] The imaging data regarding the dopamine transporter are in disagreement, as Laasonen-Balk et al[131.] found higher striatal dopamine transporter binding in depressed patients, while Meyer et al[132] found decreased dopamine transporter binding in depressives versus controls. Furthermore, Martinot et al[133] reported a specific association of

---

Box 5.3 Summary of receptor binding studies

Serotonergic system

Mixed evidence for 5-hydroxytryptamine (5-HT) transporter density and 5-HT_{2A} receptor abnormalities, but several reports of decreases following selective serotonin reuptake inhibitor (SSRI) treatment

Decreased 5-HT_{1A} receptor densities in primary unipolar depression (UP) and bipolar disorder (BP) patients, which persist in UP patients following antidepressant treatment

Dopaminergic system

Little evidence of striatal dopamine D_2 receptor abnormalities in UP patients, but densities may increase following successful SSRI treatment

Reports of increased striatal D_2 receptor density in BP with psychotic symptoms

Little evidence of abnormalities in endogenous dopamine stores in UP and BP patients, as no significant changes in D_2 receptor densities observed following an amphetamine challenge

Conflicting evidence for dopamine transporter abnormalities

Impaired presynaptic function ($[^{18}F]$fluorodopa) associated with psychomotor retardation in UP patients

Suggestion of decreased prefrontal D_1 receptor densities in BP patients

impaired striatal presynaptic dopamine function in UP patients with marked psychomotor retardation and affective flattening, as measured with [^{18}F]fluorodopa (DOPA) and PET. Also, following SSRI antidepressant treatment, Klimke et al[126] found increased D2 receptor binding in UP patients who had a successful response to treatment. Finally, Suhara et al[134] reported that the binding potential for the dopamine D1 receptor radioligand, [^{11}C]SCH-23990, was below the age-adjusted normal range in the frontal cortex in nine of 10 BP subjects scanned in a variety of mood states. This finding awaits replication using D1 receptor ligands that are more amenable to quantitation. Overall, these neuroimaging data have provided some preliminary *in vivo* evidence of dopaminergic dysfunction in mood disorders, but also suggest that there may be some specificity in its clinical associations and sites of the impairments.

Neurophysiological studies

Initial functional neuroimaging studies were typically acquired with subjects in a resting state with their eyes closed, or open, and with their ears plugged, or not. Although there has been some debate about the reproducibility of a resting state, as some authors suggest that there is significant variability in the thoughts and feelings between persons which may be reflected in cerebral activity,[135–137] meta-analyses have implicated a consistent set of regions active during a resting state in healthy individuals.[138,139] However, there may be greater variation in cognitive, behavioural and emotional states in psychiatric disorders. In order to account for such potential heterogeneity, researchers have correlated regional cerebral activity with specific symptoms, and more recent studies have utilized particular cognitive activation and mood-induction tasks. As well, several groups have begun to examine the effects of treatment, both pharmacotherapy and psychotherapy, on cerebral activity which are revealing regions that may be predictive of recovery from an illness episode. We shall review the functional neuroimaging studies in mood disorders along this outline. Again, we have highlighted the central findings but a detailed review of each study is beyond the scope of this chapter. Instead, we refer the reader to several comprehensive reviews.[94,140–143]

Resting state studies

The first studies of global cerebral activity were conducted over 20 years ago with the ^{133}Xe inhalation technique.[144,145] Subsequent investigations have used SPECT, which provides measures of relative, regional cerebral blood flow (rCBF), and PET, which can quantitatively assess glucose metabolism or rCBF. Over 20 studies have examined resting state global cerebral activity, and the majority have not observed significant differences between patients with mood disorders as compared to controls.[142]

One of the most consistent findings from resting state studies of regional cortical activity has been decreased activity in the dorsal aspects of the frontal lobes in depressed UP and BP patients, in particular the dorsolateral prefrontal cortex.[141–143,146] In contrast, ventral regions of the frontal lobes have shown increased activity, specifically the ventrolateral and orbital prefrontal cortices.[147–150] In the anterior cingulate cortex, there have been some discrepant reports, but these may be resolved when factors of treatment outcome and structural abnormalities are taken into account. In the subgenual anterior cingulate cortex, decreased activity has been observed;[42,151,152] however, as the volume of this region is also reportedly reduced in depression,[42,153,154] correcting for this partial volume effect reveals that the activity is actually increased.[155] In the pregenual anterior cingulate cortex (rostral to the corpus callosum), both increased and decreased activity has been found, which appears to be related to treatment response as patients who showed a good response had increased activity while those with a poor response showed decreased activity,[156] although this has not been consistent across all studies.[157] Mixed findings have also been reported in the temporal and parietal lobes, and there has been little evidence of resting state dysfunction in the occipital lobes.[142,143] In subcortical regions, decreased activity in the basal ganglia has been replicated across a number of studies of UP patients, but findings have been less consistent for the thalamus.[142,143,158] Accurate identification of the amygdala has been limited due to its small volume relative to the spatial resolution of current technologies, but this may be improved by combining measurements of its functional activity with specific structural localization. This method has consistently revealed increased activity in patients with familial pure depressive disease and BP depression (with a history of major depression in first-degree relatives), particularly in the left amygdala,[140,149,159] with recent studies also reporting increased activity in the right amygdala.[159,160]

Correlations with clinical symptoms

Correlations in cerebral activity with measures of depression severity have been examined in over 20 studies. Findings demonstrate a regional specificity with some regions showing no relationship to severity,[142,143] others showing

145

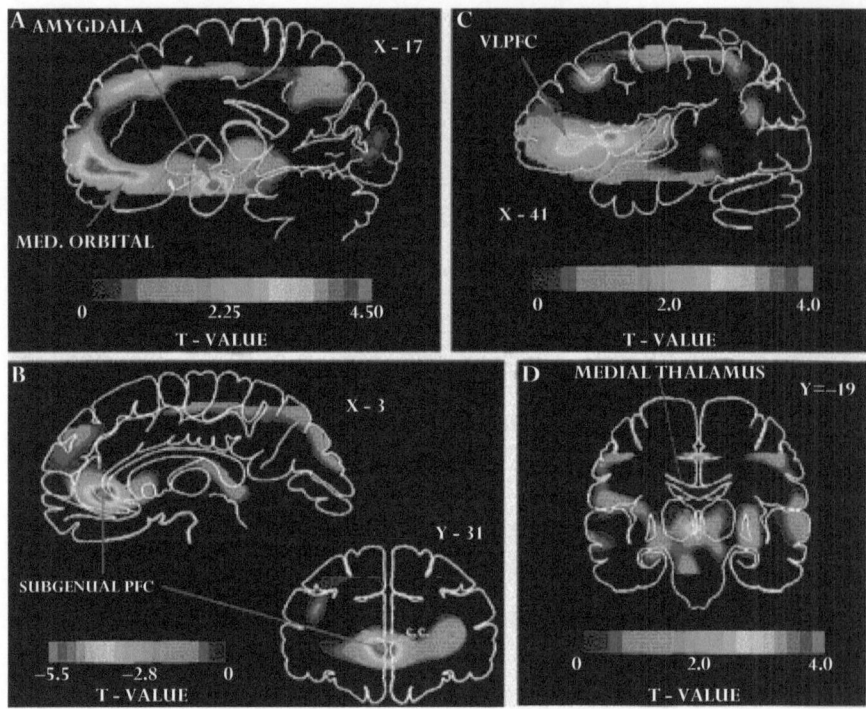

Figure 5.3   *Regions showing increased cerebral blood flow in familial major depressive disorder relative to control subjects. Increased activity was observed in the amygdala and medial orbitofrontal cortex (A), left ventrolateral prefrontal cortex (VLPFC), lateral orbital cortex and anterior insula (C), and left medial thalamus (D). Decreased activity was found in the subgenual prefrontal cortex (PFC) which was accounted for by a corresponding reduction in cortex volume (B). The colours correspond to values from unpaired t statistic comparisons between depressed and control groups. (Reproduced by permission of Elsevier Science from Drevets. Biol Psychiatry 2000; 48: 813–29.[50] Copyright 2000 by the Society of Biological Psychiatry.)*

an inverse relationship (e.g. ventrolateral prefrontal cortex[142,143,149,161,162] and still others (e.g. amygdala) demonstrating positive correlations with assessments of illness severity.[149,163–166] The few studies that have directly compared UP versus BP patients and endogenous versus non-endogenous depression have similarly reported conflicting findings.[142,143]

Correlations with clinical symptoms have indicated that psychomotor retardation shows an inverse relationship with activity in the left dorsolateral prefrontal[167] and anterior cingulate cortices,[168] and subsequent improvement in psychomotor activity has been associated with increased anterior cingulate activity.[169] Comorbid anxiety symptoms have shown a positive association with activity in the posterior cingulate and inferior

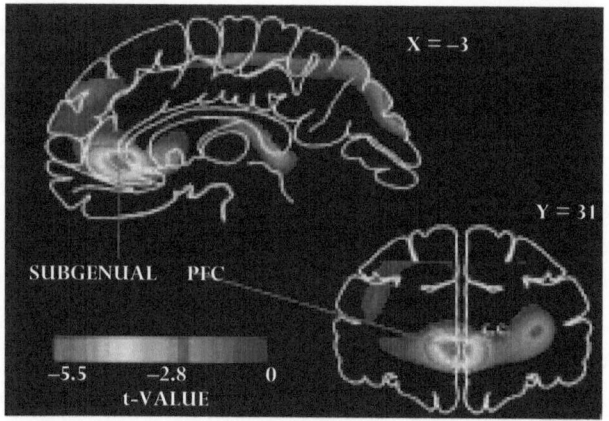

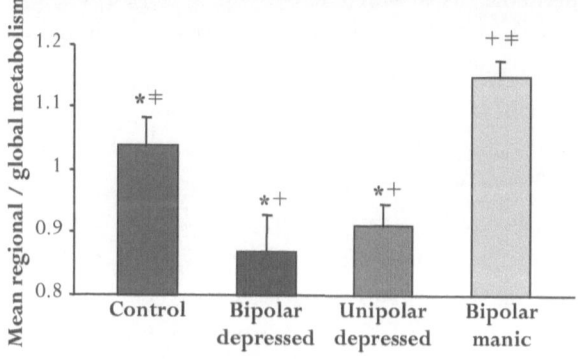

* p<0.025 control vs depressed;
+p<0.01 depressed vs manic;
‡p<0.05 control vs manic

Figure 5.4 *Altered metabolism in the prefrontal cortex (PFC) ventral to the genu of the corpus callosum (subgenual PFC) in mood disorders. The top panel shows negative voxel t-values where glucose metabolism is decreased in depressives relative to controls in coronal (31 mm anterior to the anterior commissure, or y = 31) and sagittal (3 mm left of midline, or x = −3) planes of a statistical parametric image that compares depressives relative to controls. The reduction in activity in this region appears to be accounted for by a corresponding reduction in cortex volume. In the figure, anterior or left is to the left. The bar histogram in the lower panel shows mean, normalized, glucose metabolic values in the subgenual PFC measured using MRI based region of interest analysis. Metabolism is decreased in depressed subjects who are either BD (bipolar depressed) or MDD (unipolar depressed) relative to healthy controls. In contrast, subjects scanned in the manic phase of a bipolar disorder (bipolar manic) have higher metabolism than either depressed or control subjects in this region.* * *Differences between controls and bipolar depressives significant at p<0.025;* † *difference between depressed and manic significant at p<0.01;* ‡ *difference between control and manic significant at p<0.05. CC, corpus callosum. (Reproduced from Drevets. Curr Opin Neurobiol 2002;* ***11:*** *240–9.[192])*

147

parietal cortices,[167] with a recent study reporting a positive relationship with anterior cingulate and parahippocampal activity and an inverse relationship in the temporal and parietal cortices.[166] Cognitive impairments have been associated with impaired activity in the medial prefrontal cortex[167,170] and increased activity in the posterior cingulate cortex,[164] but also no regional correlations have been observed.[168]

Cognitive activation and affect processing tasks

Correlational studies have sought to identify regions which show a significant relationship with particular symptoms or cognitive impairments. However, in order to delineate the neural correlates of a specific mood or cognitive impairment, tasks which selectively engage these processes have also been investigated in patients in comparison with matched control subjects.

Some of the early studies utilized somatosensory stimulation[171,172] and continuous performance tasks, which provide a measure of sustained attention, revealing decreased activity in the prefrontal cortex in depressed patients.[161,173,174] These tasks may seem straightforward, as they engage primary processes such as tactile sensory systems, pain pathways and attention; however, primary processes impact on more complex neurocognitive processes, which have been found to be impaired in mood disorders.[175–177] As a measure of psychomotor performance using a reaction time test, Hickie et al[178] found that depressed patients with the greatest psychomotor slowing showed the least increase in activity in the striatum. Gur et al,[179] examining both a verbal and visuospatial matching task in UP patients, found that the tasks elicited differential activations in anterior and posterior regions, and there was a further interaction by gender. However, specific cortical regions could not be identified due to the low resolution of the ^{133}Xe inhalation brain imaging technique utilized.[179] In medication-free UP depressed patients, while performing an auditory continuous performance task, Kimbrell et al[161] further correlated brain activity with scores of depression severity, finding a negative correlation in the right anterior cingulate and bilateral prefrontal cortices.

Drawing from neuropsychological studies of cognitive impairments in mood disorders, more complex activation paradigms have examined processes of response selection and inhibition (Stroop task),[180] abstract reasoning [Wisconsin Card Sorting Task (WCST)],[181] problem solving and planning (Tower of London task),[182] decision-making,[183] and word generation (verbal fluency).[184,185] Among the regions elicited by these tasks, a notable failure to recruit the anterior cingulate cortex was observed in both the Stroop and Tower of London tasks in depressed UP and BP patients.[180,186] However, no significant difference from healthy controls has been found.[181,183] In BP patients, increased activity in the anterior cingulate[183] and medial frontal cortices,[185] but decreases in the right prefrontal cortex,[183,184] have been reported as compared to controls. Although these studies have been limited by their small sample sizes, ranging from five to 11 patients in each study, and by medication confounds, with the exception of one study,[180] there is an intriguing suggestion of a differential recruitment of the anterior cingulate cortex in depressed as compared to manic patients during complex cognitive tasks.

An important consideration with cognitive tasks is whether both the patient and control groups are able to perform the task equally well in order to interpret the corresponding cerebral activity. If the patient group shows decreased regional cerebral activity in the context of a poorer behavioural performance, the impaired performance may be related to an inability to sufficiently increase cerebral activity, but alternatively the decreased cerebral activity may be related to the impaired performance. In this situation, it is difficult to distinguish between the possible interpretations. Explicit measurements of task performance and their inclusion in the data analysis are essential for understanding differences in cerebral activity.

Additional paradigms have sought to examine fundamental aspects of affective processing in mood disorders. In a fMRI study using film clips to passively induce a sad state in depressed UP patients and healthy controls, Beauregard et al[187] found that both groups showed activations in the medial prefrontal, inferior frontal and middle temporal cortices, cerebellum and caudate, but the depressed group had greater activation in the dorsal anterior cingulate and medial prefrontal cortices as compared to controls. In a PET study using autobiographical scripts, Mayberg et al[188] found that healthy subjects had increased activity in the subgenual anterior cingulate cortex, insula and cerebellum, but decreased activity in the dorsal anterior cingulate, middle prefrontal, inferior frontal and inferior parietal cortices associated with a sad state. An inverse pattern was observed in UP depressed patients who had improved following treatment, i.e. decreased activity in the subgenual anterior cingulate and insular cortices and increased activity in dorsal cortical regions.[188] Both of these studies involved the induction of a transiently sad affective state and revealed activity in similar regions.[187,188] The form of activation though, with increased activity observed in dorsal cortical regions by Beauregard et al[187] but decreased activity in these regions reported by Mayberg et al[188] in healthy controls, may reflect differences in mood induction instructions with a passive induction with video clips as compared to an active induction with autobiographical memories, respectively. Affect processing has also been examined with affective facial expressions. Increased activity in the amygdala has been reported with viewing fearful facial expressions in BP patients.[189] This activation has also been found in medication-free UP patients when the fearful face was 'masked' by a neutral face so that it was not consciously perceived.[190] In contrast, the haemodynamic response of the left amygdala to fearful faces shown for a longer stimulus duration (so that subjects are consciously aware of having seen the fearful face) is attenuated in both depressed children[191] and in depressed adults[192] in comparison to age-matched, healthy controls.

Elliott et al[193] combined a cognitive paradigm, the Tower of London problem-solving and planning task, with feedback on their performance (positive, negative or neutral), which may be considered to be an implicit modulation of affect. With feedback, either positive or negative, healthy control subjects showed increased activity in the caudate; however, depressed UP patients failed to show any changes in caudate activity with feedback. In an event-related fMRI study, Siegle et al[194] examined amygdalar activity in response to emotional adjectives and non-emotional verbal memory tasks, finding a persistence of their activation into the non-emotional trials in UP depressed patients as compared to healthy controls. Another aspect of affective and cognitive processing has been the finding of mood-congruent biases in the processing of incoming information at the psychological level in patient groups,[195] which have also been observed at the neural level.[196] Elliot et al[196] examined an inhibition and attention task in which participants had to respond to target words but inhibit a response to distractor words. A significant interaction between emotional valence and subject group was observed in the rostral anterior cingulate and medial prefrontal regions, with greater activation in healthy volunteers with happy targets but the inverse in depressed patients who showed a greater neural response to sad targets. Such studies, probing both cognition and affect, could provide important insights into the interface of these key aspects of mood disorders.

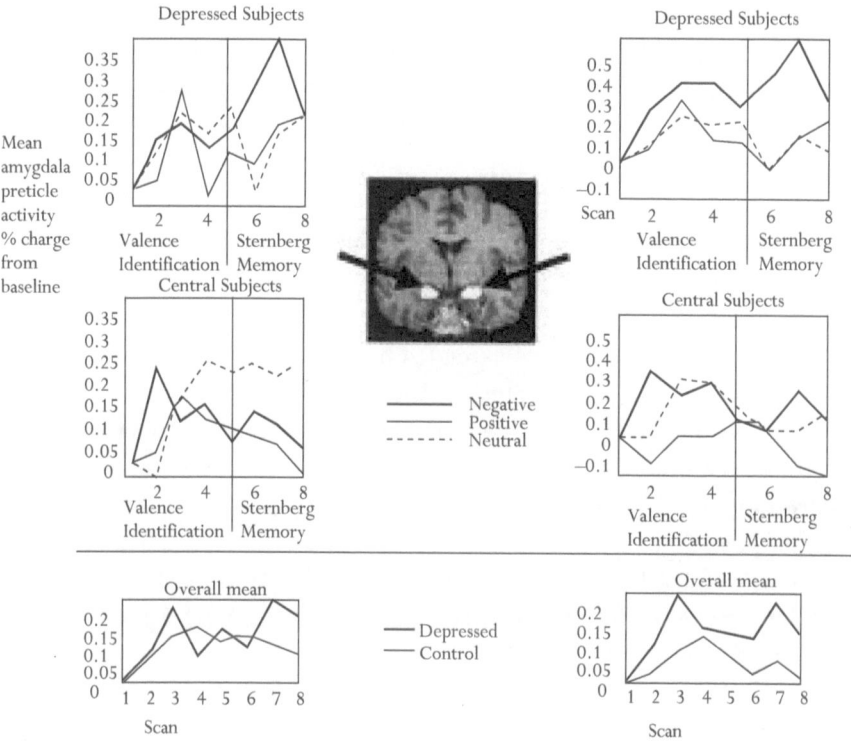

Figure 5.5 *Persistence of amygdalar activity during non-emotional verbal memory tasks In primary unipolar disorder (UP) depressed patients as compared to healthy controls in an event-related functional magnetic resonance imaging (fMRI) study examining amygdalar response to emotional and non-emotional adjectives. Numbers on left axis represent percent change in activity from baseline. Adjectives were negative, positive, or neutral in valence. (Reproduced by permission of Elsevier Science from Siegle et al. Biol Psychiatry 2002; 51: 693–707.[194] Copyright 2002 by the Society of Biological Psychiatry.)*

Treatment studies

Longitudinal studies in which image data are acquired before and during treatment have been conducted to examine the neural correlates of state and trait markers of a course of illness and to identify predictors of treatment response. The forms of treatment that have been examined include antidepressant medication, temporary sleep deprivation, electroconvulsive therapy (ECT), transcranial magnetic stimulation (TMS), and, more recently, comparisons between short-term psychotherapy and pharmacotherapy treatments.

ECT

Some of the earliest studies examined functional cerebral changes associated with ECT. Several groups have reported decreased global cerebral activity following ECT, as measured with the ^{133}Xe inhalation technique[144,197] and SPECT.[198,199] Several SPECT studies have also reported increased cerebral activity in frontal[200] and parietal regions,[201] and no changes except in responders who showed increased frontal activity.[202] Using PET, Nobler et al[203] found extensive regional decreases in glucose metabolism in medication-free UP patients following a successful treatment course of ECT. These regions extended from the prefrontal cortex, including the anterior cingulate cortex, to the posterior cingulate, bilateral parietal and left medial temporal cortices; however, increased metabolism was also observed in the occipital cortex.[203] Henry et al[204] also found decreased prefrontal cortical metabolism following ECT treatment in a medication-free depressed group, but noted increased activity in the occipital cortex and basal ganglia. It is less clear how these changes relate to baseline abnormalities, however, as comparisons with a healthy control group were not performed.[203,204]

TMS

TMS is based on the interdependent relationship between electricity and magnetism. An electrical current passing through a coil of wire generates a magnetic field and a magnetic field adjacent to a conducting medium induces an electrical current. Applying a TMS coil to the scalp can temporarily stimulate underlying neurons, causing their depolarization. TMS may be used to examine regional cortical functions and their interactions; repeated TMS is also reported to have antidepressant effects and is being investigated as an alternative therapy to ECT. For a discussion of its optimal stimulation parameters, the reader is referred to a recent review by George et al.[205] Kimbrell et al[206] found an inverse relationship between baseline regional cerebral activity and frequency of TMS stimulation; such that improvement with high-frequency (20 Hz) TMS was associated with decreased metabolism in the anterior cingulate, right prefrontal, bilateral temporal and occipital regions, while low-frequency (1 Hz) TMS improvements were associated with increased metabolism in the right prefrontal cortex. Following a series of TMS treatments over the left prefrontal cortex, high-frequency TMS was associated with widespread regional activations, which included the anterior cingulate[207,208] and prefrontal cortices,[207–209] basal ganglia, amygdala, hippocampus and cerebellum,[207] while low-frequency TMS was associated with decreased activity in the right prefrontal and left medial temporal cortices, basal ganglia and amygdala.[207] Changes in cerebral activity associated with a successful treatment response have not been identified in these preliminary studies.[207,209]

Pharmacotherapy

Medication studies have typically examined depressed patients at baseline, with recent studies including a washout period so that patients were medication-free, and following a course of treatment of several weeks or longer. Despite differences in antidepressant medication, diagnostic subtypes of depression and neuroimaging techniques between studies, some consistent findings are emerging. Comparing responders with non-responders, a successful response to antidepressant medication has been associated with increased activity in the dorsal anterior cingulate,[146,151,156,210–213] dorsolateral prefrontal[146,210,212–214] inferior parietal[146,210,212,213] and posterior cingulate[211,212] cortices; as well as decreases in the ventrolateral prefrontal cortex,[148,149,157] subgenual anterior cingulate cortex,[148,212] insula and hippocampus,[146,212] although decreases in dorsal prefrontal activity have also been reported.[148] Increased activity in the striatum has been observed in some[146,211,215] but not other studies.[151,212,216]

However, only a few studies included a healthy control group at baseline allowing comparison of post-treatment changes with pretreatment abnormalities.[146,148,210,213] Findings from those studies included decreased activity in the dorsolateral prefrontal cortex in depressed patients at baseline, which subsequently increased in patients who responded to treatment,[146,210,213] although Brody et al[148] noted a converse finding. In order to assess whether these changes reflect a normalization of pretreatment abnormalities, control subjects should ideally also undergo a follow-up scan, and the only study to have performed this to date found that elevated pretreatment activity in the ventrolateral prefrontal cortex and caudate decreased following treatment.[148]

Pharmacotherapy and psychotherapy

Two studies have recently compared the neural correlates associated with treatment with pharmacotherapy or psychotherapy.[148,215] With [18F]FDG PET, Brody et al[148] examined UP depressed patients at baseline and following 12 weeks of treatment with paroxetine or interpersonal therapy (IPT) in comparison with healthy controls who were also scanned on two occasions.

Martin et al[215] used SPECT to examine UP depressed patients at baseline and following 6 weeks of treatment with venlafaxine or IPT. Both studies found that pharmacotherapy and psychotherapy were associated with similar but distinct neural correlates. Brody et al[148] observed increased pretreatment metabolism in the prefrontal cortex, caudate and thalamus, and decreases in the temporal cortex in depressed patients as compared to controls, and these regions showed changes towards normalization following either treatment. Martin et al[215] found increased basal ganglia activity following both treatments, with greater temporal activity associated with medication but greater posterior cingulate activity with IPT. Limitations of both studies were that pharmacotherapy was more effective than psychotherapy and patients were not fully randomized in their treatment allocation. Nonetheless, these studies have provided some intriguing initial insights into the neural mechanisms underlying psychotherapy and pharmacotherapy treatments.

An important aspect of these treatment studies is their potential for identifying neural correlates that are predictive of subsequent treatment response. One of the most consistent findings has been increased baseline activity in the pregenual anterior cingulate cortex in depressed patients who subsequently respond to antidepressant medication,[146,148,149,151,156] the mood-stabilizing medication carbamazepine,[217] or sleep deprivation,[218–221] although decreased medial prefrontal activity has also been reported.[157,222] This differentiation between subsequent responders and non-responders does not seem to be evident following 1 week of treatment with fluoxetine.[212]

Conclusions

After 20 years of neuroimaging research in mood disorders, it is well established that the pathophysiology of these disorders involves both structural and functional impairments within the brain. Although valuable insights have been provided, the research is still in its early stages. A major challenge for researchers at this stage is to integrate findings from structural, ligand binding, neurochemical and functional neuroimaging studies. Moreover, research from molecular biology, genetics and cognitive neuroscience must complement neuroimaging studies and may guide subject selection and directions for investigations.

The established literature has delineated the neural structures involved in the pathophysiology of mood disorders. Mood disorders are associated with

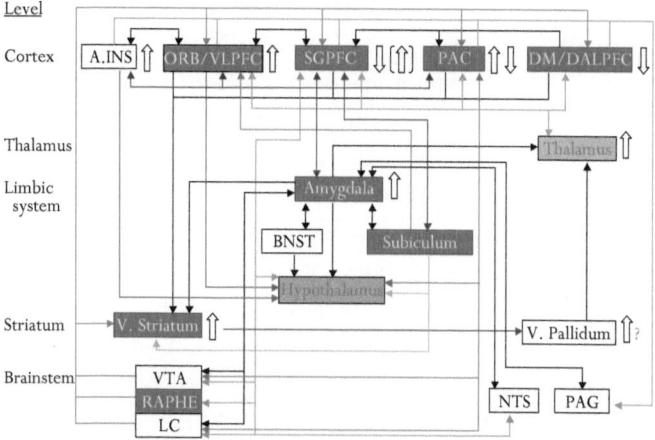

Figure 5.6 *Proposed anatomic circuit of regions implicated in the pathophysiology of depression from neuroimaging and neuropathologic studies of familial mood disorders. Regions in red have neuromorphometric and / or histopathologic abnormalities in primary unipolar disorder (UP) and / or bipolar disorder (BP). Regions in yellow have not been microscopically examined in mood disorders, but are areas where structural abnormalities are suspected based upon the finding of third ventricle enlargement in children and adults with BP. Open arrows to the right of each region indicate the direction of abnormalities in cerebral blood flow (CBF) and metabolism reported in depressives relative to control subjects (? indicates where experimental data await replication). Parenthetical open arrows indicate the direction of metabolic abnormalities after correcting the positron emission tomography (PET) measures for partial volume effects of reduced gray matter volume [(?) indicates where decreased gray matter is suspected as the explanation for reductions in CBF and metabolism, but partial-volume-corrected PET results have not been reported]. Solid lines indicate major anatomic connections between structures (e.g., weak projections, such as that from the orbital cortex back to the subiculum are not included), with closed arrowheads indicating the direction of the projecting axons (reciprocal connections have arrowheads at both line ends). Affected prefrontal cortex (PFC) areas include the ventrolateral and orbital PFC (ORB / VLPFC), the anterior (agranular) insula (A.INS), the anterior cingulate gyrus ventral and anterior to the genu of the corpus callosum [subgenual PFC (SGPFC) and pregenual anterior cingulate (PAC), respectively], and the dorsomedial / dorsal anterolateral PFC (DM / DALPFC). The parts of the striatum under consideration are the ventromedial caudate and nucleus accumbens, which particularly project to the ventral pallidum. AINS, anterior insula; ORB, orbitofrontal cortex; VLPFC, ventrolateral prefrontal cortex; SGPFC, subgenual prefrontal cortex; PAC, pregenual anterior cingulate; DM / DLPFC, dorsomedial / dorsolateral prefrontal cortex; BNST, bed nucleus of the stria terminalis; V, ventral; VTA, ventral tegmental area; LC, locus coeruleus; NTS, nucleus tractus solitarius; PAG, periaqueductal grey. (Adapted by permission of Elsevier Science from Drevets. Biol Psychiatry 2000; 48: 813–29.[150] Copyright 2000 by the Society of Biological Psychiatry.)*

impairments in an interacting network of regions, rather than as a consequence of a single depressive region. Researchers have proposed various neural circuits,[142,223–227] which have implicated some similar regions, including the anterior cingulate, dorsolateral and ventrolateral prefrontal cortices, basal ganglia, thalamus and amygdala. Consistent abnormalities from structural, receptor mapping and functional neuroimaging studies have been reported in these regions, providing support for these neuroanatomic models. Furthermore, the subgenual anterior cingulate cortex has shown a pattern of activity in correspondence with the insula and other regions during mood induction tasks.[188] Yet, to describe these regions as a neural network will require evidence of specific interactions between regions from analyses of effective connectivity.[228]

The advent of neuroimaging has provided unprecedented insights into the neural correlates underlying mood disorders. Ongoing research includes family and prospective studies to identify neurobiological risk factors of mood disorders and neural markers that may be apparent prior to the onset of clinical symptoms. Fundamental questions on the relationship between mood disorders and normal fluctuations in affective states are also being investigated. With genetic markers, it may be possible identify particular neurocognitive impairments or dysfunction of neurotransmitter systems for individual patients, thus offering greater specificity within the heterogeneity of mood disorders. Further innovations in technology and experimental design, along with integration of neuroimaging findings with neuropsychological impairments, will continue to expand our understanding of the pathophysiology of mood disorders.

References

1. Cummings JL. Depression and Parkinson's disease: a review. *Am J Psychiatry* 1992; **149**: 443–54.
2. Cummings JL. Behavioral and psychiatric symptoms associated with Huntington's disease. *Adv Neurol* 1995; **65**: 179–86.
3. Carota A, Staub F, Bogousslavsky J. Emotions, behaviours and mood changes in stroke. *Curr Opin Neurol* 2002; **15**: 57–69.
4. Gainotti G, Marra C. Determinants and consequences of post-stroke depression. *Curr Opin Neurol* 2002; **15**: 85–9.
5. Morris PL, Robinson RG, Raphael B, Hopwood MJ. Lesion location and poststroke depression. *J Neuropsychiatry Clin Neurosci* 1996; **8**: 399–403.

6. Drevets WC. Prefrontal cortical–amygdalar metabolism in major depression. *Ann NY Acad Sci* 1999; **877:** 614–37.

7. Jeste DV, Lohr JB, Goodwin FK. Neuroanatomical studies of major affective disorders. A review and suggestions for further research. *Br J Psychiatry* 1988; **153:** 444–59.

8. Nasrallah HA, Coffman JA, Olson SC. Structural brain-imaging findings in affective disorders: an overview. *J Neuropsychiatry Clin Neurosci* 1989; **1:** 21–6.

9. Norris SD, Krishnan KR, Ahearn E. Structural changes in the brain of patients with bipolar affective disorder by MRI: a review of the literature. *Prog Neuropsychopharmacol Biol Psychiatry* 1997; **21:** 1323–37.

10. Soares JC, Mann JJ. The anatomy of mood disorders – review of structural neuro-imaging studies. *Biol Psychiatry* 1997; **41:** 86–106.

11. Elkis H, Friedman L, Wise A, Meltzer HY. Meta-analyses of studies of ventricular enlargement and cortical sulcal prominence in mood disorders. Comparisons with controls or patients with schizophrenia. *Arch Gen Psychiatry* 1995; **52:** 735–46.

12. Raz S, Raz N. Structural brain abnormalities in the major psychoses: a quantitative review of the evidence from computerized imaging. *Psychol Bull* 1990; **108:** 93–108.

13. Videbech P. MRI findings in patients with affective disorder: a meta-analysis. *Acta Psychiatr Scand* 1997; **96:** 157–68.

14. Wright IC, Rabe-Hesketh S, Woodruff PW, David AS, Murray RM, Bullmore ET. Meta-analysis of regional brain volumes in schizophrenia. *Am J Psychiatry* 2000; **157:** 16–25.

15. Elkis H, Friedman L, Buckley PF et al. Increased prefrontal sulcal prominence in rela-tively young patients with unipolar major depression. *Psychiatry Res* 1996; **67:** 123–34.

16. Jacoby RJ, Levy R. Computed tomography in the elderly. 3. Affective disorder. *Br J Psychiatry* 1980; **136:** 270–5.

17. Luchins DJ, Lewine RR, Meltzer HY. Lateral ventricular size, psychopathology, and medication response in the psychoses. *Biol Psychiatry* 1984; **19:** 29–44.

18. Pearlson GD, Garbacz DJ, Tompkins RH et al. Clinical correlates of lateral ventricular enlargement in bipolar affective disorder. *Am J Psychiatry* 1984; **141:** 253–6.

19. Dolan RJ, Calloway SP, Mann AH. Cerebral ventricular size in depressed subjects. *Psychol Med* 1985; **15:** 873–8.

20. Strakowski SM, DelBello MP, Sax KW et al. Brain magnetic resonance imaging of structural abnormalities in bipolar disorder. *Arch Gen Psychiatry* 1999; **56:** 254–60.

21. Bremner JD, Vythilingam M, Vermetten E et al. Reduced volume of orbitofrontal cortex in major depression. *Biol Psychiatry* 2002; **51:** 273–9.

22. Videbech P, Ravnkilde B, Fiirgaard B et al. Structural brain abnormalities in unselected in-patients with major depression. *Acta Psychiatr Scand* 2001; **103:** 282–6.

23. Pillay SS, Yurgelun-Todd DA, Bonello CM, Lafer B, Fava M, Renshaw PF. A quan-titative magnetic resonance imaging study of cerebral and cerebellar gray matter volume in primary unipolar major depression: relationship to treatment response and clinical severity. *Biol Psychiatry* 1997; **42:** 79–84.

24. Dupont RM, Butters N, Schafer K, Wilson T, Hesselink J, Gillin JC. Diagnostic specificity of focal white matter abnormalities in bipolar and unipolar mood disorder. *Biol Psychiatry* 1995; **38:** 482–6.

25. Harvey I, Persaud R, Ron MA, Baker G, Murray RM. Volumetric MRI measurements in bipolars compared with schizophrenics and healthy controls. *Psychol Med* 1994; **24:** 689–99.

26. Pearlson GD, Barta PE, Powers RE et al. Ziskind-Somerfeld Research Award 1996. Medial and superior temporal gyral volumes and cerebral asymmetry in schizophrenia versus bipolar disorder. *Biol Psychiatry* 1997; **41:** 1–14.

27. Schlaepfer TE, Harris GJ, Tien AY et al. Decreased regional cortical gray matter volume in schizophrenia. *Am J Psychiatry* 1994; **151:** 842–8.

28. Strakowski SM, Woods BT, Tohen M, Wilson DR, Douglass AW, Stoll AL. MRI subcortical signal hyperintensities in mania at first hospitalization. *Biol Psychiatry* 1993; **33:** 204–6.

29. Zipursky RB, Seeman MV, Bury A, Langevin R, Wortzman G, Katz R. Deficits in gray matter volume are present in schizophrenia but not bipolar disorder. *Schizophr Res* 1997; **26:** 85–92.

30. Lim KO, Rosenbloom MJ, Faustman WO, Sullivan EV, Pfefferbaum A. Cortical gray matter deficit in patients with bipolar disorder. *Schizophr Res* 1999; **40:** 219–27.

31. Awad IA, Spetzler RF, Hodak JA, Awad CA, Carey R. Incidental subcortical lesions identified on magnetic resonance imaging in the elderly. I. Correlation with age and cerebrovascular risk factors. *Stroke* 1986; **17:** 1084–9.

32. Fazekas F, Kleinert R, Offenbacher H et al. Pathologic correlates of incidental MRI white matter signal hyperintensities. *Neurology* 1993; **43:** 1683–9.

33. Dupont RM, Jernigan TL, Butters N et al. Subcortical abnormalities detected in bipolar affective disorder using magnetic resonance imaging. Clinical and neuropsychological significance. *Arch Gen Psychiatry* 1990; **47:** 55–9.

34. Moore PB, Shepherd DJ, Eccleston D et al. Cerebral white matter lesions in bipolar affective disorder: relationship to outcome. *Br J Psychiatry* 2001; **178:** 172–6.

35. Ahearn EP, Jamison KR, Steffens DC et al. MRI correlates of suicide attempt history in unipolar depression. *Biol Psychiatry* 2001; **50:** 266–70.

36. Altshuler LL, Curran JG, Hauser P, Mintz J, Denicoff K, Post R. T2 hyperintensities in bipolar disorder: magnetic resonance imaging comparison and literature meta-analysis. *Am J Psychiatry* 1995; **152:** 1139–44.

37. Stoll AL, Renshaw PF, Yurgelun-Todd DA, Cohen BM. Neuroimaging in bipolar disorder: what have we learned? *Biol Psychiatry* 2000; **48:** 505–17.

38. Steffens DC, Krishnan KR. Structural neuroimaging and mood disorders: recent findings, implications for classification, and future directions. *Biol Psychiatry* 1998; **43:** 705–12.

39. Lewine RR, Hudgins P, Brown F, Caudle J, Risch SC. Differences in qualitative brain morphology findings in schizophrenia, major depression, bipolar disorder, and normal volunteers. *Schizophr Res* 1995; **15:** 253–9.

40. Swayze VW, Andreasen NC, Alliger RJ, Ehrhardt JC, Yuh WT. Structural brain abnormalities in bipolar affective disorder. Ventricular enlargement and focal signal hyperintensities. *Arch Gen Psychiatry* 1990; **47:** 1054–9.

41. Bremner JD, Narayan M, Anderson ER, Staib LH, Miller HL, Charney DS. Hippocampal volume reduction in major depression. *Am J Psychiatry* 2000; **157:** 115–18.

42. Drevets WC, Price JL, Simpson Jr JR et al. Subgenual prefrontal cortex abnormalities in mood disorders. *Nature* 1997; **386:** 824–7.

43. Hirayasu Y, Shenton ME, Salisbury DF et al. Lower left temporal lobe MRI volumes in patients with first-episode schizophrenia compared with psychotic patients with first-episode affective disorder and normal subjects. *Am J Psychiatry* 1998; **155:** 1384–91.

44. Altshuler LL, Bartzokis G, Grieder T, Curran J, Mintz J. Amygdala enlargement in bipolar disorder and hippocampal reduction in schizophrenia: an MRI study demonstrating neuroanatomic specificity. *Arch Gen Psychiatry* 1998; **55:** 663–4.

45. Roy PD, Zipursky RB, Saint-Cyr JA, Bury A, Langevin R, Seeman MV. Temporal horn enlargement is present in schizophrenia and bipolar disorder. *Biol Psychiatry* 1998; **44:** 418–22.

46. Axelson DA, Doraiswamy PM, McDonald WM et al. Hypercortisolemia and hippocampal changes in depression. *Psychiatry Res* 1993; **47:** 163–73.

47. Swayze VW, Andreasen NC, Alliger RJ, Yuh WT, Ehrhardt JC. Subcortical and temporal structures in affective disorder and schizophrenia: a magnetic resonance imaging study. *Biol Psychiatry* 1992; **31:** 221–40.

48. Sheline YI, Wang PW, Gado MH, Csernansky JG, Vannier MW. Hippocampal atrophy in recurrent major depression. *Proc Natl Acad Sci USA* 1996; **93:** 3908–13.

49. Sheline YI, Sanghavi M, Mintun MA, Gado MH. Depression duration but not age predicts hippocampal volume loss in medically healthy women with recurrent major depression. *J Neurosci* 1999; **19:** 5034–43.

50. Sheline YI. 3D MRI studies of neuroanatomic changes in unipolar major depression: the role of stress and medical comorbidity. *Biol Psychiatry* 2000; **48:** 791–800.

51. Ashtari M, Greenwald BS, Kramer-Ginsberg E et al. Hippocampal/amygdala volumes in geriatric depression. *Psychol Med* 1999; **29:** 629–38.

52. Hauser P, Altshuler LL, Berrettini W, Dauphinais ID, Gelernter J, Post RM. Temporal lobe measurement in primary affective disorder by magnetic resonance imaging. *J Neuropsychiatry Clin Neurosci* 1989; **1:** 128–34.

53. Pantel J, Schroder J, Essig M et al. Quantitative magnetic resonance imaging in geriatric depression and primary degenerative dementia. *J Affect Disord* 1997; **42:** 69–83.

54. Vakili K, Pillay SS, Lafer B et al. Hippocampal volume in primary unipolar major depression: a magnetic resonance imaging study. *Biol Psychiatry* 2000; **47:** 1087–90.

55. von Gunten A, Fox NC, Cipolotti L, Ron MA. A volumetric study of hippocampus and amygdala in depressed patients with subjective memory problems. *J Neuropsychiatry Clin Neurosci* 2000; **12:** 493–8.

56. Kemmerer M, Nasrallah HA, Sharma S, Olson SC, Martin R, Lynn MB. Increased hippocampal volume in bipolar disorder. *Biol Psychiatry* 1994; **35:** 626.

57. Noga JT, Vladar K, Torrey EF. A volumetric magnetic resonance imaging study of monozygotic twins discordant for bipolar disorder. *Psychiatry Res* 2001; **106:** 25–34.

58. Altshuler LL, Bartzokis G, Grieder T et al. An MRI study of temporal lobe structures in men with bipolar disorder or schizophrenia. *Biol Psychiatry* 2000; **48:** 147–62.

59. Sheline YI, Gado MH, Price JL. Amygdala core nuclei volumes are decreased in recurrent major depression. *Neuroreport* 1998; **9:** 2023–8.

60. Mervaala E, Fohr J, Kononen M et al. Quantitative MRI of the hippocampus and amygdala in severe depression. *Psychol Med* 2000; **30:** 117–25.

61. Frodl T, Meisenzahl E, Zetzsche T et al. Enlargement of the amygdala in patients with a first episode of major depression. *Biol Psychiatry* 2002; **51**: 708–14.

62. Brierley B, Shaw P, David AS. The human amygdala: a systematic review and meta-analysis of volumetric magnetic resonance imaging. *Brain Res Rev* 2002; **39**: 84–105.

63. Husain MM, McDonald WM, Doraiswamy PM et al. A magnetic resonance imaging study of putamen nuclei in major depression. *Psychiatry Res* 1991; **40**: 95–9.

64. Krishnan KR, McDonald WM, Escalona PR et al. Magnetic resonance imaging of the caudate nuclei in depression. Preliminary observations. *Arch Gen Psychiatry* 1992; **49**: 553–7.

65. Parashos IA, Tupler LA, Blitchington T, Krishnan KR. Magnetic-resonance morphometry in patients with major depression. *Psychiatry Res* 1998; **84**: 7–15.

66. Dupont RM, Jernigan TL, Heindel W et al. Magnetic resonance imaging and mood disorders. Localization of white matter and other subcortical abnormalities. *Arch Gen Psychiatry* 1995; **52**: 747–55.

67. Greenwald BS, Kramer-Ginsberg E, Bogerts B et al. Qualitative magnetic resonance imaging findings in geriatric depression. Possible link between later-onset depression and Alzheimer's disease? *Psychol Med* 1997; **27**: 421–31.

68. Lenze EJ, Sheline YI. Absence of striatal volume differences between depressed subjects with no comorbid medical illness and matched comparison subjects. *Am J Psychiatry* 1999; **156**: 1989–91.

69. Pillay SS, Renshaw PF, Bonello CM, Lafer BC, Fava M, Yurgelun-Todd D. A quantitative magnetic resonance imaging study of caudate and lenticular nucleus gray matter volume in primary unipolar major depression: relationship to treatment response and clinical severity. *Psychiatry Res* 1998; **84**: 61–74.

70. Axelson DA, Doraiswamy PM, Boyko OB et al. In vivo assessment of pituitary volume with magnetic resonance imaging and systematic stereology: relationship to dexamethasone suppression test results in patients. *Psychiatry Res* 1992; **44**: 63–70.

71. Krishnan KR, Doraiswamy PM, Lurie SN et al. Pituitary size in depression. *J Clin Endocr Metab* 1991; **72**: 256–9.

72. Sassi RB, Nicoletti M, Brambilla P et al. Decreased pituitary volume in patients with bipolar disorder. *Biol Psychiatry* 2001; **50**: 271–80.

73. DelBello MP, Strakowski SM, Zimmerman ME, Hawkins JM, Sax KW. MRI analysis of the cerebellum in bipolar disorder: a pilot study. *Neuropsychopharmacology* 1999; **21**: 63–8.

74. Charney DS, Drevets WC. The neurobiological basis of anxiety disorders. In: (Davis K, Charney DS, Coyle J, Nemeroff CB, eds) *Psychopharmacology: The Fifth Generation of Progress.* (Lippincott: 2002.)

75. Desmond JE, Fiez JA. Neuroimaging studies of the cerebellum: language, learning and memory. *Trends Cogn Sci* 1998; **2**: 355–62.

76. Schmahmann JD, Sherman JC. The cerebellar cognitive affective syndrome. *Brain* 1998; **121**: 561–79.

77. Middleton FA, Strick PL. Cerebellar projections to the prefrontal cortex of the primate. *J Neurosci* 2001; **21**: 700–12.

78. Petrie RX, Reid IC, Stewart CA. The N-methyl-D-aspartate receptor, synaptic plasticity, and depressive disorder. A critical review. *Pharmacol Ther* 2000; **87**: 11–25.

79. Maes M, Meltzer H. The serotonin hypothesis of major depression. In: (Bloom FE, Kupfer DJ, eds) *Psychopharmacology: The Fourth Generation of Progress.* (Raven Press: New York, 1995) 933–44.

80. Mann JJ. Role of the serotonergic system in the pathogenesis of major depression and suicidal behavior. *Neuropsychopharmacology* 1999; **21:** 99S–105S.

81. Tork I. Anatomy of the serotonergic system. *Ann NY Acad Sci* 1990; **600:** 9–34.

82. Bonvento G, Mackensie E. *Serotonin and the Cerebral Circulation.* (CRC Press: Boca Raton, Florida, 1997.)

83. D'haenen H, Bossuyt A, Mertens J, Bossuyt-Piron C, Gijsemans M, Kaufman L. SPECT imaging of serotonin2 receptors in depression. *Psychiatry Res* 1992; **45:** 227–37.

84. Biver F, Wikler D, Lotstra F, Damhaut P, Goldman S, Mendlewicz J. Serotonin 5-HT2 receptor imaging in major depression: focal changes in orbito-insular cortex. *Br J Psychiatry* 1997; **171:** 444–8.

85. Meltzer CC, Price JC, Mathis CA et al. PET imaging of serotonin type 2A receptors in late-life neuropsychiatric disorders. *Am J Psychiatry* 1999; **156:** 1871–8.

86. Attar-Levy D, Martinot JL, Blin J et al. The cortical serotonin2 receptors studied with positron-emission tomography and [18F]-setoperone during depressive illness and antidepressant treatment with clomipramine. *Biol Psychiatry* 1999; **45:** 180–6.

87. Yatham LN, Liddle PF, Shiah IS et al. Brain serotonin2 receptors in major depression: a positron emission tomography study. *Arch Gen Psychiatry* 2000; **57:** 850–8.

88. Meyer JH, Kapur S, Houle S et al. Prefrontal cortex 5-HT2 receptors in depression: an [18F]setoperone PET imaging study. *Am J Psychiatry* 1999; **156:** 1029–34.

89. Massou JM, Trichard C, Attar-Levy D et al. Frontal 5-HT2A receptors studied in depressive patients during chronic treatment by selective serotonin reuptake inhibitors. *Psychopharmacology (Berl)* 1997; **133:** 99–101.

90. Yatham LN, Liddle PF, Dennie J et al. Decrease in brain serotonin 2 receptor binding in patients with major depression following desipramine treatment: a positron emission tomography study with fluorine-18-labeled setoperone. *Arch Gen Psychiatry* 1999; **56:** 705–11.

91. Meyer JH, Kapur S, Eisfeld B et al. The effect of paroxetine on 5-HT(2A) receptors in depression: an [(18)F]setoperone PET imaging study. *Am J Psychiatry* 2001; **158:** 78–85.

92. Zanardi R, Artigas F, Moresco R et al. Increased 5-hydroxytryptamine-2 receptor binding in the frontal cortex of depressed patients responding to paroxetine treatment: a positron emission tomography scan study. *J Clin Psychopharmac* 2001; **21:** 53–8.

93. Drevets WC, Frank E, Price JC et al. PET imaging of serotonin 1A receptor binding in depression. *Biol Psychiatry* 1999; **46:** 1375–87.

94. Drevets WC, Gadde KM, Krishnan R. Neuroimaging studies of depression. In: (Charney DS, Nestler EJ, Bunney BJ, eds) *The Neurobiological Foundation of Mental Illness.* (Oxford University Press: New York, 2003).

95. Parsey RV, Oquendo MA, Simpson NR et al. Altered serotonin 1A binding in major depression: a [11C]WAY100635 PET Study. *Biol Psychiatry* 2002; **51:** 106S.

96. Fujita M, Charney DS, Innis RB. Imaging serotonergic neurotransmission in depression: hippocampal pathophysiology may mirror global brain alterations. *Biol Psychiatry* 2000; **48:** 801–12.

97. Sargent PA, Kjaer KH, Bench CJ et al. Brain serotonin1A receptor binding measured by positron emission tomography with [11C]WAY-100635: effects of depression and antidepressant treatment. *Arch Gen Psychiatry* 2000; **57**: 174–80.

98. Drevets WC, Frank E, Price JC, Kupfer DJ, Greer PJ, Mathis C. Serotonin type-1A receptor imaging in depression. *Nucl Med Biol* 2000; **27**: 499–507.

99. Artigas F, Romero L, de Montigny C, Blier P. Acceleration of the effect of selected antidepressant drugs in major depression by 5-HT1A antagonists. *Trends Neurosci* 1996; **19**: 378–83.

100. Andree B, Thorberg SO, Halldin C, Farde L. Pindolol binding to 5-HT1A receptors in the human brain confirmed with positron emission tomography. *Psychopharmacology (Berl)* 1999; **144**: 303–5.

101. Martinez D, Broft A, Laruelle M. Pindolol augmentation of antidepressant treatment: recent contributions from brain imaging studies. *Biol Psychiatry* 2000; **48**: 844–53.

102. Rabiner EA, Gunn RN, Castro ME et al. Beta-blocker binding to human 5-HT(1A) receptors in vivo and in vitro: implications for antidepressant therapy. *Neuropsychopharmacology* 2000; **23**: 285–93.

103. Nyberg L, Persson J, Habib R et al. Large scale neurocognitive networks underlying episodic memory. *J Cogn Neurosci* 2000; **12**: 163–73.

104. Pilowsky LS. Probing targets for antipsychotic drug action with PET and SPET receptor imaging. *Nucl Med Commun* 2001; **22**: 829–33.

105. Malison RT, Price LH, Berman R et al. Reduced brain serotonin transporter availability in major depression as measured by [123I]-2 beta-carbomethoxy-3 beta-(4-iodophenyl)tropane and single photon emission computed tomography. *Biol Psychiatry* 1998; **44**: 1090–8.

106. Pirker W, Asenbaum S, Kasper S et al. Beta-CIT SPECT demonstrates blockade of 5HT-uptake sites by citalopram in the human brain in vivo. *J Neural Transmem Gen Sect* 1995; **100**: 247–56.

107. Meyer JH, Wilson AA, Ginovart N et al. Occupancy of serotonin transporters by paroxetine and citalopram during treatment of depression: a [(11)C]DASB PET imaging study. *Am J Psychiatry* 2001; **158**: 1843–9.

108. Ichimiya T, Suhara T, Sudo Y et al. Serotonin transporter binding in patients with mood disorders: a PET study with [11C](+)McN5652. *Biol Psychiatry* 2002; **51**: 715–22.

109. Leake A, Fairbairn AF, McKeith IG, Ferrier IN. Studies on the serotonin uptake binding site in major depressive disorder and control post-mortem brain: neurochemical and clinical correlates. *Psychiatry Res* 1991; **39**: 155–65.

110. Mann JJ, Huang YY, Underwood MD et al. A serotonin transporter gene promoter polymorphism (5-HTTLPR) and prefrontal cortical binding in major depression and suicide. *Arch Gen Psychiatry* 2000; **57**: 729–38.

111. Perry EK, Marshall EF, Blessed G, Tomlinson BE, Perry RH. Decreased imipramine binding in the brains of patients with depressive illness. *Br J Psychiatry* 1983; **142**: 188–92.

112. Mann JJ, Malone KM, Diehl DJ, Perel J, Cooper TB, Mintun MA. Demonstration in vivo of reduced serotonin responsivity in the brain of untreated depressed patients. *Am J Psychiatry* 1996; **153**: 174–82.

113. Meyer JH, Kennedy S, Brown GM. No effect of depression on [(15)O]H2O PET response to intravenous d-fenfluramine. *Am J Psychiatry* 1998; **155**: 1241–6.

114. van Praag HM, Lemus C, Kahn R. The pitfalls of serotonin precursors as challengers in hormonal probes of central serotonin activity. *Psychopharmac Bull* 1986; **22**: 565–70.

115. Agren H, Reibring L, Hartvig P et al. Low brain uptake of L-[11C]5-hydroxytryptophan in major depression: a positron emission tomography study on patients and healthy volunteers. *Acta Psychiatr Scand* 1991; **83**: 449–55.

116. Bremner JD, Innis RB, Salomon RM et al. Positron emission tomography measurement of cerebral metabolic correlates of tryptophan depletion-induced depressive relapse. *Arch Gen Psychiatry* 1997; **54**: 364–74.

117. Smith KA, Morris JS, Friston KJ, Cowen PJ, Dolan RJ. Brain mechanisms associated with depressive relapse and associated cognitive impairment following acute tryptophan depletion. *Br J Psychiatry* 1999; **174**: 525–9.

118. Cooper JR, Bloom FE, Roth RH. *The Biochemical Basis of Neuropharmacology*, 7th edn. (Oxford University Press: New York, 1996.)

119. Schatzberg AF, Schildkraut JJ. Recent studies on norepinephrine systems in mood disorders. In: (Bloom FE, Kupfer DJ, eds) *Pharmacology: The Fourth Generation of Progress*. (Raven Press: New York, 1995) 911–20.

120. Fu CH, Reed LJ, Meyer JH et al. Noradrenergic dysfunction in the prefrontal cortex in depression: a [15O]H2O PET study of the neuromodulatory effects of clonidine. *Biol Psychiatry* 2001; **49**: 317–25.

121. Rampello L, Nicoletti G, Raffaele R. Dopaminergic hypothesis for retarded depression: a symptom profile for predicting therapeutical responses. *Acta Psychiatr Scand* 1991; **84**: 552–4.

122. Randrup L, Munkvald J, Fog R, Gerlach J, Molander L, Kjeillberg B. Mania, depression and brain dopamine. In: (Essman WB, Valizelli L, eds) *Current Developments in Psychopharmacology*. (Spectrum: New York, 1975) 206–48.

123. van Praag HM, Korf J. A pilot study of some kinetic aspects of the metabolism of 5-hydroxytryptamine in depressive patients. *Biol Psychiatry* 1971; **3**: 105–12.

124. D'Haenen HA, Bossuyt A. Dopamine D2 receptors in depression measured with single photon emission computed tomography. *Biol Psychiatry* 1994; **35**: 128–32.

125. Ebert D, Feistel H, Loew T, Pirner A. Dopamine and depression – striatal dopamine D2 receptor SPECT before and after antidepressant therapy. *Psychopharmacology (Berl)* 1996; **126**: 91–4.

126. Klimke A, Larisch R, Janz A, Vosberg H, Muller-Gartner HW, Gaebel W. Dopamine D2 receptor binding before and after treatment of major depression measured by [123I]IBZM SPECT. *Psychiatry Res* 1999; **90**: 91–101.

127. Parsey RV, Oquendo MA, Zea-Ponce Y et al. Dopamine D(2) receptor availability and amphetamine-induced dopamine release in unipolar depression. *Biol Psychiatry* 2001; **50**: 313–22.

128. Shah PJ, Ogilvie AD, Goodwin GM, Ebmeier KP. Clinical and psychometric correlates of dopamine D2 binding in depression. *Psychol Med* 1997; **27**: 1247–56.

129. Pearlson GD, Wong DF, Tune LE et al. In vivo D2 dopamine receptor density in psychotic and nonpsychotic patients with bipolar disorder. *Arch Gen Psychiatry* 1995; **52**: 471–7.

130. Anand A, Verhoeff P, Seneca N et al. Brain SPECT imaging of amphetamine-induced dopamine release in euthymic bipolar disorder patients. *Am J Psychiatry* 2000; **157:** 1108–14.

131. Laasonen-Balk T, Kuikka J, Viinamaki H, Husso-Saastamoinen M, Lehtonen J, Tiihonen J. Striatal dopamine transporter density in major depression. *Psychopharmacology (Berl)* 1999; **144:** 282–5.

132. Meyer JH, Kruger S, Wilson AA et al. Lower dopamine transporter binding potential in striatum during depression. *Neuroreport* 2001; **12:** 4121–5.

133. Martinot M, Bragulat V, Artiges E et al. Decreased presynaptic dopamine function in the left caudate of depressed patients with affective flattening and psychomotor retardation. *Am J Psychiatry* 2001; **158:** 314–16.

134. Suhara T, Nakayama K, Inoue O et al. D1 dopamine receptor binding in mood disorders measured by positron emission tomography. *Psychopharmacology (Berl)* 1992; **106:** 14–18.

135. Andreasen NC, O'Leary DS, Cizadlo T et al. Remembering the past: two facets of episodic memory explored with positron emission tomography. *Am J Psychiatry* 1995; **152:** 1576–85.

136. Mazziotta JC, Phelps ME, Carson RE, Kuhl DE. Tomographic mapping of human cerebral metabolism: sensory deprivation. *Ann Neurol* 1982; **12:** 435–44.

137. McGuire PK, Paulesu E, Frackowiak RS, Frith CD. Brain activity during stimulus independent thought. *Neuroreport* 1996; **7:** 2095–9.

138. Mazoyer B, Zago L, Mellet E et al. Cortical networks for working memory and executive functions sustain the conscious resting state in man. *Brain Res Bull* 2001; **54:** 287–98.

139. Shulman GL, Corbetta M, Buckner RL et al. Top-down modulation of early sensory cortex. *Cereb Cortex* 1997; **7:** 193–206.

140. Drevets WC. Functional anatomical abnormalities in limbic and prefrontal cortical structures in major depression. *Prog Brain Res* 2000; **126:** 413–31.

141. Fu CH, McGuire PK. Functional neuroimaging in psychiatry. *Phil Trans R Soc Lond B Biol Sci* 1999; **354:** 1359–70.

142. Soares JC, Mann JJ. The functional neuroanatomy of mood disorders. *J Psychiatr Res* 1997; **31:** 393–432.

143. Videbech P. PET measurements of brain glucose metabolism and blood flow in major depressive disorder: a critical review. *Acta Psychiatr Scand* 2000; **101:** 11–20.

144. Johanson M, Risberg J, Silverskiold P. Regional cerebral blood flow related to acute memory disturbance following electroconvulsive therapy in depression. *Acta Neurol Scand* 1979; **60:** 534–5.

145. Mathew RJ, Meyer JS, Francis DJ, Semchuk KM, Mortel K, Claghorn JL. Cerebral blood flow in depression. *Am J Psychiatry* 1980; **137:** 1449–50.

146. Kennedy SH, Evans KR, Kruger S et al. Changes in regional brain glucose metabolism measured with positron emission tomography after paroxetine treatment of major depression. *Am J Psychiatry* 2001; **158:** 899–905.

147. Biver F, Goldman S, Delvenne V et al. Frontal and parietal metabolic disturbances in unipolar depression. *Biol Psychiatry* 1994; **36:** 381–8.

148. Brody AL, Saxena S, Mandelkern MA, Fairbanks LA, Ho ML, Baxter LR. Brain metabolic changes associated with symptom factor improvement in major depressive disorder. *Biol Psychiatry* 2001; **50:** 171–8.

149. Drevets WC, Videen TO, Price JL, Preskorn SH, Carmichael ST, Raichle ME. A functional anatomical study of unipolar depression. *J Neurosci* 1992; **12:** 3628–41.

150. Drevets WC. Neuroimaging studies of mood disorders. *Biol Psychiatry* 2000; **48:** 813–29.

151. Buchsbaum MS, Wu J, Siegel BV et al. Effect of sertraline on regional metabolic rate in patients with affective disorder. *Biol Psychiatry* 1997; **41:** 15–22.

152. Kegeles LS, Malone KM, Slifstein M et al. Response of cortical metabolic deficits to serotonergic challenge in familial mood disorders. *Am J Psychiatry* 2003; **160:** 76–82.

153. Botteron KN, Raichle ME, Drevets WC, Heath AC, Todd RD. Volumetric reduction in left subgenual prefrontal cortex in early onset depression. *Biol Psychiatry* 2002; **51:** 342–4.

154. Hirayasu Y, Shenton ME, Salisbury DF et al. Subgenual cingulate cortex volume in first-episode psychosis. *Am J Psychiatry* 1999; **156:** 1091–3.

155. Drevets WC, Price JC, Kupfer DJ et al. PET measures of amphetamine-induced dopamine release in ventral versus dorsal striatum. *Neuropsychopharmacology* 1999; **21:** 694–709.

156. Mayberg HS, Brannan SK, Mahurin RK et al. Cingulate function in depression: a potential predictor of treatment response. *Neuroreport* 1997; **8:** 1057–61.

157. Brody AL, Saxena S, Silverman DH et al. Brain metabolic changes in major depressive disorder from pre- to post-treatment with paroxetine. *Psychiatry Res* 1999; **91:** 127–39.

158. Brody AL, Barsom MW, Bota RG, Saxena S. Prefrontal–subcortical and limbic circuit mediation of major depressive disorder. *Semin Clin Neuropsychiatry* 2001; **6:** 102–12.

159. Drevets WC, Price JL, Bardgett ME, Reich T, Todd RD, Raichle ME. Glucose metabolism in the amygdala in depression: relationship to diagnostic subtype and plasma cortisol levels. *Pharmac Biochem Behav* 2002; **71:** 431–47.

160. Ketter TA, Kimbrell TA, George MS et al. Effects of mood and subtype on cerebral glucose metabolism in treatment-resistant bipolar disorder. *Biol Psychiatry* 2001; **49:** 97–109.

161. Kimbrell TA, Ketter TA, George MS et al. Regional cerebral glucose utilization in patients with a range of severities of unipolar depression. *Biol Psychiatry* 2002; **51:** 237–52.

162. Saxena S, Brody AL, Ho ML et al. Cerebral metabolism in major depression and obsessive–compulsive disorder occurring separately and concurrently. *Biol Psychiatry* 2001; **50:** 159–70.

163. Abercrombie HC, Schaefer SM, Larson CL et al. Metabolic rate in the right amygdala predicts negative affect in depressed patients. *Neuroreport* 1998; **9:** 3301–7.

164. Austin MP, Dougall N, Ross M et al. Single photon emission tomography with 99mTc-exametazime in major depression and the pattern of brain activity underlying the psychotic/neurotic continuum. *J Affect Disord* 1992; **26:** 31–43.

165. Galynker II, Cai J, Ongseng F, Finestone H, Dutta E, Serseni D. Hypofrontality and negative symptoms in major depressive disorder. *J Nucl Med* 1998; **39:** 608–12.

166. Osuch EA, Ketter TA, Kimbrell TA et al. Regional cerebral metabolism associated with anxiety symptoms in affective disorder patients. *Biol Psychiatry* 2000; **48:** 1020–3.

167. Bench CJ, Friston KJ, Brown RG, Frackowiak RS, Dolan RJ. Regional cerebral blood flow in depression measured by positron emission tomography: the relationship with clinical dimensions. *Psychol Med* 1993; **23:** 579–90.

168. Mayberg HS, Lewis PJ, Regenold W, Wagner Jr HN. Paralimbic hypoperfusion in unipolar depression. *J Nucl Med* 1994; **35:** 929–34.

169. Brody AL, Saxena S, Fairbanks LA et al. Personality changes in adult subjects with major depressive disorder or obsessive-compulsive disorder treated with paroxetine. *J Clin Psychiatry* 2000; **61:** 349–55.

170. Dolan RJ, Bench CJ, Brown RG, Scott LC, Frackowiak RS. Neuropsychological dysfunction in depression: the relationship to regional cerebral blood flow. *Psychol Med* 1994; **24:** 849–57.

171. Buchsbaum MS, Wu J, DeLisi LE et al. Frontal cortex and basal ganglia metabolic rates assessed by positron emission tomography with [18F]2-deoxyglucose in affective illness. *J Affect Disord* 1986; **10:** 137–52.

172. Post RM, DeLisi LE, Holcomb HH, Uhde TW, Cohen R, Buchsbaum MS. Glucose utilization in the temporal cortex of affectively ill patients: positron emission tomography. *Biol Psychiatry* 1987; **22:** 545–53.

173. Cohen RM, Semple WE, Gross M et al. Evidence for common alterations in cerebral glucose metabolism in major affective disorders and schizophrenia. *Neuropsychopharmacology* 1989; **2:** 241–54.

174. Hagman JO, Buchsbaum MS, Wu JC, Rao SJ, Reynolds CA, Blinder BJ. Comparison of regional brain metabolism in bulimia nervosa and affective disorder assessed with positron emission tomography. *J Affect Disord* 1990; **19:** 153–62.

175. Burt DB, Zembar MJ, Niederehe G. Depression and memory impairment: a meta-analysis of the association, its pattern, and specificity. *Psychol Bull* 1995; **117:** 285–305.

176. Veiel HO. A preliminary profile of neuropsychological deficits associated with major depression. *J Clin Exp Neuropsychol* 1997; **19:** 587–603.

177. Wilkins AJ, Shallice T, McCarthy R. Frontal lesions and sustained attention. *Neuropsychologia* 1987; **25:** 359–65.

178. Hickie I, Ward P, Scott E et al. Neo-striatal rCBF correlates of psychomotor slowing in patients with major depression. *Psychiatry Res* 1999; **92:** 75–81.

179. Gur RE, Skolnick BE, Gur RC et al. Brain function in psychiatric disorders. II. Regional cerebral blood flow in medicated unipolar depressives. *Arch Gen Psychiatry* 1984; **41:** 695–9.

180. George MS, Ketter TA, Parekh PI et al. Blunted left cingulate activation in mood disorder subjects during a response interference task (the Stroop). *J Neuropsychiatry Clin Neurosci* 1997; **9:** 55–63.

181. Berman KF, Doran AR, Pickar D, Weinberger DR. Is the mechanism of prefrontal hypofunction in depression the same as in schizophrenia? Regional cerebral blood flow during cognitive activation. *Br J Psychiatry* 1993; **162:** 183–92.

182. Elliott R, Baker SC, Rogers RD et al. Prefrontal dysfunction in depressed patients performing a complex planning task: a study using positron emission tomography. *Psychol Med* 1997; **27**: 931–42.

183. Rubinsztein JS, Fletcher PC, Rogers RD et al. Decision-making in mania: a PET study. *Brain* 2001; **124**: 2550–63.

184. Blumberg HP, Stern E, Ricketts S et al. Rostral and orbital prefrontal cortex dysfunction in the manic state of bipolar disorder. *Am J Psychiatry* 1999; **156**: 1986–8.

185. Curtis VA, Dixon TA, Morris RG et al. Differential frontal activation in schizophrenia and bipolar illness during verbal fluency. *J Affect Disord* 2001; **66**: 111–21.

186. Elliott R, Sahakian BJ, Herrod JJ, Robbins TW, Paykel ES. Abnormal response to negative feedback in unipolar depression: evidence for a diagnosis specific impairment. *J Neurol Neurosurg Psychiatry* 1997; **63**: 74–82.

187. Beauregard M, Leroux JM, Bergman S et al. The functional neuroanatomy of major depression: an fMRI study using an emotional activation paradigm. *Neuroreport* 1998; **9**: 3253–8.

188. Mayberg HS, Liotti M, Brannan SK et al. Reciprocal limbic–cortical function and negative mood: converging PET findings in depression and normal sadness. *Am J Psychiatry* 1999; **156**: 675–82.

189. Yurgelun-Todd DA, Gruber SA, Kanayama G, Killgore WD, Baird AA, Young AD. fMRI during affect discrimination in bipolar affective disorder. *Bipolar Disord* 2000; **2**: 237–48.

190. Sheline YI, Barch DM, Donnelly JM, Ollinger JM, Snyder AZ, Mintun MA. Increased amygdala response to masked emotional faces in depressed subjects resolves with antidepressant treatment: an fMRI study. *Biol Psychiatry* 2001; **50**: 651–8.

191. Thomas KM, Drevets WC, Dahl RE et al. Amygdala response to fearful faces in anxious and depressed children. *Arch Gen Psychiatry* 2001; **58**: 1057–63.

192. Drevets WC. Neuroimaging and neuropathological studies of depression: implications for the cognitive–emotional features of mood disorders. *Curr Opin Neurobiol* 2001; **11**: 240–9.

193. Elliott R, Sahakian BJ, Michael A, Paykel ES, Dolan RJ. Abnormal neural response to feedback on planning and guessing tasks in patients with unipolar depression. *Psychol Med* 1998; **28**: 559–71.

194. Siegle GJ, Steinhauer SR, Thase ME, Stenger VA, Carter CS. Can't shake that feeling: event-related fMRI assessment of sustained amygdala activity in response to emotional information in depressed individuals. *Biol Psychiatry* 2002; **51**: 693–707.

195. Murphy FC, Sahakian BJ. Neuropsychology of bipolar disorder. *Br J Psychiatry* 2001; **41 (Suppl):** s120–s127.

196. Elliott R, Rubinsztein JS, Sahakian BJ, Dolan RJ. The neural basis of mood-congruent processing biases in depression. *Arch Gen Psychiatry* 2002; **59**: 597–604.

197. Nobler MS, Sackeim HA, Prohovnik I et al. Regional cerebral blood flow in mood disorders, III. Treatment and clinical response. *Arch Gen Psychiatry* 1994; **51**: 884–97.

198. Rosenberg R, Vorstrup S, Andersen A, Bolwig TG. Effect of ECT on cerebral blood flow in melancholia assessed with SPECT. *Convuls Ther* 1988; **4:** 62–73.

199. Scott AI, Dougall N, Ross M et al. Short-term effects of electroconvulsive treatment on the uptake of 99mTc-exametazime into brain in major depression shown with single photon emission tomography. *J Affect Disord* 1994; **30:** 27–34.

200. Bonne O, Krausz Y, Shapira B et al. Increased cerebral blood flow in depressed patients responding to electroconvulsive therapy. *J Nucl Med* 1996; **37:** 1075–80.

201. Mervaala E, Kononen M, Fohr J et al. SPECT and neuropsychological performance in severe depression treated with ECT. *J Affect Disord* 2001; **66:** 47–58.

202. Milo TJ, Kaufman GE, Barnes WE et al. Changes in regional cerebral blood flow after electroconvulsive therapy for depression. *J ECT* 2001; **17:** 15–21.

203. Nobler MS, Oquendo MA, Kegeles LS et al. Decreased regional brain metabolism after ect. *Am J Psychiatry* 2001; **158:** 305–8.

204. Henry ME, Schmidt ME, Matochik JA, Stoddard EP, Potter WZ. The effects of ECT on brain glucose: a pilot FDG PET study. *J ECT* 2001; **17:** 33–40.

205. George MS, Lisanby SH, Sackeim HA. Transcranial magnetic stimulation: applications in neuropsychiatry. *Arch Gen Psychiatry* 1999; **56:** 300–11.

206. Kimbrell TA, Little JT, Dunn RT et al. Frequency dependence of antidepressant response to left prefrontal repetitive transcranial magnetic stimulation (rTMS) as a function of baseline cerebral glucose metabolism. *Biol Psychiatry* 1999; **46:** 1603–13.

207. Speer AM, Kimbrell TA, Wassermann EM et al. Opposite effects of high and low frequency rTMS on regional brain activity in depressed patients. *Biol Psychiatry* 2000; **48:** 1133–41.

208. Zheng XM. Regional cerebral blood flow changes in drug-resistant depressed patients following treatment with transcranial magnetic stimulation: a statistical parametric mapping analysis. *Psychiatry Res* 2000; **100:** 75–80.

209. Catafau AM, Perez V, Gironell A et al. SPECT mapping of cerebral activity changes induced by repetitive transcranial magnetic stimulation in depressed patients. A pilot study. *Psychiatry Res* 2001; **106:** 151–60.

210. Bench CJ, Frackowiak RS, Dolan RJ. Changes in regional cerebral blood flow on recovery from depression. *Psychol Med* 1995; **25:** 247–61.

211. Goodwin GM, Austin MP, Dougall N et al. State changes in brain activity shown by the uptake of 99mTc-exametazime with single photon emission tomography in major depression before and after treatment. *J Affect Disord* 1993; **29:** 243–53.

212. Mayberg HS, Brannan SK, Tekell JL et al. Regional metabolic effects of fluoxetine in major depression: serial changes and relationship to clinical response. *Biol Psychiatry* 2000; **48:** 830–43.

213. Ogura A, Morinobu S, Kawakatsu S, Totsuka S, Komatani A. Changes in regional brain activity in major depression after successful treatment with antidepressant drugs. *Acta Psychiatr Scand* 1998; **98:** 54–9.

214. Martinot JL, Hardy P, Feline A et al. Left prefrontal glucose hypometabolism in the depressed state: a confirmation. *Am J Psychiatry* 1990; **147:** 1313–17.

215. Martin SD, Martin E, Rai SS, Richardson MA, Royall R. Brain blood flow changes in depressed patients treated with interpersonal psychotherapy or venlafaxine hydrochloride: preliminary findings. *Arch Gen Psychiatry* 2001; **58:** 641–8.

216. Brody AL, Saxena S, Stoessel P et al. Regional brain metabolic changes in patients with major depression treated with either paroxetine or interpersonal therapy: preliminary findings. *Arch Gen Psychiatry* 2001; **58**: 631–40.

217. Ketter TA, Kimbrell TA, George MS et al. Baseline cerebral hypermetabolism associated with carbamazepine response, and hypometabolism with nimodipine response in mood disorders. *Biol Psychiatry* 1999; **46**: 1364–74.

218. Ebert D, Feistel H, Barocka A. Effects of sleep deprivation on the limbic system and the frontal lobes in affective disorders: a study with Tc-99m-HMPAO SPECT. *Psychiatry Res* 1991; **40**: 247–51.

219. Ebert D, Feistel H, Kaschka W, Barocka A, Pirner A. Single photon emission computerized tomography assessment of cerebral dopamine D2 receptor blockade in depression before and after sleep deprivation – preliminary results. *Biol Psychiatry* 1994; **35**: 880–5.

220. Wu J, Buchsbaum MS, Gillin JC et al. Prediction of antidepressant effects of sleep deprivation by metabolic rates in the ventral anterior cingulate and medial prefrontal cortex. *Am J Psychiatry* 1999; **156**: 1149–58.

221. Wu JC, Gillin JC, Buchsbaum MS, Hershey T, Johnson JC, Bunney Jr WE. Effect of sleep deprivation on brain metabolism of depressed patients. *Am J Psychiatry* 1992; **149**: 538–43.

222. Little JT, Ketter TA, Kimbrell TA et al. Venlafaxine or bupropion responders but not nonresponders show baseline prefrontal and paralimbic hypometabolism compared with controls. *Psychopharmac Bull* 1996; **32**: 629–35.

223. Davidson RJ, Pizzagalli D, Nitschke JB, Putnam K. Depression: perspectives from affective neuroscience. *Ann Rev Psychol* 2002; **53**: 545–74.

224. Depue RA, Iacono WG. Neurobehavioral aspects of affective disorders. *Ann Rev Psychol* 1989; **40**: 457–92.

225. Drevets WC, Raichle ME. Neuroanatomical circuits in depression: implications for treatment mechanisms. *Psychopharmac Bull* 1992; **28**: 261–74.

226. Mayberg HS. Limbic–cortical dysregulation: a proposed model of depression. *J Neuropsychiatry Clin Neurosci* 1997; **9**: 471–81.

227. Swerdlow NR, Koob GF. Dopamine, schizophrenia, mania and depression: toward a unified hypothesis of cortico–striato–pallido–thalamic function. *Behav Brain Sci* 1987; **10**: 197–245.

228. Friston KJ. Imaging neuroscience: principles or maps? *Proc Natl Acad Sci USA* 1998; **95**: 796–802.

6. NEUROIMAGING AND EATING DISORDERS

Rudolf Uher, Janet Treasure

Eating disorders: a spectrum of varied conditions

Eating disorders (ED) constitute a group of conditions in which abnormal eating behaviour negatively influences the psychosocial functioning of an individual. Attitudes towards food and eating and the perception of the patient's own body are also disturbed. ED include a range of conditions, which are grouped under the diagnoses of anorexia nervosa (AN), bulimia nervosa (BN), ED not otherwise specified (EDNOS), binge eating disorder (BED) and simple obesity (OB). Within the current conceptualizations, AN and BN are classified as psychiatric diseases, whereas OB is considered to be a somatic medical condition and its inclusion into ED is controversial. The distinctions between individual diagnoses are often arbitrary, e.g. a body mass index (BMI) of 17.5 constitutes the boundary between AN and BN, the frequency of binging–purging behaviour determines the distinction between BN and EDNOS etc. To avoid confusion it is helpful to consider ED as a continuous spectrum ranging from restrictive AN to OB (Figure 6.1). The subjective importance of eating is common to all these disorders, but the drive to eat, the perception of hunger/satiety and actual body weight vary on a continuum along the spectrum.[1]

Although major advances have been made in the research on the physiology of eating and its disorders, the etiology and pathogenesis of ED is far from clear. Genetic, neurodevelopmental, early and immediate environmental factors are all implicated in the genesis and maintenance of these diseases. This chapter will review the contribution of neuroimaging research to the ongoing discussion on ED pathogenesis.

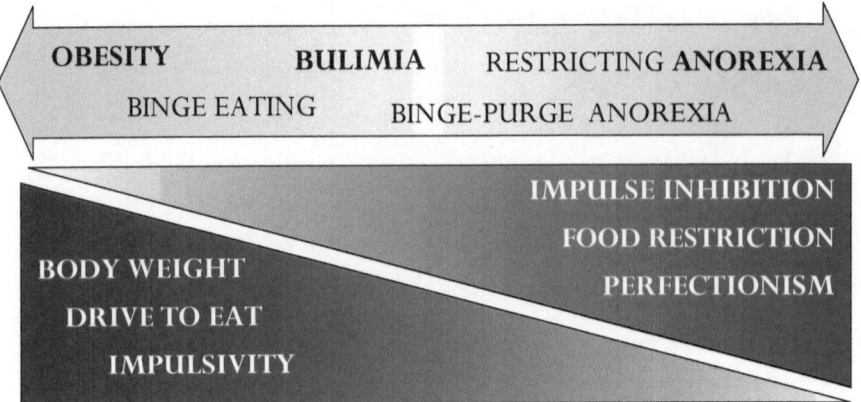

Figure 6.1 *Eating disorders lie on a continuum without clear boundaries between the diagnostic categories. Obesity with high drive to eat represents one extreme of the spectrum, binge-eating disorder and bulimia nervosa follow, both characterized by high impulsivity. The other extreme is represented by restricting anorexia nervosa with perfectionist self-control, inhibition of feelings and impulses, and extremely low body weight.*

What does the brain look like?

Gross anatomical findings

Historically, AN has been grouped with somatic illness, often as a form of endocrine disorder, e.g. a condition caused by a hormone-producing tumour.[2] Indeed brain lesions and tumours associated with syndromes similar to AN or BN have been described.[3–5] On the other hand food restriction alone can produce many of the behavioural symptoms of AN and BN. Thus the distinction between psychological or somatic etiology was unclear and a quest for a macroscopical or microscopical substrate in the brain constituted an essential part of the etiological investigation of ED.

Today, the results of neuroimaging and post-mortem neuroanatomical studies clearly indicate that there is no macroscopical brain lesion in most cases of AN.[6–8] On the other hand there is evidence suggesting that perinatal hypoxic injury can contribute to the development of AN. Perinatal factors (e.g. birth injury or being small for date) are linked to an increased risk of developing AN,[9–11] and authors of early neuropsychological and neuroimaging studies claimed that their findings were consistent with a perinatal injury in a substantial proportion (up to 60%) of AN patients.[12–14]

BN was more readily accepted as being primarily a psychogenic disorder and its somatic correlates have been studied less extensively. Echoing the results from studies of AN, the available studies indicate an absence of macroscopic focal brain damage in BN. In summary, neuroimaging together with neuropathological investigations contributed to the exclusion of macroscopic organic causes for the vast majority of ED cases, and thus helped to focus the research on functional and pharmacological aspects of ED pathophysiology.

The brain is atrophic

The assumption that the emaciated body of AN patients would harbour an emaciated brain has been confirmed by a large number of structural neuro-imaging studies. Using computer tomography (CT), brain shrinkage in AN was visualized as widening of the cerebral and cerebellar cortical sulci and enlargement of the ventricles.[12,14–16] As many of these changes tended to resolve with recovery of normal body weight,[12,17–19] the term pseudo-atrophy was coined to emphasize the reversibility of the process.[20] More recently, it has been established that even adult brain neurons can regenerate and therefore even 'true' atrophy, meaning loss of neurons, may be reversible. The distinction between atrophy and a pseudoatrophy has thus become less meaningful, and atrophy is used further in this text.

The initial CT findings were later confirmed with magnetic resonance imaging (MRI).[7,21,22] The thalamus and midbrain areas were both reported to be significantly smaller in AN patients compared to healthy controls.[23] The possible links with endocrine dysfunction have further focused the attention on the pituitary (significantly smaller in AN patients)[6] and to the hippocampus–amygdala formation, which is also reduced in size.[24] MRI also brought the possibility of objective brain volume measurements with distinction between white matter (mainly the myelinated axons) and grey matter (cell bodies of neurons and glial cells). Although both white and grey matter volumes are significantly decreased in acute AN patients,[25] the potential for reversibility may be different for these two compartments. People recovered from AN have normal white matter volume but their grey matter volume remains significantly decreased 1–3 years after recovery.[26,27] A question remains whether there is an irreversible loss of grey matter, possibly corresponding to neuronal loss, or the grey matter restoration only occurs on a more protracted timescale. Proton magnetic resonance spec-troscopy (^{1}H MRS), a method visualizing brain metabolic components *in vivo*, showed decreases in lipid signal, but not in the neuronal marker NA

(*N*-acetylated compounds) in ED patients; these findings are consistent with nutrient deficit and testify against neuronal loss in ED.[28,29]

Widening of cerebral sulci (cortical atrophy) and decreased size of the pituitary were also reported in normal weight patients suffering from BN; on the other hand BN patients have normal sized ventricles, thalamus and midbrain areas.[6,30,31] One study found that the atrophy in BN selectively affected the inferior frontal lobe cortex.[30] To our knowledge, there are no data on brain structure abnormalities in BED or OB.

To summarize the established facts: (1) the brain in AN and BN patients is atrophic; (2) atrophy in AN is widespread, afflicting both grey and white matter, both cortex and subcortical regions; (3) the atrophy is partially reversible with recovery of normal body weight and eating habits; (4) there is a significant grey matter deficit persisting beyond recovery from AN; (5) the atrophy in BN may be different in distribution, affecting mainly the cerebral cortex.

Next we will consider two essential questions linked to the structural brain findings in ED: what is the mechanism mediating the brain atrophy? What is the functional significance of the brain atrophy?

Lack of nutrients or excess cortisol are possible mechanisms of atrophy

Atrophic brain changes are present very early in the course of AN, correlate significantly with the BMI and partial restoration is already evident after a few months of appropriate nutrition.[17,25,26,32] Moreover, reversible enlargement of cerebrospinal fluid spaces and cortical sulci widening were also noted in malnourished children with kwashiorkor.[33] All these data indicate that brain atrophy may correspond to the decreased nutrient supply in the state of starvation, but sufficiency of this simple explication was put in question by the findings of cortical atrophy in normal weight BN patients: why should the brain in BN be smaller if the body is of normal size? In the search for other causal mechanisms of the brain atrophy in ED, neuroendocrine abnormalities, most notably hypercortisolaemia, seem to be the most plausible candidates. They are supported by the following evidence: (1) elevated levels of cortisol are found consistently in AN;[34–36] (2) hypercortisolaemia in other conditions [e.g. Cushing's syndrome, exogenous corticoid administration, post-traumatic stress disorder (PTSD) and depression] is associated with brain atrophic changes;[37] (3) the noxious effect of elevated cortisol on neural cells has been demonstrated on cellular level;[37] (4) measures of cortisol secretion correlate with the degree of brain atrophy in AN.[25,32] Thus cortisol has been proposed to be a noxious agent, mediating the decrease in brain mass in ED.[32] Nevertheless, much remains to be explained, as there are two important caveats to the cortisol theory. First, in some hypercortisolaemic states, such as Cushing's syndrome or PTSD, there is a more or less selective atrophy of the hippocampi, rich in glucocorticoid receptors, with little or no changes in the total brain volume,[37] whereas in AN (and also in depression) the atrophy seems to be rather generalized. Second, cortisol levels in BN do not seem to be consistently elevated[38–40] and so the explanation of atrophy, especially in BN, will require further investigations. Other possible mechanisms may be decreased thyroid function (levels of triodothyronine correlated negatively with ventricular enlargement in AN[41]), dehydration or salt and water imbalance caused by vomiting.

Does atrophy matter?

Are the atrophic changes in the brain just insignificant epiphenomenona of starvation? Or do they have functional relevance? Do they contribute to the maintenance of the disease? Answering these questions will require: (1) defining a specific functional deficit and (2) linking it to morphological or functional findings in specific brain structures. The available research aiming at these goals will now be reviewed.

People with ED are characterized as rigid and inflexible; on the other hand many of these patients are high achieving academically and intellectually, even in the gruesome condition of anorexic wasting. Standard tools measuring general intelligence often give unremarkable results and specific test batteries are necessary to capture the nature of the cognitive impairment in ED. Furthermore, the diagnostic categories may be not homogeneous enough to provide significant results, e.g. only about 40% of AN patients seem to be significantly affected in cognitive performance.[42,43] Having said this, we may summarize that there is a general cognitive deficit in attention and concentration in AN patients.[13,42] In addition there may be some more specific deficits in spatial processing[7,44] and in the flexibility of cognitive set shifting.[7,45,46] Such findings are suggestive of impairment of parietal and prefrontal cortical circuits.[47]

To investigate the links between brain structure and cognitive function in AN, two studies combined brain CT[8] or MRI[7] with neuropsychological testing. In the first, impaired performance in a symbol digit test (assesses mainly perceptual–motor speed) correlated significantly with a cumulative measure of cortical atrophy and external cerebrospinal fluid spaces enlargement (cortical score); but in most tests, patients performed in normal range.[8] The second study used MRI and an extensive battery of neuropsychological tests on a relatively large sample (46 AN patients and 41 healthy controls); although both brain atrophic changes and cognitive performance (in attention, visuospatial skills, memory and flexibility) correlated with body weight deficit and improved with treatment, the correlations between them were weak.[7]

Thus, although both cognitive deficit and structural brain changes are present, the relationship between these two has not yet been sufficiently clarified. As the cognitive impairment in ED is relatively mild, structural imaging is perhaps not the appropriate tool to detect its neural correlates. The combination of functional neuroimaging with on-line neuropsychological testing may help to elucidate this brain–performance relationship in future.

How does the brain work?

ED, among other psychiatric diseases, are now regarded as functional disorders of the brain and dysfunctions of specific neural circuits have been proposed to underlie the ED pathology.[47–49] Visualization of *in vivo* brain metabolism or blood flow with functional neuroimaging methods, such as positron emission tomography (PET), single photon emission computed tomography (SPECT) and functional MRI (fMRI), provide tools to test such theories.

Imaging the resting brain activity

In 1987, Herholz and collaborators published the first functional neuroimaging study in ED patients. Using PET, they found significantly increased metabolism in the caudate nucleus in a group of five acute AN patients and this abnormality normalized with weight gain.[50] As the caudate nucleus is involved in the feeding behaviour of primates and obsessive–compulsive behaviour in humans, this study opened a large space for hypotheses and further experiments. The original finding of caudate hypermetabolism was not replicated in some of the later studies;[41,51] however, there is some consistency in the findings which can be summarized into an emerging pattern of brain function in AN.[49,52,53] The brain as a whole seems to work less intensely in AN patients than in healthy persons, and this hypofunction is most pronounced in the frontal and parietal regions;[49,51–54] on the other hand the basal ganglia may be hyperactive in AN patients.[50,52] Takano et al[49] also reported increased perfusion in the thalamus and in the hippocampo–amygdalar complex. In a recent PET study the medial temporal region, comprising the parahippocampal gyrus and hippocampus bilaterally, was also significantly more activated in the AN patients, irrespective of specific paradigm.[55] Global brain hypometabolism, most pronounced in the temporoparietal and frontal regions, has been shown to persist after weight-restoration in AN.[56]

Brain function in BN has been investigated in several PET and SPECT studies. Parietal hypometabolism[52] and inferior temporal lobe hypermetabolism,[57] as well as a loss of normal right–left asymmetry of glucose brain metabolism during the continuous performance test,[57,58] have been reported. As depressed mood is a regular part of BN symptomatology, analogies with affective disorders were also examined. As in major depression, left prefrontal metabolism levels correlated negatively with depressive symptoms measured by the Hamilton scale,[57] but a direct comparison between BN and depressed patients showed distinct patterns of activation in these two disorders.[59]

The interpretation of resting brain activity studies can be difficult because many of the somatic consequences of eating disorders (low blood pressure and heart rate, anaemia, hypoglycaemia, ketone bodies) may confound the results. Furthermore, the uncontrolled nature of a resting condition does not allow specific interpretations. However, these studies provide a basis for further studies in which defined aspects of brain function are investigated under specific conditions.

Brain response to food challenge

We now know that there are differences in brain structure, metabolism and blood flow between ED patients and healthy people. To assess the functional significance of these data, we need to know which brain circuits are involved in the genesis and maintenance of the disease and its specific symptoms. This can be achieved by recording the brain activity under controlled conditions, which are relevant to ED psychopathology. The ED specific paradigms may involve food, eating or body image; relevant also are conditions related to emotions, anxiety, depression and obsessive–compulsive symptoms. So far, several studies have been published, investigating brain activity in AN, BN and OB when eating or looking at food. To better appreciate these studies we will first review the functional neuroanatomy of normal eating.

Neural basis of eating

The central control of eating behaviour is disrupted in all eating disorders. However, it is not known whether the abnormality is the primary cause or a secondary consequence. Neural mechanisms involved in the response to food and its modulation by hunger and satiation have been extensively investigated with single neuron activity mapping in primates.[60] It has been established that taste, olfactory and visual pathways that process food-related stimuli converge on the amygdala and the caudal orbitofrontal cortex, where the reward value is appraised and a choice is made whether to engage in action aimed at ingesting the potential food. Whereas the amygdala provides a relatively slow and rigid mechanism of learned stimulus–reinforcement associations, the hierarchically superior orbitofrontal cortex adds the flexibility necessary to rapidly adapt the behaviour to a changing environment. Information on the organism's energy needs is conveyed from the hypothalamus, and in both the caudal orbitofrontal cortex and in the lateral hypothalamus the representation of food-related stimuli depends on whether the organism is hungry or satiated. The ventral striatum is implicated in the representation of reward value of food-related stimuli and also constitutes a link to the motor system. In the head of the caudate nucleus, which receives a direct input from the orbitofrontal cortex, an appropriate behavioural (motor) response is selected, once the decision is made. For a detailed review of findings in primates, see Rolls.[60] (see also Figure 6.2.)

Human neuroimaging studies suggest that the neural circuitry involved in eating might be more widespread than suggested by primate studies. In the human amygdala, parahippocampal gyrus and anterior fusiform gyrus, neural activity in response to visual food-related cues was found to be hunger dependent.[61] Several loci in the orbitofrontal and medial prefrontal cortex are activated by food stimuli in a sensory specific manner, i.e. they are activated only to food that has not been eaten to satiety.[62] A PET study in healthy men identified the hypothalamus, posterior orbitofrontal cortex, anterior cingulate cortex and insular cortex, but also the hippocampus, precuneus, caudate nucleus, putamen and cerebellum as being activated in a hungry state (36 h fasting) compared to the state of satiety.[63] Satiation on the other hand was associated with increased neural activity in the dorsolateral and anterior ventromedial prefrontal cortices and left inferior parietal lobule, whereas the activity in the hypothalamus, orbitofrontal cortex and insula decreased.[63] The influence of satiety on eating-related brain processing has been further investigated in a study where chocolate was eaten to satiety and beyond, so that its reward value gradually diminished and even became negative. The activity [measured as regional cerebral blood flow (rCBF) with ^{15}O H$_2$O PET] in response to eating another piece of chocolate gradually decreased in the subcallosal and medial orbitofrontal cortex, insula, striatum and midbrain, whereas lateral orbitofrontal, prefrontal and parahippocampal regions became activated with increasing satiety.[64]

The human central appetite control system is comprised of an orexigenic (i.e. appetite-promoting) network and an inhibitory control (or anorexigenic) circuit; the balance between these two subsystems determines eating behaviour.[63,65] The orexigenic paralimbic network (consisting of the orbitofrontal and insular cortices, hypothalamus, parts of striatum and hippocampal formation) activates with fasting and it promotes feeding behaviour. The inhibitory anorexigenic circuit consists of anterior ventromedial and dorsolateral prefrontal cortices and acts to terminate eating, probably by direct inhibition of the orexigenic system.[63–68]

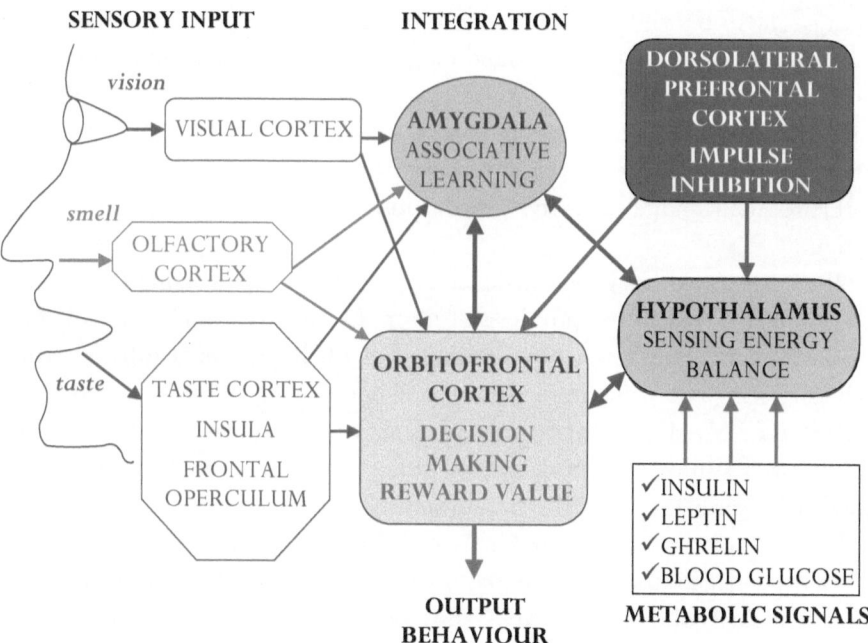

Figure 6.2 *Model of cerebral food intake regulation: food-related signals from different sensory modalities converge to the orbitofrontal cortex, the amygdala and the hypothalamus, which are major constituents of the orexigenic circuit, important for the initiation of eating behaviour. The hypothalamus receives blood metabolic signals, informing on body nutritional status. The dorsolateral prefrontal cortex may be the basis of a circuit with inhibitory, anorexigenic influence.*

Food as a behavioural challenge

Eating or viewing food are the most natural conditions provoking symptoms of ED. The first specific-challenge neuroimaging study, using SPECT, reported significant increases in perfusion of the frontal lobes in reaction to eating a cake in AN patients.[69] When both BN and AN patients were tested using this cake-eating paradigm, there were inverse patterns of rCBF changes in these two diagnostic groups. In BN there was increased frontotemporal perfusion in the rest state and the rCBF in these areas decreased upon eating a cake; in the AN group a decreased perfusion at rest contrasted with an increase of perfusion with eating (again most importantly in the frontal and temporal lobes).[54] These findings may correspond to the well-known differences between these two disorders: BN patients often feel a high urge to eat, which drives them into bingeing and overeating, whereas restricting AN patients do not feel any need to eat at all and experience a great distress when forced to eat normally. The increased frontotemporal activity would then correspond to the high distress state in each disorder (not eating in BN and eating in AN); other interpretations are also possible.

A recent SPECT study separated diagnostic subgroups of binge–purging anorexia nervosa (BPAN) and restricting anorexia nervosa (RAN). BPAN but not RAN showed increases in glucose metabolism in the right prefrontal and parietal regions in response to visualizing custard cake.[70] The authors interpret their findings as activity corresponding to the recall of experienced binging.

Recently, fMRI has been introduced in ED research, bringing the potential of better spatio-temporal resolution. In an fMRI study, the medial orbitofrontal cortex was activated in AN patients but not in healthy controls when viewing colour photographs of food and drink.[71] As the orbitofrontal cortex is involved in the appraisal and processing of subjectively salient and self-related stimuli, this activity may reflect the subjective importance of food and drink for AN patients, as well as the biological need for food. Labelled caloric drinks elicited activity in the limbic structures, including the amygdala and insula, which may correspond to a strong emotional reaction – caloric phobia – in AN.[72] But when $O^{15} CO_2$ PET was used to measure the rCBF while viewing low-/high-calorie foods in seven AN patients, none of the limbic/paralimbic regions were significantly more activated in response to high-calorie food and only the visual–associative cortices showed significant food-related activity in the AN group.[55] Nevertheless, the failure to confirm the hypothesis in the latter study may be due to the modest sample size.

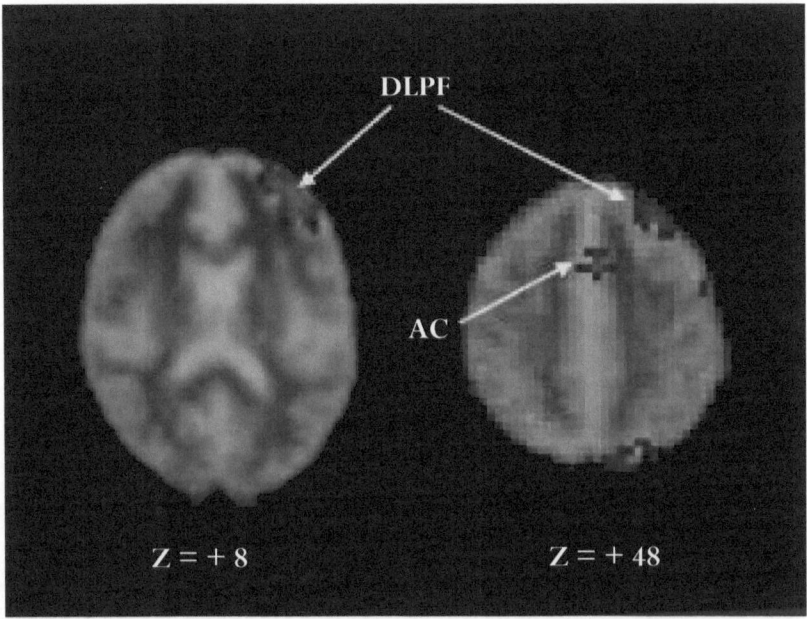

Figure 6.3 *Brain response to viewing pictures of food as it was registered by functional magnetic resonance imaging in a group of patients with anorexia nervosa. Anterior cingulate (AC) activity may be linked to the emotional conflict related to food, whereas the dorsolateral prefrontal cortex (DLPF) is likely to represent inhibitory control (unpublished results).*

When interpreting these results, it is important to consider that visualizing or viewing food in some studies[70–73] is different from actual eating,[54,69] in that it may intensify the craving for food without satisfying it. Thus rather than the food stimulus being rewarding, it elicits mixed emotional responses, including frustration, in hungry people.[74] Similarly, unlike actual eating, viewing food pictures may be relatively safe and non-threatening in AN patients, who refuse eating.

Imaging brain chemistry

Disturbances of specific neuromediator systems may play a key part in the predisposition to and the development of ED. In particular, serotonin and dopamine signalling exert strong influences on eating and appetite. Studies measuring levels of neuromediator metabolites in cerebrospinal fluid as well as investigating the effects of drugs mimicking or antagonizing neuromedia-tors' effects provided the basis for influential theories of ED. With recent advances in neuroimaging, notably PET technology, it has become possible to investigate these neuromediator systems *in vivo*, opening a new field of exciting possibilities in ED research.

Serotonin

From the raphe nuclei of the brainstem, serotonin [or 5-hydroxytryptamine (5-HT)] is diffusely distributed throughout the central nervous system; among other functions it stimulates satiety and decreases food intake. Levels of serotonin metabolites in the cerebrospinal fluid also correlate positively with personality traits characteristic for AN, such as perfectionism, harm avoidance and compulsive behaviours. These facts together with investiga-tions of serotonin metabolites and serotonergic drug effects in eating disor-ders led to the development of the serotonergic theory of ED. According to this theory, low serotonin levels constitute a trait predisposing to AN whereas increased serotonin leads to overeating and bingeing, characteristi-cally on carbohydrate, and thus BN or OB. Food restriction or overeating modifies the supply of tryptophan – the precursor of serotonin – and, in this way, ED patients self-medicate themselves against their endogenous sero-tonin signalling levels.[75–77] Neuroimaging, notably PET and SPECT with radiolabelled ligands to serotonin receptors or transporter proteins, has been instrumental in verifying this theory and further specifying the nature of serotonin abnormality in ED. A particularly important aspect of this research is a focus on people recovered from ED rather than acutely ill patients. Traits predisposing to the development of ED are present in recov-ered people without the confounding secondary effects of malnutrition and abnormal eating habits.[78,79]

Using PET, reduced 5-HT_{2A} receptor activity, especially in mesial tempo-ral regions, was found in women recovered from AN.[78] This finding is of particular interest because the 5-HT_{2A} receptors are implicated in the mod-ulation of feeding and mood. It remains to be explained whether these receptor changes constitute an adaptation to chronic excess in serotonin sig-nalling. In women recovered from BN, 5-HT_{2A} receptor binding was significantly reduced, specifically in the medial orbitofrontal cortex.[79] The similarity of findings in recovered AN and BN patients apparently contra-dicts the hypothesis, according to which the opposite finding would be expected in BN and AN. It is therefore probable that the original hypothesis will require modification, e.g. inclusion of common aspects for AN and BN or specifying the brain regions and circuits rather then increases or decreases in the whole serotonergic system.

As antidepressants inhibiting the serotonin transporter are effective in reducing BN symptoms, the study of their target protein in BN is of particular interest. Using SPECT, the serotonin transporter density was found to be significantly decreased in the thalamic and hypothalamic regions in BN patients.[80] Similar findings were obtained in people with seasonal affective disorder[81] and may be associated with the depressive symptoms of BN.

These results are the first examples indicating the possibilities of neuro-mediator system imaging in ED. Further work is currently in progress and the serotonin hypothesis of ED cannot be considered confirmed or refuted at this stage.

Dopamine

Dopamine supplied from the mesencephalic tegmental nuclei to the ventral striatum is a pleasure messenger, signalling rewarding and novel stimuli. Eating is a naturally pleasurable stimulus and triggers dopaminergic firing in this pathway. An abnormality in this reward circuit can make people vulnerable to pathological pleasure-seeking behaviours such as drinking alcohol, smoking, sniffing cocaine, taking heroin, gambling, compulsive shopping or overeating. This abnormality has been identified at the molecular level: the A1 and B1 alleles of the dopaminergic receptor D2 (DRD2), associated with decreased levels of this receptor, are convicted culprits in this case. Some studies report the prevalence of the A1 allele of the DRD2 in OB is increased to 45.2% (compared to 15.7% in dependency-free healthy controls) – a level comparable to severe alcoholism or other substance abuse.[82,83] The A1 allele is also associated with increased carbohydrate craving.

It is in keeping with this background evidence that a PET study revealed decreased availability of D2 receptors in the striatum of obese people.[84] The decrease in D2 binding correlated with the BMI of the obese participants, as it did in normal weight individuals,[85] further confirming the dopaminergic contribution to OB.

Clinical implications

We have reviewed the development of brain research in ED from the initial search for AN causing tumours, through the establishment of brain atrophy as a part of AN and BN symptomatology, to the quest for dysfunctional brain circuits or neuromediator systems. Although we are not able to draw a final conclusion as to the nature of neural mechanisms of ED there are data that can already improve the approach to ED patients: (1) the brain suffers from inadequate nutrition but, fortunately, much of the damage is reversible, i.e. it is well worth trying to restore healthy food intake as soon as possible; (2) there is an abnormality in brain function that very probably precedes the onset of ED and renders some people more vulnerable to AN, BN or OB – i.e. eating disorders are real diseases with a biological basis and not just adolescent whims. Neuroimaging research has not yet had any major repercussions in the treatment of ED, but perhaps these also may be forthcoming. As a promising example, transcranial magnetic stimulation (TMS) provides the means to stimulate specific brain regions, shown to be deactivated in neuroimaging studies. This new technique has recently been successfully used in depression and its application in ED may not take long to come: could right parietal or left frontal TMS stimulation help to reverse AN? Further, the evolving field of neurochemical imaging holds a promise for a more sophisticated administration of specific pharmacotherapy, perhaps complementing a biochemical disturbance in a given individual. If any of these dreams come true, our early efforts at neuroimaging in ED will have been worthwhile.

Summary

- Eating disorders are a continuous spectrum of diseases characterized by preoccupation and distress related to eating and body shape with anorexia nervosa and obesity being the two extreme conditions
- Brain is atrophic in anorexia and bulimia nervosa. White matter atrophy is reversible with recovery but grey matter atrophy may be irreversible.
- The brain in anorexia nervosa is less active, especially the frontal and parietal lobes.
- The cerebral processing of food-related stimuli is abnormal in eating disorders patients, with excessive involvement of prefrontal cortical areas.
- Availability or sensitivity of neuromediator receptors may predispose to eating disorders: serotonin receptors are implicated in anorexia and bulimia nervosa, dopamine receptors in obesity.

References

1. Treasure J, Collier D. The spectrum of eating disorders. In: (Owen JB, Treasure J, Collier D, eds) *Animal Models – Disorders of Eating Behaviour and Body Composition*. (Dordrecht, The Netherlands: Kluwer Academic Publishers, 2001.)

2. Lewin K, Mattingly D, Millis RR. Anorexia nervosa associated with hypothalamic tumour. *Br Med J* 1972; **2:** 629–30.

3. Chipkevitch E. Brain tumors and anorexia nervosa syndrome. *Brain Dev* 1994; **16:** 175–9.

4. Griffith JL, Hochberg FH. Anorexia and weight loss in glioma patients. *Psychosomatics* 1988; **29:** 335–7.

5. Ward A, Tiller J, Treasure J, Russell G. Eating disorders: psyche or soma? *Int J Eat Disord* 2000; **27:** 279–87.

6. Doraiswamy PM, Krishnan KR, Figiel GS et al. A brain magnetic resonance imaging study of pituitary gland morphology in anorexia nervosa and bulimia. *Biol Psychiatry* 1990; **28:** 110–16.

7. Kingston K, Szmukler G, Andrewes D et al. Neuropsychological and structural brain changes in anorexia nervosa before and after refeeding. *Psychol Med* 1996; **26:** 15–28.

8. Palazidou E, Robinson P, Lishman WA. Neuroradiological and neuropsychological assessment in anorexia nervosa. *Psychol Med* 1990; **20:** 521–7.

9. Cnattingius S, Hultman CM, Dahl M, Sparen P. Very preterm birth, birth trauma, and the risk of anorexia nervosa among girls. *Arch Gen Psychiatry* 1999; **56:** 634–8.

10. Eagles JM, Andrew JE, Johnston MI et al. Season of birth in females with anorexia nervosa in Northeast Scotland. *Int J Eat Disord* 2001; **30:** 167–75.

11. Foley DL, Thacker LR, Aggen SH et al. Pregnancy and perinatal complications associated with risks for common psychiatric disorders in a population-based sample of female twins. *Am J Med Genet* 2001; **105:** 426–31.

12. Artmann H, Grau H, Adelmann M, Schleiffer R. Reversible and non-reversible enlargement of cerebrospinal fluid spaces in anorexia nervosa. *Neuroradiology* 1985; **27:** 304–12.

13. Hamsher K, Halmi KA, Benton AL. Prediction of outcome of anorexia nervosa from neuropsychological status. *Psychiatry Research* 1981; **4:** 79–88.

14. Lankenau H, Swigar ME, Bhimani S et al. Cranial CT scans in eating disorder patients and controls. *Comp Psychiatry* 1985; **26:** 136–47.

15. Datlof S, Coleman PD, Forbes GB, Kreipe RE. Ventricular dilation on CAT scans of patients with anorexia nervosa. *Am J Psychiatry* 1986; **143:** 96–8.

16. Enzmann DR, Lane B. Cranial computed tomography findings in anorexia nervosa. *J Comput Assist Tomogr* 1977; **1:** 410–14.

17. Dolan RJ, Mitchell J, Wakeling A. Structural brain changes in patients with anorexia nervosa. *Psychol Med* 1988; **18:** 349–53.

18. Heinz ER, Martinez J, Haenggeli A. Reversibility of cerebral atrophy in anorexia nervosa and Cushing's syndrome. *J Comput Assist Tomogr* 1977; **1:** 415–18.

19. Kohlmeyer K, Lehmkuhl G, Poutska F. Computed tomography of anorexia nervosa. *Am J Neuroradiol* 1983; **4:** 437–8.

20. Sein P, Searson S, Nicol AR, Hall K. Anorexia nervosa and pseudo-atrophy of the brain. *Br J Psychiatry* 1981; **139:** 257–8.

21. Hoffman GW, Ellinwood Jr EH, Rockwell WJ et al. Cerebral atrophy in anorexia nervosa: a pilot study. *Biol Psychiatry* 1989; **26:** 321–4.

22. Kornreich L, Shapira A, Horev G et al. CT and MR evaluation of the brain in patients with anorexia nervosa. *Am J Neuroradiol* 1991; **12:** 1213–16.

23. Husain MM, Black KJ, Doraiswamy PM et al. Subcortical brain anatomy in anorexia and bulimia. *Biol Psychiatry* 1992; **31:** 735–8.

24. Giordano GD, Renzetti P, Parodi RC et al. Volume measurement with magnetic resonance imaging of hippocampus–amygdala formation in patients with anorexia nervosa. *J Endocr Invest* 2001; **24:** 510–14.

25. Katzman DK, Lambe EK, Mikulis DJ et al. Cerebral gray matter and white matter volume deficits in adolescent girls with anorexia nervosa. *J Pediatr* 1996; **129:** 794–803.

26. Katzman DK, Zipursky RB, Lambe EK, Mikulis DJ, A longitudinal magnetic resonance imaging study of brain changes in adolescents with anorexia nervosa. *Arch Pediatr Adolesc Med* 1997; **151:** 793–7.

27. Lambe EK, Katzman DK, Mikulis DJ et al. Cerebral gray matter volume deficits after weight recovery from anorexia nervosa. *Arch Gen Psychiatry* 1997; **54:** 537–42.

28. Roser W, Bubl R, Buergin D et al. Metabolic changes in the brain of patients with anorexia and bulimia nervosa as detected by proton magnetic resonance spectroscopy. *Int J Eat Disord* 1999; **26:** 119–36.

29. Schlemmer HP, Mockel R, Marcus A et al. Proton magnetic resonance spectroscopy in acute, juvenile anorexia nervosa. *Psychiatry Res* 1998; **82:** 171–9.

30. Hoffman GW, Ellinwood EH Jr, Rockwell WJ et al. Cerebral atrophy in bulimia. *Biol Psychiatry* 1989; **25:** 894–902.

31. Krieg JC, Backmund H, Pirke KM, Cranial computed tomography findings in bulimia. *Acta Psychiatr Scand* 1987; **75:** 144–9.

32. Katzman DK, Christensen B, Young AR, Zipursky RB. Starving the brain: Structural abnormalities and cognitive impairment in adolescents with anorexia nervosa. *Semin Clin Neuropsychiatry* 2001; **6:** 146–52.

33. Gunston GD, Burkimsher D, Malan H, Sive AA, Reversible cerebral shrinkage in kwashiorkor: an MRI study. *Arch Dis Child* 1992; **67:** 1030–2.

34. Boyar RM, Hellman L, Roffwarg H et al. Cortisol secretion and metabolism in anorexia nervosa. *N Engl J Med* 1977; **296:** 190–3.

35. Doerr P, Fichter M, Pirke KM, Lund R, Relationship between weight gain and hypothalamic pituitary adrenal function in patients with anorexia nervosa. *J Steroid Biochem* 1980; **13:** 529–37.

36. Walsh BT, Katz JL, Levin J et al. Adrenal activity in anorexia nervosa. *Psychosom Med* 1978; **40:** 499–506.

37. Sapolsky RM, Glucocorticoids and hippocampal atrophy in neuropsychiatric disorders. *Arch Gen Psychiatry* 2000; **57:** 925–35.

38. Coiro V, Volpi R, Marchesi C et al. Abnormal growth hormone and cortisol, but not thyroid-stimulating hormone, responses to an intravenous glucose tolerance test in normal-weight, bulimic women. *Psychoneuroendocrinology* 1992; **17:** 639–45.

39. Connan F, Treasure J, Neuroendocrinology of eating disorders. In: (D'haenen H, den Boer JA, Willner P, eds) *Biological Psychiatry*. (Chichester: Wiley and Sons, 2002.)

40. Fichter MM, Pirke KM, Pollinger J et al. Disturbances in the hypothalamo-pituitary-adrenal and other neuroendocrine axes in bulimia. *Biol Psychiatry* 1990; **27:** 1021–37.

41. Krieg JC, Lauer C, Leinsinger G et al. Brain morphology and regional cerebral blood flow in anorexia nervosa. *Biol Psychiatry* 1989; **25:** 1041–8.

42. Lauer C, Neuropsychology findings. In: (D'haenen H, den Boer JA, Willner P, eds) *Biological Psychiatry*. 2002.

43. Lauer CJ, Gorzewski B, Gerlinghoff M et al. Neuropsychological assessments before and after treatment in patients with anorexia nervosa and bulimia nervosa. *J Psychiatr Res* 1999; **33:** 129–38.

44. Szmukler GI, Andrewes D, Kingston K et al. Neuropsychological impairment in anorexia nervosa: before and after refeeding. *J Clin Exp Neuropsychol* 1992; **14:** 347–52.

45. Tchanturia K, Serpell L, Troop N, Treasure J, Perceptual illusions in eating disorders: rigid and fluctuating styles. *J Behavioral Therapy* 2001; **32:** 107–15.

46. Tchanturia K, Morris RG, Surguladze S, Treasure J. An examination of perceptual and cognitive set shifting tasks in acute anorexia nervosa and following recovery. *Eating and Weight Disorders* 2002; **7:** 312–15.

47. Uher R, Treasure J, Campbell CI, Neuroanatomical bases of eating disorders. In: (D'haenen, den Boer JA, Willner P, eds) *Biological Psychiatry*. (Chichester: John Wiley and Sons, 2002.)

48. Braun CM, Chouinard MJ, Is anorexia nervosa a neuropsychological disease? *Neuropsychol Rev* 1992; **3:** 171–212.

49. Takano A, Shiga T, Kitagawa N et al. Abnormal neuronal network in anorexia nervosa studied with I-123-IMP SPECT. *Psychiatry Res* 2001; **107:** 45–50.

50. Herholz K, Krieg JC; Emrich HM et al. Regional cerebral glucose metabolism in anorexia nervosa measured by positron emission tomography. *Biol Psychiatry* 1987; **22:** 43–51.

51. Delvenne V, Lotstra F, Goldman S et al. Brain hypometabolism of glucose in anorexia nervosa: a PET scan study. *Biol Psychiatry* 1995; **37:** 161–9.

52. Delvenne V, Goldman S, De MV, Lotstra F, Brain glucose metabolism in eating disorders assessed by positron emission tomography. *Int J Eat Disord* 1999; **25:** 29–37.

53. Naruo T, Nakabeppu Y, Sagiyama K et al. Decreases in blood perfusion of the anterior cingulate gyri in Anorexia Nervosa Restricters assessed by SPECT image analysis. *BMC Psychiatry* 2001; **1:** 2.

54. Nozoe S, Naruo T, Yonekura R et al. Comparison of regional cerebral blood flow in patients with eating disorders. *Brain Res Bull* 1995; **36:** 251–5.

55. Gordon CM, Dougherty DD, Fischman AJ et al. Neural substrates of anorexia nervosa: a behavioral challenge study with positron emission tomography. *J Pediatr* 2001; **139:** 51–7.

56. Rastam M, Bjure J, Vestergren E et al. Regional cerebral blood flow in weight-restored anorexia nervosa: a preliminary study. *Dev Med Child Neurol* 2001; **43:** 239–42.

57. Andreason PJ, Altemus M, Zametkin AJ et al. Regional cerebral glucose metabolism in bulimia nervosa. *Am J Psychiatry* 1992; **149:** 1506–13.

58. Wu JC, Hagman J, Buchsbaum MS et al. Greater left cerebral hemispheric metabolism in bulimia assessed by positron emission tomography. *Am J Psychiatry* 1990; **147:** 309–12.

59. Hagman JO, Buchsbaum MS, Wu JC et al. Comparison of regional brain metabolism in bulimia nervosa and affective disorder assessed with positron emission tomography. *J Affect Disord* 1990; **19:** 153–62.

60. Rolls ET. *Brain and Emotions* (Oxford: Oxford University Press, 1999.)

61. LaBar KS, Gitelman DR, Parrish TB et al. Hunger selectively modulates corticolimbic activation to food stimuli in humans. *Behav Neurosci* 2001; **115:** 493–500.

62. O'Doherty J, Rolls ET, Francis S et al. Sensory-specific satiety-related olfactory activation of the human orbitofrontal cortex. *Neuroreport* 2000; **11:** 399–403.

63. Tataranni PA, Gautier JF, Chen K et al. Neuroanatomical correlates of hunger and satiation in humans using positron emission tomography. *Proc Natl Acad Sci U S A* 1999; **96:** 4569–74.

64. Small DM, Zatorre RJ, Dagher A et al. Changes in brain activity related to eating chocolate: From pleasure to aversion. *Brain* 2001; **124:** 1720–33.

65. Gautier JF, Chen K, Uecker A et al. Regions of the human brain affected during a liquid-meal taste perception in the fasting state: a positron emission tomography study. *Am J Clin Nutr* 1999; **70:** 806–10.

66. Karhunen LJ, Lappalainen RI, Vanninen EJ et al. Regional cerebral blood flow during food exposure in obese and normal-weight women. *Brain* 1997; **120 (Pt 9):** 1675–84.

67. Gautier JF, Chen K, Salbe AD et al. Differential brain responses to satiation in obese and lean men. *Diabetes* 2000; **49:** 838–46.

68. Karhunen LJ, Vanninen EJ, Kuikka JT et al. Regional cerebral blood flow during exposure to food in obese binge eating women. *Psychiatry Res* 2000; **99:** 29–42.

69. Nozoe S, Naruo T, Nakabeppu Y et al. Changes in regional cerebral blood flow in patients with anorexia nervosa detected through single photon emission tomography imaging. *Biol Psychiatry* 1993; **34:** 578–80.

70. Naruo T, Nakabeppu Y, Sagiyama K et al. Characteristic regional cerebral blood flow patterns in anorexia nervosa patients with binge/purge behavior. *Am J Psychiatry* 2000; **157:** 1520–2.

71. Uher R, Murphy T, Ng V et al. Perception of food and emotional stimuli in anorexia nervosa. *Neuroimage* 2001; **13:** S1022.

72. Ellison Z, Foong J, Howard R et al. Functional anatomy of calorie fear in anorexia nervosa. *Lancet* 1998; **352:** 1192.

73. Gordon CM, Dougherty DD, Fischman AJ et al. Neuroanatomy of human appetitive function: A positron emission tomography investigation. *Int J Eat Disord* 2000; **27:** 163–71.

74. Drobes DJ, Miller EJ, Hillman CH et al. Food deprivation and emotional reactions to food cues: implications for eating disorders. *Biol Psychol* 2001; **57:** 153–77.

75. Brewerton TD, Toward a unified theory of serotonin dysregulation in eating and related disorders. *Psychoneuroendocrinology* 1995; **20:** 561–90.

76. Ericsson M, Poston WS, Foreyt JP, Common biological pathways in eating disorders and obesity. *Addict Behav* 1996; **21:** 733–43.

77. Kaye WH, Gendall K, Kye C, The role of the central nervous system in the psycho-neuroendocrine disturbances of anorexia and bulimia nervosa. *Psychiatr Clin North Am* 1998; **21:** 381–96.

78. Frank GK, Kaye WH, Meltzer CC et al. Reduced 5-HT2A receptor binding after recovery from anorexia nervosa. *Biol Psychiatry* 2002; **52:** 896–906.

79. Kaye WH, Frank GK, Meltzer CC et al. Altered serotonin 2A receptor activity in women who have recovered from bulimia nervosa. *Am J Psychiatry* 2001; **158:** 1152–5.

80. Tauscher J, Pirker W, Willeit M et al. [123I]beta-CIT and single photon emission computed tomography reveal reduced brain serotonin transporter availability in bulimia nervosa. *Biol Psychiatry* 2001; **49:** 326–32.

81. Willeit M, Praschak-Rieder N, Neumeister A et al. [123I]-beta-CIT SPECT imaging shows reduced brain serotonin transporter availability in drug-free depressed patients with seasonal affective disorder. *Biol Psychiatry* 2000; **47:** 482–9.

82. Noble EP, St Jeor ST, Ritchie T et al. D2 dopamine receptor gene and obesity. *Int J Eat Disord* 1994; **15:** 205–17.

83. Noble EP, Addiction and its reward process through polymorphisms of the D2 dopamine receptor gene: a review. *Eur Psychiatry* 2000; **15:** 79–89.

84. Wang GJ, Volkow ND, Logan J et al. Brain dopamine and obesity. *Lancet* 2001; **357:** 354–7.

85. Yasuno F, Suhara T, Sudo, Y et al. Relation among dopamine D(2) receptor binding, obesity and personality in normal human subjects. *Neurosci Lett* 2001; **300:** 59–61.

7. Neuroimaging and the Pathophysiology of Obsessive-Compulsive Disorder (OCD)

Sanjaya Saxena

Introduction

Obsessive-compulsive disorder (OCD) is a common neuropsychiatric illness characterized by intrusive, repetitive thoughts and ritualistic behaviors that cause marked distress. Common symptoms include harm-related fears with checking compulsions; contamination fears with cleaning compulsions; symmetry obsessions with arranging and repeating compulsions; and hoarding and saving compulsions. OCD affects 2–3% of the population worldwide[1] and can cause significant disability and functional impairment.[2] Effective treatments for OCD include serotonin reuptake inhibitor (SRI) medications[3] and cognitive–behavioral therapy (CBT).[4] Because OCD symptoms tend to be chronic, relatively consistent over time, and reliably reproducible, it has been possible to study them with a variety of neuroimaging techniques in an effort to determine how the brain mediates their expression.[5]

This chapter provides an updated review and analysis of the neuroimaging studies in OCD published to date. It first reviews studies of brain structure in OCD using computerized tomography (CT) and magnetic resonance imaging (MRI), then moves to studies of brain function using single photon emission computed tomography (SPECT), positron emission tomography (PET), functional MRI (fMRI), and magnetic resonance spectroscopy (MRS). As functional imaging studies have provided the most consistent and informative data about the pathophysiology of OCD, they are examined in greater detail. Then follows a discussion of the functional neuroanatomy of frontal–subcortical brain circuits elucidated by basic research. Finally, a theoretical model of the pathophysiology of OCD that is supported both by neuroimaging findings and basic research is presented. This model describes how the symptomatic expression of OCD may be mediated by abnormally elevated activity along specific frontal–subcortical brain circuits,[6] and how successful treatments may ameliorate symptoms. Of necessity, this review repeats much from earlier reviews.[7–12]

Studies of brain structure in obsessive-compulsive disorder (OCD) patients

CT studies of OCD

CT studies were the first to suggest brain abnormalities in OCD but did not provide consistent findings (see Table 7.1). Two CT studies[13,14] found that OCD patients had a significantly larger ventricle: brain matter ratio (VBR) – an index of brain atrophy – than controls, while one study found no differences in ventricular volumes between groups.[15] Another CT study found that the volume of the caudate nucleus was significantly smaller in male adolescents with childhood-onset OCD subjects than in male controls,[16] a finding that would later be replicated by some, but not all, MRI studies of OCD.

MRI studies of OCD

Compared with CT, MRI provides superior spatial resolution, distinction between gray and white matter, and visualization of neuroanatomical structures in multiple planes. As with CT, few consistent findings have emerged from MRI studies of OCD (see Table 7.1 for summary), although several studies have found abnormalities in the basal ganglia, orbitofrontal cortex (OFC), anterior cingulate gyrus (AC), and thalamus, structures also implicated in the pathophysiology of OCD by functional neuroimaging studies.

Several MRI studies have found abnormal volumes of basal ganglia structures in OCD patients compared with normal controls, including greater volumes of the right caudate nucleus and a loss of the normal left–right caudate asymmetry,[17] smaller caudate nucleus volumes and enlarged ventricles,[18] and smaller putamen volumes and larger third ventricles.[19] Decreased striatal volumes have been found to correlate with OCD symptom severity.[19] However, two other MRI studies found no differences in caudate volumes between OCD subjects and controls.[20,21]

The heterogeneity of structural neuroimaging findings in OCD may reflect heterogeneity in the disorder itself. Recent studies suggest that the discrepant basal ganglia volume findings in OCD may be due to different

Table 7.1 Structural imaging studies in obsessive-compulsive disorder (OCD)

Author and year (ref)	Technique	Subjects	Results
Insel et al 1983 (13)	CT	10 OCD patients 10 normal controls	OCD = controls
Behar et al 1984 (14)	CT	17 OCD patients 16 controls	VBR larger in OCD subjects
Luxenberg et al 1988 (16)	CT	10 male OCD adolescents 10 male control adolescents	Decreased caudate volume in OCD
Stein et al 1993 (15)	CT	24 patients	Increased ventricular volume in OCD
Garber et al 1989 (27)	MRI	32 treated OCD patients 14 normal controls	T1 abnormalities in anterior cingulate gyrus
Kellner et al 1991 (20)	MRI	12 OCD subjects 12 matched controls	Caudate volume in OCD = controls
Scarone et al 1992 (17)	MRI	20 treated OCD patients 16 normal controls	Increased right caudate volume in OCD
Robinson et al 1995 (18)	MRI	26 OCD patients 26 healthy controls	Decreased caudate volume in OCD
Aylward et al 1996 (21)	MRI	24 OCD patients 21 controls	OCD = controls for all structures
Jenike et al 1996 (28); and Grachev et al 1998 (29)	MRI	10 female OCD patients 10 female controls	Increased total cortex volume and decreased white matter in OCD Right frontal cortex volumes negatively correlated with non-verbal recall
Rosenberg et al 1997 (19)	MRI	19 children with OCD 19 healthy controls	Decreased striatal volume and larger third ventricles in OCD
Rosenberg et al 1997 (34); MacMaster et al 1999 (35)	MRI	21 children with OCD 21 healthy controls	Enlarged corpus callosum in OCD Decreased signal intensity in anterior corpus callosum

Table 7.1 Structural imaging studies in obsessive-compulsive disorder (OCD) – *Continued*

Author and year (ref)	Technique	Subjects	Results
Szezko et al 2000 (31)	MRI	26 OCD patients 26 healthy controls	Decreased orbitofrontal cortex and right amygdala volumes in OCD
Giedd et al 2000 (23)	MRI	34 children with streptococcus-related OCD and/or tics 82 healthy children	Larger caudate, putamen, and globus pallidus in streptococcus-related OCD/tics
Peterson et al 2000 (24)	MRI	113 patients with OCD, ADHD, or tic disorder 34 healthy controls	Anti-streptococcal antibody titers predicted higher putamen and globus pallidus volumes in OCD and ADHD
Gilbert et al 2000 (33)	MRI	21 never-treated children with OCD 10 OCD after paroxetine treatment 21 healthy controls	Larger thalamic volume in OCD; decreased after paroxetine treatment
Rosenberg et al 2000 (36)	MRI	11 children with OCD, before and after CBT	No change in thalamic volumes with treatment
Kim et al 2001 (32)	MRI	25 OCD patients 25 healthy controls	Increased gray matter density in left orbitofrontal cortex, thalamus, hypothalamus, and right insula in OCD

ADHD, Attention deficit hyperactivity disorder; CBT, cognitive–behavioral therapy; CT, computerized tomography; MRI, magnetic resonance imaging; VBR, ventricle: brain matter ratio.

etiologies in different subgroups of OCD patients. It has been suggested that there is a distinct subgroup of patients whose OCD is a pediatric auto-immune neuropsychiatric disorder associated with streptococcal infection (PANDAS),[22] and that this subgroup has basal ganglia enlargement due to antibody-mediated inflammation. Enlarged caudate, putamen, and globus pallidus volumes have been seen in children with streptococcus-related OCD,[23] and larger volumes of putamen and globus pallidus have been associated with higher antistreptolysin O antibody titers in subjects with OCD and/or attention deficit hyperactivity disorder (ADHD).[24] Conversely, those structural imaging studies of OCD patients that found *decreased* caudate volumes might have included more patients with comorbid tic disorders such as Tourette's syndrome (TS) or childhood-onset OCD, who may have more developmental brain abnormalities than other OCD patients. Some studies have found reduced caudate volumes in patients with TS,[25,26] and since patients with tic disorders have not always been excluded from imaging studies of OCD, they may have skewed their findings.

MRI studies have also found various abnormalities in cerebral cortical structures, the thalamus, and limbic structures in OCD patients, including T1-mapping abnormalities in the AC,[27] greater total cerebral cortical volumes,[28,29] enlarged AC volumes,[30] reduced OFC (including gray and white matter) and right amygdala volumes,[31] reduction in the normal right–left asymmetry in amygdala volumes,[31] increased gray matter density in multiple cortical regions,[32] and enlarged thalami.[33] These abnormalities might indicate widespread alteration of the programmed neuronal death that normally occurs during brain development, or reduced myelination in the brains of patients with OCD.[28] Abnormalities have also been found in white matter structures, including significantly lower volumes of total cerebral and cerebellar white matter,[28] but enlarged volumes[28,34] and decreased signal intensities in the corpus callosum (CC),[35] indicating increased myelination and greater concentration of white matter in the CC of OCD patients.

A few recent studies have investigated whether structural abnormalities seen in OCD patients change with successful treatment. In children with OCD, thalamic volumes have been found to decline significantly after 12 weeks of paroxetine treatment,[33] but not after treatment with CBT.[36] In patients with refractory OCD treated with anterior cingulotomy, caudate volumes decreased after surgery.[37] These results suggest that even short-term medication and surgical treatment can produce structural changes in the size of brain structures.

Functional imaging techniques

Four different functional neuroimaging study designs have been used to investigate the pathophysiology of OCD: (1) measuring cerebral activity in OCD patients versus normal controls with functional brain imaging scans done in neutral or baseline states; (2) scanning OCD patients before and after treatment to measure cerebral activity changes that correspond to treatment response; (3) scanning patients while actively provoking their OCD symptoms; and (4) scanning OCD patients while they perform a cognitive activation task.

Most early functional neuroimaging studies of OCD used PET or SPECT, which employ radioisotope-labeled tracers to measure glucose metabolism or blood flow. PET, which offers better spatial resolution than SPECT, employs the radiolabeled tracers [^{18}F]fluorodeoxyglucose (FDG) and [^{11}C]deoxyglucose to measure glucose uptake and metabolism, and ^{15}O CO_2 or H_2O for regional cerebral blood flow (rCBF). In non-starvation conditions, glucose is by far the predominant energy substrate in the human brain, and its uptake has been shown to be a highly sensitive indicator of cerebral function. Under most circumstances, rCBF is highly correlated with glucose metabolism. SPECT uses tracers to estimate rCBF, including technetium-99m (Tc-99m)-d,l-hexamethylpropyleneamineoxime (HMPAO), Tc-99m-ethylcisteinate dimer (ECD), and the inhaled gas xenon-133 (^{133}Xe). Although HMPAO uptake usually is interpreted as a valid method of estimating the blood flow of one brain structure relative to that of another, HMPAO uptake is not consistently correlated with rCBF, especially in the basal ganglia.[38] Readers interested in more detail are referred to Chapter 1 and elsewhere.[39,40] Recent functional neuroimaging studies of OCD have employed magnetic resonance techniques such as MRS and fMRI. MRS measures concentrations of large molecules, such as N-acetylaspartate (NAA), glutamate, myoinositol, and choline in brain tissue by acquiring proton (^{1}H) spectra from these molecules following a magnetic resonance pulse.[41] fMRI measures correlates of regional brain activation by detecting changes in the blood oxygen-level dependent (BOLD) signal in the brain during different clinical states or cognitive tasks.

Functional neuroimaging studies comparing obsessive-compulsive disorder (OCD) patients to normal controls at baseline

Nine PET studies to date have compared subjects with OCD to controls (see Table 7.2 for details). Five of the nine studies found elevated metabolism or rCBF in the OFC (Figure 7.1),[42–46] while three found elevated activity in the basal ganglia,[42,43,47] three found increased thalamic activity,[45,47,48] and two found elevated metabolism in the AC.[45,47] Elevated activity has also been found in other parts of the prefrontal cortex.[42–46] One study had results at

Table 7.2 Baseline functional neuroimaging studies of obsessive-compulsive disorder (OCD) patients versus normal controls

Author and year (ref)	Subjects	Technique	Results in OCD
Baxter et al 1985 (42)	14 OCD (nine with depression) 14 depressed 14 controls	FDG-PET	Increased orbital gyri and caudate in OCD
Baxter et al 1988 (43)	10 non-depressed OCD 10 controls	FDG-PET	Increased orbital gyri and caudate in OCD
Nordahl et al 1989 (44)	Eight OCD 30 controls	FDG-PET	Increased orbitofrontal, decreased parietal . cortex
Swedo et al 1989 (45)	18 OCD childhood onset 18 controls	FDG-PET	Increased orbitofrontal, prefrontal, anterior cingulate right thalamus, cerebellum
Martinot et al 1990 (49)	16 OCD Eight controls	FDG-PET	Decreased lateral prefrontal cortex in OCD
Sawle et al 1991 (46)	Six with obsessional slowness Six controls	^{15}O H_2O-PET	Increased orbitofrontal, and premotor cortex
Perani et al 1995 (47)	11 OCD 15 controls	FDG-PET	Increased cingulate, lenticular nuclei, and thalamus in OCD
Saxena et al 2001 (48)	27 OCD alone 17 OCD + depression 27 depression alone 17 controls	FDG-PET	Increased thalamus in OCD alone; decreased left hippocampus in depression alone and OCD + depression
Machlin et al 1991 (57)	10 OCD Eight controls	HMPAO-SPECT	Increased medial frontal cortex in OCD
Rubin et al 1992 (38)	10 OCD 10 controls	^{133}Xe-SPECT and HMPAO-SPECT	Xe: OCD = control HMPAO: increased parietal and frontal cortex, decreased caudate

Table 7.2 Baseline functional neuroimaging studies of obsessive-compulsive disorder (OCD) patients versus normal controls – *Continued*

Author and year (ref)	Subjects	Technique	Results in OCD
Adams et al 1989 (53)	11 OCD	HMPAO-SPECT	Decreased left basal ganglia
Edmonstone et al 1994 (52)	12 OCD 12 depressed 12 controls	HMPAO-SPECT	Decreased basal ganglia in OCD
Lucey et al 1995 (54)	30 OCD 30 controls	HMPAO-SPECT	Decreased superior frontal, inferior frontal, temporal, parietal cortex, right caudate, and right thalamus in OCD
Lucey et al 1995 (54) and 1997 (55)	15 OCD 16 PTSD 15 panic 15 controls	HMPAO-SPECT	Decreased right caudate and bilateral superior frontal cortex in OCD and PTSD
Crespo-Facorro et al 1999 (56)	27 OCD (seven with tics) 16 controls	HMPAO-SPECT	Decreased right OFC in OCD without tics
Busatto et al 2000 (59)	26 OCD (13 early onset, 13 later onset) 22 controls	ECD-SPECT	Decreased right OFC and left DLPFC, but OFC activity correlated with OCD severity. Decreased left AC, right OFC, and right thalamus in early onset OCD
Alptekin et al 2001 (58)	Nine OCD Six controls	HMPAO-SPECT	Increased right thalamus, left frontotemporal cortex, and bilateral OFC
Ebert et al 1996 (67)	12 OCD Six controls	MRS	Decreased NAA in right striatum and right AC
Bartha et al 1998 (68)	13 OCD 13 controls	MRS	Decreased NAA in left striatum
Ohara et al 1999	12 OCD 12 controls	MRS	OCD = control in lenticular nuclei NAA

Table 7.2 Baseline functional neuroimaging studies of obsessive-compulsive disorder (OCD) patients versus normal controls – Continued

Author and year (ref)	Subjects	Technique	Results in OCD
Fitzgerald et al 2000 (70); Rosenberg et al 2001 (69)	11 OCD children 11 control children	MRS	Increased choline (Cho) and decreased NAA/Cho in bilateral medial thalamus

AC, Anterior cingulate gyrus; DLPFC, dorsolateral prefrontal cortex; ECD, Tc-99m-ethylcisteinate dimer; FDG, [¹⁸F]-fluorodeoxyglucose; HMPAO, d,l-hexamethylpropyleneamineoxime; MRS, magnetic resonance spectroscopy; NAA, N-acetylaspartate; OFC, orbitofrontal cortex; PET, position emission tomography; PTSD, post-traumatic stress disorder; SPECT, single photon emission computed tomography; ¹³³Xe, xenon-133.

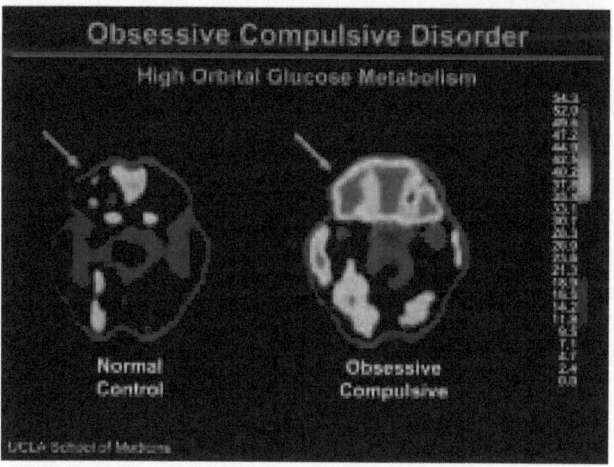

Figure 7.1 *Positron emission tomography (PET) images showing significantly elevated glucose metabolism in the orbitofrontal cortex in OCD patients, compared with normal controls. (Reproduced from Baxter et al. Arch Gen Psychiatry 1985; **44:** 211–18.[42])*

odds with those of the above PET studies, finding *lower* absolute metabolic rates in OCD subjects than in controls in all brain regions examined, including the lateral prefrontal cortex.[49] These results resemble PET findings in depressed OCD subjects[48,50] and may have been due to significant depressive symptoms in their patient sample.[51] Depressive symptoms strongly influence cerebral activity in OCD patients and are associated with *reduced* metabolism in caudate, thalamus, and limbic structures.[48]

SPECT studies of OCD have been less consistent than PET studies in finding increased activity compared to normal controls (Table 7.2). In the SPECT studies published to date that have compared OCD patients to normal controls at baseline, the most common finding has been *decreased* HMPAO uptake in the basal ganglia.[38,52–56] Comparisons of prefrontal cortical and thalamic perfusion have shown both increased[38,57,58] and decreased[56,57,59] HMPAO uptake. Some of the variability in the results of the SPECT studies of OCD may be due to differences in rates of comorbid depression between studies. Several of the studies included patients with major depression,[56,59] and depression severity was significantly negatively correlated with caudate activity.[48,55] Another important factor contributing to findings of caudate hypoperfusion in SPECT studies may be the presence of TS, other tic disorders, or comorbid ADHD in OCD subjects, since ventral striatal hypometabolism, hypoperfusion, and low HMPAO uptake have been found in several SPECT studies of TS and ADHD.[60–65] Caution must be exercised before equating HMPAO uptake with rCBF or abnormal glucose metabolism in a pathologic state such as OCD, in which the blood–brain barrier could be abnormal, causing dissociation of perfusion and metabolism.

Most MRS studies of OCD have measured NAA, thought to be a marker of neuronal density that is reduced in disease states that involve neuronal loss or dysfunction.[66] Low relative levels of NAA have been found in the striatum[67,68] and AC[68] in OCD patients compared with normal control subjects, while elevated choline concentrations[69] and reduced NAA/choline ratios[70] correlating with OCD severity have been found in the medial thalami of children with OCD. Elevated glutamate concentrations have also been found in the caudate nuclei of pediatric OCD patients.[71] Thus, MRS studies have found neurochemical abnormalities in the very same brain structures found to have structural and functional alterations in OCD.

The various baseline studies of OCD patients compared to normal controls consistently indicate elevated activity in the OFC, with less consistent abnormalities in the caudate nuclei, thalamus, and AC, which also show neurochemical alterations suggestive of neuronal dysfunction.

Cerebral correlates of obsessive-compulsive disorder (OCD) symptom factors

Although standard diagnostic classifications consider OCD to be a single diagnostic entity, it has become clear that several different OCD symptom factors exist.[72,73] Large factor analyses of OCD symptoms[73] have yielded four principal symptom factors: (1) aggressive, sexual, and religious obsessions with checking compulsions; (2) symmetry obsessions with ordering, arranging, and repeating compulsions; (3) contamination obsessions with washing and cleaning compulsions; and (4) hoarding, saving, and collecting symptoms. These symptom factors appear to show different inheritance patterns. Despite this phenotypic heterogeneity, virtually all prior neurobiological and treatment studies of OCD have grouped patients with diverse symptom patterns together.

Very few neuroimaging studies have examined the neural correlates of specific OCD symptom factors. Rauch et al[74] found that the severity of factor 1 symptoms correlated significantly with rCBF in the bilateral striatum, while factor 2 symptoms had a trend toward *negative* correlation with rCBF in the right striatum. Factor 3 symptoms correlated with rCBF in the bilateral AC, left OFC, and other cortical areas. Saxena et al (unpublished data) found decreased cingulate gyrus metabolism in OCD patients with the compulsive hoarding syndrome, and found that AC metabolism was negatively correlated with the severity of factor 4 symptoms. Although these were preliminary results, they suggest that different OCD symptom clusters are mediated by quite different patterns of brain activity, raising the question of whether the heterogeneity in the findings of previous functional imaging studies of OCD could be accounted for by phenotypic variations between their subject pools. Moreover, patients with primary hoarding/saving symptoms have been underrepresented in most studies of OCD,[75] potentially skewing their results.

Functional neuroimaging studies of obsessive-compulsive disorder (OCD) patients before and after treatment

Functional neuroimaging studies done before and after treatment test hypotheses about the brain mediation of psychiatric symptoms by determining what changes in regional brain activity occur when patients respond to treatment, and what regional changes correlate best with symptomatic improvement. Such studies can also reveal differences in cerebral mechanisms of action between treatments. PET has been used to study OCD patients before and after treatment with SRIs, CBT, and neurosurgery. Of the 10 pre- and post-treatment PET studies of OCD published to date, eight have found pre- to post-treatment decreases in the OFC and/or caudate nuclei in responders to treatment,[76–83] while a few have found decreases in the AC[47,83] and thalamus[82]

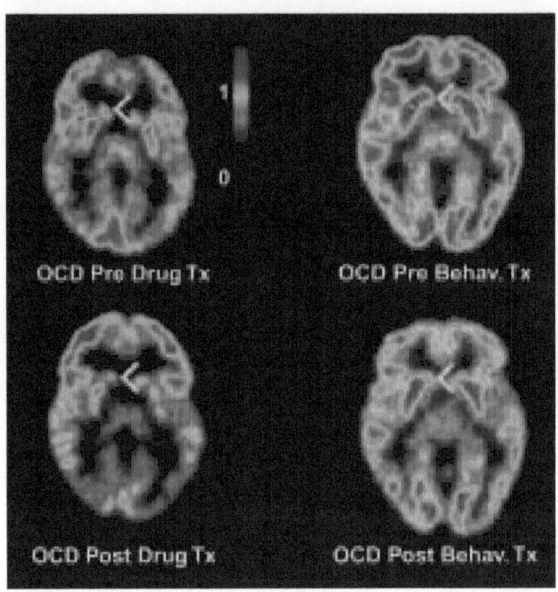

Figure 7.2 *Pre- and post-treatment positron emission tomography (PET) images of OCD patients treated with fluoxetine (left), and OCD patients treated with cognitive-behavioral therapy (right). Both patient groups showed similar significant decreases in right caudate metabolism with response to treatment. (Reproduced from Baxter et al. Arch Gen Psychiatry 1992; 49: 681–9.[80])*

(Table 7.3). These changes have generally not been seen in non-responders to treatment. SPECT studies of OCD patients before and after treatment have also shown significant decreases in frontal cortex activity after treatment with SRI medications.[84–86] The changes most strongly associated with OCD treatment response are decreases in the right caudate nucleus[80–83] and right antero-lateral OFC.[76,78] Moreover, these changes are specific to OCD and do not occur in patients with major depression[82] or other disorders treated with similar medications. MRS studies[71,87] found striking drops in glutamate resonance in the left caudate in 11 children with OCD after successful treatment with paroxetine. These changes are consistent with the glucose metabolic decreases seen with paroxetine treatment in FDG-PET studies of OCD,[82,83] and suggest that glutamate–serotonin interactions in the caudate may play a role in the pathophysiology and treatment of OCD. Thus, regardless of the type of imaging modality or the type of treatment used, pre- to post-treatment studies of OCD have consistently shown that OFC and caudate activity decreases with effective treatment.

A seminal study by Baxter et al[80] compared brain metabolic changes in OCD patients before and after treatment with either fluoxetine or CBT. In

Table 7.3 Pre- and post-treatment imaging studies in obsessive-compulsive disorder (OCD)

Author and year (ref)	Subjects/treatment	Technique	Results with treatment
Benkelfat et al 1990 (76)	Eight treated with clomipramine	FDG-PET	Decreased left caudate and OFC areas
Mindus et al 1991 (79)	Five treated with anterior capsulotomy	¹¹C-Glc-PET	Decreased caudate and OFC
Swedo et al 1992 (77)	13 subjects (eight on clomipramine, two on fluoxetine and three off medicine)	FDG-PET	Decreased bilateral OFC
Baxter et al 1992 (80)	Nine with fluoxetine, Nine with behavior therapy	FDG-PET	Decreased right caudate in responders to either treatment; loss of pathological correlations between OFC, caudate and thalamus
Perani et al 1995 (47)	Four with fluvoxamine, Two with fluoxetine Three with clomipramine	FDG-PET	Decreased cingulate
Schwartz et al 1996 (81)	18 treated with behavior therapy	FDG-PET	Decreased bilateral caudate in responders; loss of correlations between OFC, caudate, and thalamus
Saxena et al 1999 (78)	20 with paroxetine	FDG-PET	Decreased right caudate and right anterolateral OFC in responders
Saxena et al 2002 (82)	25 OCD 25 depression 16 OCD + depression (all treated with paroxetine) 16 controls	FDG-PET	OCD: decreased OFC, thalamus, right caudate Depress decreased VLPFC OCD + Depression increased caudate and putamen

Table 7.3 Pre- and post-treatment imaging studies in obsessive-compulsive disorder (OCD) – *Continued*

Author and year (ref)	Subjects/treatment	Technique	Results with treatment
Hansen et al 2002 (83)	20 OCD with paroxetine	FDG-PET	Decreased right caudate
Hoehn-Saric et al 1991 (84)	Six with fluoxetine	HMPAO-SPECT	Decreased medial frontal to whole cortex ratio
Rubin et al 1995 (85)	10 with clomipramine	^{133}Xe-SPECT and HMPAO-SPECT	Decreased cortical HMPAO uptake
Hoehn-Saric et al 2001 (86)	16 OCD + depression (nine with sertraline, seven with desipramine)	HMPAO-SPECT	Diffuse prefrontal decreases in responders
Rosenberg et al 2000 (71)	11 children with paroxetine	MRS	Decreased glutamate in left caudate

FDG, [^{18}F]-fluorodeoxyglucose; Glc, glucose; HMPAO, d,l-hexamethylpropyleneamineoxime; MRS, magnetic resonance spectroscopy; OFC, orbitofrontal cortex; PET, positron emission tomography; SPECT, single photon emission computed tomography; VLPFC, ventrolateral prefrontal cortex; ^{133}Xe, xenon-133.

both treatment groups, right caudate metabolic rates decreased significantly in responders but not in non-responders (Figure 7.2), showing that both pharmacological and non-pharmacological treatments can have significant effects on brain activity patterns that mediate neuropsychiatric disorders. When all responders to treatment were lumped together, significant correlations between metabolism in the right OFC, AC, caudate nucleus, and thalamus were found *before, but not after, treatment*. These correlations were not found in patients with unipolar depression or normal control subjects, suggesting that treatment-responsive OCD is characterized by abnormal, disease-specific, functional relationships between these brain regions only in the symptomatic state.[80] Successful treatment appears to disrupt the linkage of regional activity that existed before treatment.[76,80,81]

Pretreatment PET predictors of response to treatment

Functional imaging data has also been examined to determine if pretreatment regional brain metabolism predicts treatment response. Lower pretreatment glucose metabolism in the OFC has been associated with better responses to the SRI clomipramine,[77] fluoxetine,[88] and paroxetine.[78] Response to paroxetine has also been correlated with higher pretreatment metabolism[89] and elevated glutamate concentrations[71] in the caudate nuclei. In contrast, higher pretreatment left OFC metabolism has been correlated with a response to CBT,[88] while higher pretreatment glucose metabolism in the right posterior cingulate cortex was associated with eventual improvement of OCD symptoms in patients who underwent anterior cingulotomy.[90] Taken together, these results suggest that OCD patients with different patterns of brain metabolism respond differentially to specific types of treatment (SRI versus CBT versus neurosurgery).

Neuroimaging studies of obsessive-compulsive disorder (OCD) symptom provocation

Perhaps the most direct information about brain–behavior relationships in OCD comes from symptom provocation studies that reveal patterns of brain activation occurring in real time, while patients are actively experiencing obsessions, anxiety, and urges to perform compulsive rituals. Symptom provocation studies have been conducted using two main methods: (1) comparing functional brain imaging scans acquired during exposure to a stimulus tailored specifically to induce each patient's OCD symptoms to scans acquired during exposure to an innocuous control stimulus, and (2) measuring changes in brain activity after exacerbating OCD symptoms with pharmacological challenges.

Exposure-based symptom provocation studies with PET[91–93] and fMRI[94,95] have consistently found increases in glucose metabolism or rCBF in the OFC, caudate, AC, and thalamus during the provoked state (Figure 7.3), more in patients than in controls, with less consistent activation of other cerebral cortical regions and limbic structures such as the amygdala,[94] hippocampus,[92,95] and insula[94] (see Table 7.4 for details). In some studies, OCD symptom severity correlated with activation of the OFC,[91,93,95] but different directions of correlation were found in different subregions of the OFC, suggesting that different subregions might play opposing roles in mediating and suppressing OCD symptoms, respectively.[91]

Symptom provocation studies using SPECT have yielded less consistent findings. One found that rCBF was somewhat increased during imaginal flooding, but decreased significantly during *in vivo* exposure to stimuli that induced OCD symptoms in superior cortical regions.[96] Two SPECT studies have measured changes in brain activity after exacerbating OCD symptoms

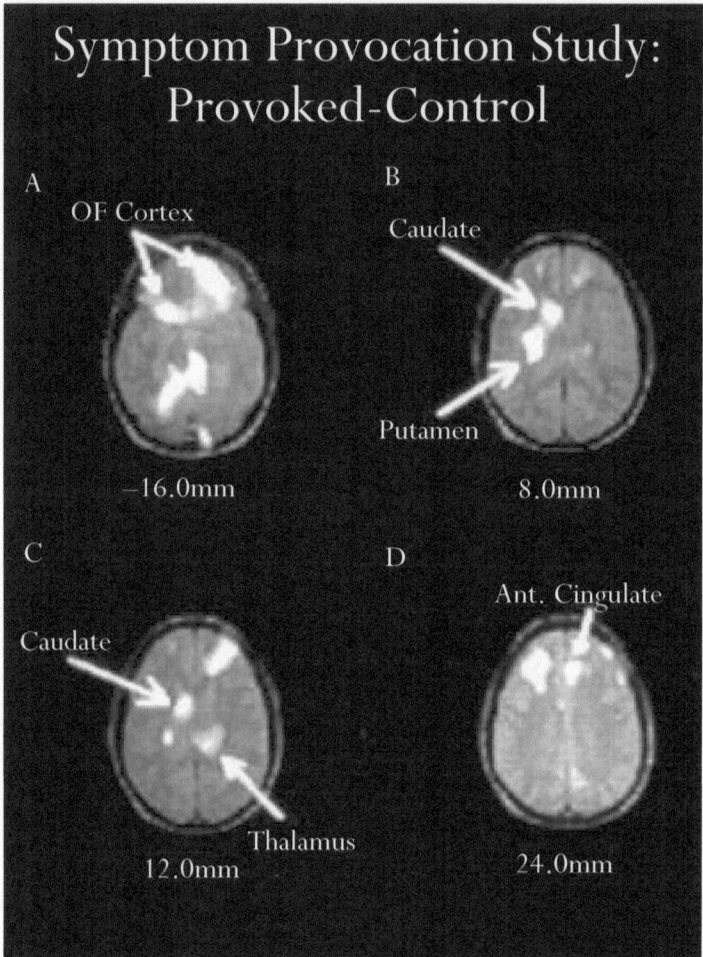

Figure 7.3 *Positron emission tomography (PET) images showing areas of significant activation of orbitofrontal cortex, caudate, putamen, thalamus, and anterior cingulate gyrus during OCD symptom provocation, compared to the control (resting) state. (Reproduced from Rauch et al. Arch Gen Psychiatry 1994; **51:** 62–70.[91])*

with pharmacological challenges with variable results: one used oral *m*-chlorophenylpiperazine (m-CPP)[97] (a serotonin receptor agonist), and the other used sumatriptan[98] (a serotonin 1d agonist). Again, the results of these SPECT studies are difficult to interpret because of the inherent limitations of the SPECT techniques used.

Taken together, the studies of OCD symptom provocation strongly link the expression of OCD symptoms with activation of the same brain areas

Table 7.4 Obsessive-compulsive disorder (OCD) symptom provocation studies

Author and year (ref)	Subjects	Technique	Results
Zohar et al 1989 (96)	10 OCD	^{133}Xe-SPECT	Increased rCBF in cortex with imaginal flooding, and decreased with in vivo exposure
Rauch et al 1994 (91)	8 OCD	^{15}O-CO$_2$-PET	Increased rCBF in R caudate, bilateral orbitofrontal, and left anterior cingulate
McGuire et al 1994 (92)	Four OCD	^{15}O CO$_2$-PET	OCD symptoms correlated with increased inferior frontal, posterior cingulate, striatum, GP, thalamus, hippocampus; decreased dorsal prefrontal and parietal-temporal cortex
Cottraux et al 1996 (93)	10 OCD 10 controls	^{15}O H$_2$O-PET	Greater increases in bilateral OFC in OCD than normals. Greater increases in thalamus and putamen in normals
Breiter et al 1996 (94)	13 OCD Six Controls	fMRI	Activation of bilateral OFC, anterior cingulate, frontal, and temporal cortex, amygdala, insula, lenticular nuclei, and right caudate
Adler et al 2000 (95)	Seven OCD	fMRI	Activation of OFC, DLPFC, temporal cortex, amygdala, hippocampus, and right AC
Hollander et al 1995 (97)	14 OCD challenged with m-CPP	^{133}Xe-SPECT	Increased global cortical perfusion
Stein et al 1999 (98)	14 OCD challenged with sumatriptan	HMPAO-SPECT	Increased right thalamus and putamen, decreased right caudate; symptom exacerbation associated with increased right cerebellum and decreased left inferior frontal and mid-frontal areas

AC, Anterior cingulate gyrus; DLPFC, dorsolateral prefrontal cortex; fMRI, functional magnetic resonance imaging; GP, globus pallidus; m-CPP, m-chlorophenylpiperazine; OFC, orbitofrontal cortex; PET, positron emission tomography; rCBF, regional cerebral blood flow; SPECT, single positron emission computed tomography; ^{133}Xe, xenon-133.

found to be overactive at baseline. These studies strengthen the hypothesis that OCD symptoms are mediated by increased activity in the frontal–subcortical circuits connecting these structures to one another.

Neuroimaging studies of cognitive activation in obsessive-compulsive disorder (OCD)

Cognitive activation studies attempt to delineate the pathophysiology of a disorder by finding abnormalities in regional brain activation during specific cognitive tasks. All cognitive activation studies comparing OCD patients to controls published thus far have shown abnormal brain activation patterns in OCD patients (Table 7.5). PET[99] and fMRI[100] studies of OCD patients

Table 7.5 Cognitive activation studies in obsessive-compulsive disorder (OCD)

Author and year (ref)	Subjects/task	Tracer	Results
Rauch et al 1997 (99)	Nine females with OCD Nine female controls Implicit sequence learning	^{15}O CO_2-PET and fMRI	Controls activated inferior striatum; but OCD patients activated medial temporal lobe
Lucey et al 1997 (102)	19 OCD 19 controls	HMPAO-SPECT	Null sorts correlated with rCBF in left inferior frontal cortex and caudate
Pujol et al 1999 (103)	20 OCD 20 controls	fMRI	Greater left inferior frontal cortex activation and defective suppression of activation in OCD
Rauch et al 2001 (100)	Six females with OCD 10 female controls	fMRI	Controls activated inferior striatum; OCD patients activated medial temporal lobe

fMRI, Functional magnetic resonance imaging; HMPAO, d, l-hexamethylpropyleneamineoxime; PET, positron emission tomography; rCBF, regional cerebral blood flow; SPECT, single positron emission computed tomography.

versus control subjects performing an implicit (procedural) sequence learning task have found that controls activated the bilateral inferior striatum and deactivated the thalamus, whereas OCD patients showed no changes in either the inferior striatum or thalamus, but instead showed bilateral mesial temporal activation. These results suggest that OCD patients have cortico–striatal–thalamic dysfunction, and so access brain systems involved in explicit memory[101] for tasks that normal controls would process implicitly, without conscious awareness. Another study showed that OCD patients made more errors than controls during performance of the Wisconsin Card Sort Task (WCST), which tests the ability to shift cognitive set and executive functions. The number of errors was significantly correlated with the rCBF in the left inferior frontal cortex and left caudate.[102] OCD patients were also found to have significantly greater frontal cortical activation than controls during a phonologically guided word-generation task, and a defective suppression of this activation during the following rest period.[103] This area of investigation into OCD is in its infancy and much more research will be required to reveal consistent links between symptoms, cognitive deficits, and brain activity abnormalities in OCD.

Summary of functional neuroimaging findings in obsessive-compulsive disorder (OCD)

Although not all studies agree, review of the OCD functional brain imaging literature reveals a remarkable amount of data suggesting abnormalities in OFC, caudate nuclei, and thalamus, linked by well-described neuroanatomical circuits.[104] The great majority of studies provide evidence for elevated activity in these structures in the untreated state that consistently decreases with response to treatment but is increased with symptom provocation. Several studies suggest a preferential role for the right caudate nucleus in mediating OCD symptoms and/or the response to pharmacotherapy. The caudate nucleus has been found to have baseline structural, neurochemical, and functional abnormalities in OCD. Caudate activity decreased after treatment of OCD with CMI (clomipramine), fluoxetine, paroxetine, CBT, and neurosurgery, but increased with symptom provocation. Further, recent studies have shown a failure of caudate activation during implicit sequence learning in OCD. Pathological correlations of glucose metabolic rates (or rCBF rates) in the caudate, OFC and thalamus characterize the symptomatic state of OCD, and are abolished by successful treatment. Although less consistently, functional neuroimaging data also support the involvement of the AC, amygdala, and related limbic structures in OCD. Differences between studies may be due to symptomatic differences between subject pools, differences between the treatments used, different duration of treatment, different scanning conditions, and different methods of localizing brain regions.

Neuroanatomy of frontal–subcortical brain circuits

Alexander et al[104] described a series of discrete, parallel, neuroanatomical circuits connecting the prefrontal cortex, basal ganglia, and thalamus. Many frontal–subcortical circuits exist, originating in nearly every part of the cerebral cortex and projecting through different subcompartments of the basal ganglia and thalamus. The various frontal–subcortical circuits subserve different behavioral functions and appear to mediate the symptomatic expression of several neuropsychiatric syndromes.[6,7]

Figure 7.4(a) presents a diagram of the classical conceptualization of frontal–subcortical circuitry. Classically, each of these circuits was described as having two loops: a direct pathway and an indirect pathway. In primates, the direct pathway projects from the cerebral cortex to the striatum to the internal segment of the globus pallidus/substantia nigra, [the pars reticulata complex (GPi/SNr)] – the main output station of the basal ganglia – then to the thalamus, and back to the cortex. The indirect pathway has a similar origin from the cortex to the striatum, but then projects from the striatum to the external segment of the globus pallidus (GPe) and then to the subthalamic nucleus before projecting to the GPi/SNr complex, where it rejoins the common pathway to the thalamus and back to the cortex. The prefrontal cortex and thalamus also reciprocally activate each other. Impulses along the direct pathway (with two inhibitory connections) 'disinhibit' the thalamus and activate the system in a positive feedback loop, while activity along the indirect pathway (with three inhibitory connections) would provide negative feedback, inhibiting the thalamus. Thus, the direct and indirect pathways appear to balance each other, allowing for both facilitation and suppression of complex motor programs, via their opposite effects on thalamo-cortical activation.[105]

Recent evidence suggests that the indirect pathway has interactions with the direct pathway that are much more complex than those envisioned in the classic model.[106] Researchers agree, however, that whatever the exact cir-

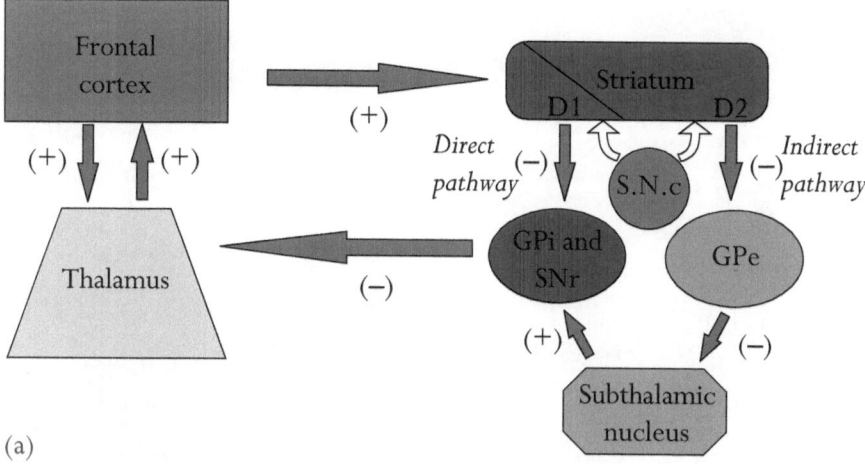

(a)

Figure 7.4 (a) Classic conception of direct and indirect frontal–basal
ganglia–thalamo–cortical pathways. The frontal–subcortical circuit originates in the
frontal cortex, which projects to striatum. The **direct** pathway projects from striatum
to the globus pallidus interna (GPi) substantia nigra, pars reticulata (SNr) complex
(the main output station of the basal ganglia), which projects to the thalamus, and
which has reciprocal, excitatory projections to and from the cortical site of origin.
This pathway contains two excitatory and two inhibitory projections, making it a net
positive-feedback loop. The **indirect** pathway also originates in the frontal cortex
and projects to the striatum, but then projects to the globus pallidus externa (GPe),
then to the subthalamic nucleus, then back to the GPi/SNr complex, prior to
returning to the thalamus and, finally, back to the frontal cortex. This indirect circuit
has three inhibitory connections, making it a net negative-feedback loop.

cuitry of the indirect pathway, activity through it results in increased activity
in the GPi/SNr complex, thereby strengthening the inhibition of the thalamus.[107] Our current conceptualization of frontal–subcortical circuitry
(Figure 7.4b) acknowledges the present uncertainties by referring to the
indirect pathway elements as the indirect basal ganglia control system. In
these frontal–subcortical circuits, excitatory projections predominantly use
glutamate as a neurotransmitter, while inhibitory ones mainly employ
gamma-aminobutyric acid (GABA). Several peptide transmitters also have
important roles within these pathways.[108] Other neurotransmitters
(dopamine, serotonin, acetylcholine, etc) modify the activity of projections
between these structures.

The connections between cortex and striatum have been described as 'a
common substrate for movement and thought'.[109] The striatum, and the
caudate nucleus in particular, is involved in processing cortical information

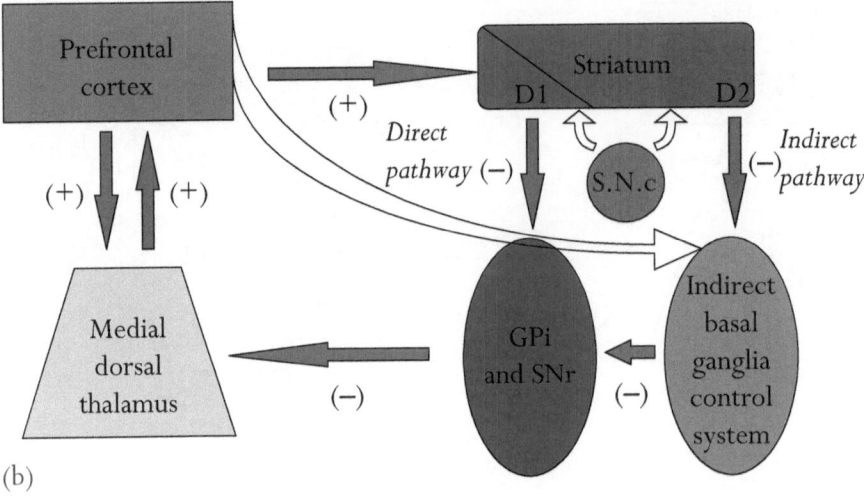

(b)

Figure 7.4 *Continued (b) Current conceptualization of prefrontal–basal ganglia–thalamo–cortical circuitry. Recent anatomical studies have called into question previous views of basal ganglia circuitry. Here, we refer to an indirect basal ganglia control system that consists of the GPe and the subthalamic nucleus. Connections within these structures are more complex than previously thought. The prefrontal cortex has excitatory projections to indirect pathway structures. In addition, the GPe directly projects to the GPi/SNr complex. Nevertheless, the net effect of activity in the indirect circuit still appears to be inhibition of the thalamus, thereby decreasing thalamo-cortical drive. The frontal–subcortical circuits originating in the lateral prefrontal cortex, the orbitofrontal cortex, and the anterior cingulate gyrus, all pass through subcompartments of the medial dorsal nucleus of the thalamus.*

for the initiation of behavioral responses and also plays an important role in procedural learning – the acquisition of new habits and skills which require minimal conscious awareness.[110] Conventionally, the striatum is divided into the caudate nucleus, putamen, and nucleus accumbens (see Figure 7.5). Different regions of the striatum receive input from different cortical regions.[104] The OFC, a paralimbic isocortical area, projects to the ventromedial caudate nucleus, while the dorsolateral prefrontal cortex (an associative neocortical area) projects to the dorsolateral caudate, and the anterior cingulate gyrus and hippocampal formation (limbic areas) project to the nucleus accumbens (see Figure 7.5). Circuits involved in motor programming travel through the putamen. These topographical representations are maintained in a related, but distinct, topology through the globus pallidus, subthalamic nucleus, and thalamus, creating relatively segregated, closed loops.[104] Direct and indirect pathways are present in each of the loops – motor, associative, and limbic.[111–113] Several different thalamic nuclei are involved in these circuits, but those originating in limbic and association cortex areas all pass through subregions of the medial dorsal nucleus of the thalamus.[114]

A function of the frontal–subcortical circuits passing through the striatum is the execution of pre-packaged, complex, sequence-critical, response behaviors (macros) that, to be adaptive, must be executed quickly in response to specific stimuli, to the exclusion of other responses dictated by interfering stimuli.[7,8] Naturally occurring activity along the direct pathway would tend to rivet behavior to the execution of the appropriate macros, until the need is judged to have passed. Conversely, activation of the indirect pathway may have as part of its function the suppression of direct pathway-driven behaviors when it is time to switch to another behavior – something OCD patients have difficulty doing.

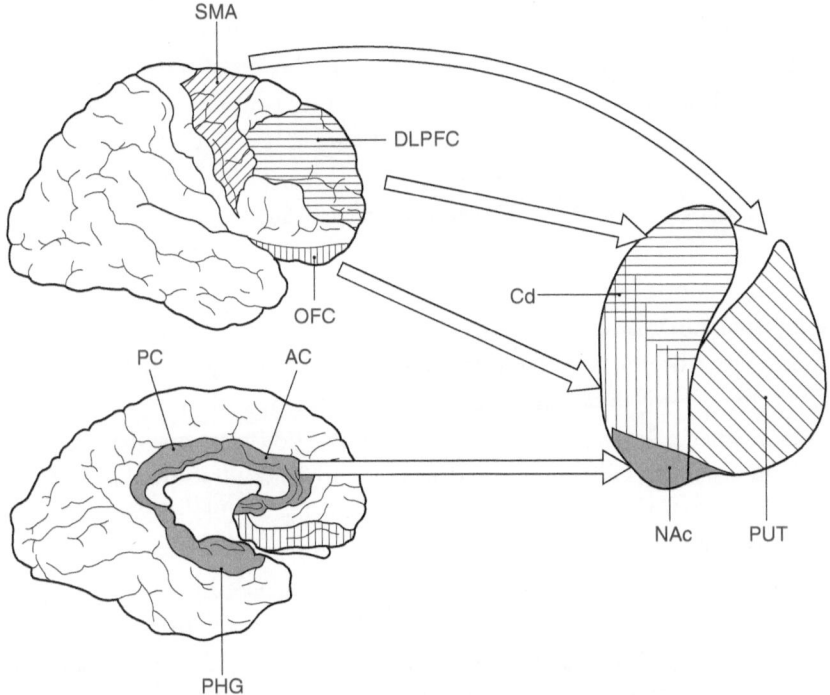

Figure 7.5 *Frontal–striatal projections. Illustration of regional distribution of cortical projections to separate striatal subcompartments. The supplementary motor areas (SMA; slanted lines) projects to the putamen (PUT), the dorsolateral prefrontal cortex (DLPFC; horizontal lines) projects to the dorsolateral head of the caudate nucleus (Cd), the orbitofrontal cortex (OFC; vertical lines) projects to the ventromedial head of the caudate, and the anterior cingulate gyrus (AC); posterior cingulate gyrus (PC), and parahippocampal gyrus (PHG) (all shaded areas) project to the nucleus accumbens (NAc). Though there may be slight overlap, cortical projection fields within the striatum are topographically distinct.*

A model of the pathophysiology of obsessive-compulsive disorder (OCD)

Imbalance of direct–indirect pathway tone in the orbitofrontal–subcortical circuit

Functional neuroimaging data clearly support pathophysiological theories put forward previously[115–119] regarding the role of the OFC, basal ganglia, and frontal–subcortical circuits in OCD. The present working model of the pathophysiology of OCD expands upon earlier theories and incorporates newer data regarding the neuroanatomy and function of frontal–subcortical brain circuits, as well as a proposed mechanism for symptom reduction with treatment.

This pathophysiological model posits that in persons with OCD there is a response bias toward stimuli relating to socio-territorial concerns about danger, violence, hygiene, order, sex, etc – the themes of most obsessions in patients with OCD – mediated by frontal–subcortical circuits involving the OFC.[7,80] There is much experimental and clinical evidence that the OFC is involved in the mediation of emotional responses to biologically significant stimuli, anticipatory anxiety, detection of errors, and social–affiliative behavior.[120] The orbitofrontal–subcortical circuit appears to mediate voluntary, prospective control of behavior influenced by affectively charged memories and internal information. In normal individuals, socio-territorial concerns and responses to stimuli perceived as dangerous may be mediated by activity through the orbitofrontal–subcortical direct pathway, with appropriate inhibition from the indirect pathway. OCD patients, however, may have a lower threshold for system activation by socio-territorial stimuli, as well as impaired inhibition of cortical–subcortical activity.[121] This could be due to excess tone in the direct relative to the indirect orbitofrontal–subcortical pathway (Figure 7.6), allowing concerns about danger, violence, hygiene, order, sex, etc, to rivet attention to themselves, compelling patients to respond with ritualistic behavior, and resulting in an inability to switch to other behaviors. Such an imbalance of direct–indirect pathway tone would produce the hyperactive circuit seen in functional neuroimaging studies of OCD that, in turn, mediates the repetitive, fixed behaviors relating to socio-territorial concerns in OCD.

It is unknown which brain structures may contain neuronal abnormalities that give rise to orbitofrontal–subcortical hyperactivity in OCD patients, but some evidence points to the striatum.[67,68,71] It is possible that, in patients with OCD, there may be dysfunction involving the intrinsic structure of the striatum, which is divided neurochemically into striosome and matrix compartments.[122,123] Striosomes receive preferential input from the OFC and AC,[124] and are involved in negative feedback control of activity in the frontal–subcortical circuits.[123] Abnormal development, loss, or dysfunction involving striosomes in the ventromedial caudate might result in an imbalance between direct and indirect pathways in the orbitofrontal–subcortical circuit, resulting in the symptoms of OCD. Damage to striosomes or other areas of the striatum could potentially be produced by post-infectious anti-neuronal autoantibodies, thought to be implicated in at least a subset of patients with OCD.[125,126] Orbitofrontal–subcortical hyperactivity in OCD may also be the result of abnormal neuroanatomical development of these structures, or a failure of pruning of neuronal connections between them.[28,30]

Mechanism of action of SRI in OCD

Currently, drugs that strongly inhibit serotonin reuptake are the only medications consistently proven effective in the treatment of OCD. It has been hypothesized that SRI medications decrease activity in the orbitofrontal–subcortical circuit, possibly by changing the relative balance of

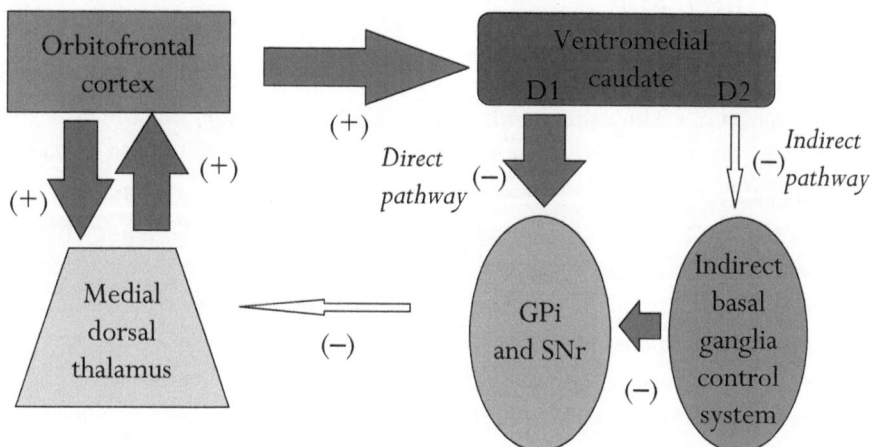

Figure 7.6 *Model of obsessive-compulsive disorder (OCD) pathophysiology. OCD symptomatology may be the result of a captured signal in the direct orbitofrontal–subcortical pathway, a positive-feedback loop. This could be due to excess tone in the direct (large arrows) relative to the indirect (small arrows) orbitofrontal–subcortical pathway, resulting in increased activity in the orbitofrontal cortex, the ventromedial caudate, and the medial dorsal thalamus. This orbitofrontal–subcortical hyperactivity would allow concerns about danger, violence, hygiene, order, sex, etc, to rivet attention to themselves, compelling patients to respond with ritualistic behavior, and resulting in an inability to switch to other behaviors.*

activity through the indirect versus direct frontal–subcortical pathways.[7–12,127] The serotonergic innervation of the striatum is heavily concentrated in the ventromedial caudate and nucleus accumbens, precisely those subcompartments that receive input from the OFC and AC.[127,128] Serotonergic pathways from the midbrain also project strongly to the subthalamic nucleus and globus pallidus,[129] key structures for the control of basal ganglia output.[107] Serotonergic drugs may also exert their effect in the OFC. Recent work has demonstrated differential effects of SRI drugs in OFC versus the dorsal prefrontal cortex, in a time course that corresponds to the effects of these medications on OCD symptoms versus depressive symptoms. SRIs have been found both to enhance serotonin release and to desensitize serotonin autoreceptors in the OFC after 8 weeks, but not 3 weeks, whereas effects in the dorsal prefrontal cortex occur after 3 weeks.[130,131] The glucose metabolic decreases in the OFC and caudate seen after successful treatment may reflect decreased release of excitatory neurotransmitters such as glutamate in these regions.[132]

Future directions

Functional neuroimaging studies have advanced our understanding of brain–behavior relationships with respect to OCD greatly, but much is still unknown. No post-mortem neuroanatomical studies of OCD exist to delineate its pathophysiology. The roles of various neurochemical systems in OCD are similarly unclear. Although there is some indirect evidence suggesting serotonergic abnormalities in OCD, there is no direct evidence demonstrating any such abnormalities, or whether they are primary or secondary phenomena in OCD. Phenotypic heterogeneity could account for many of the inconsistencies among previous neuroimaging studies of OCD. Current studies are seeking to find the neurobiological and genetic substrates of specific OCD symptom factors, as well as predictors of treatment response.

Acknowledgments

I wish to thank several colleagues, especially Lewis R Baxter Jr, who developed many of the concepts and theories presented here, as well as Arthur L Brody, Elyse Katz, and Tokuzo Matsui, for their assistance, suggestions, and careful review of this manuscript.

References

1. Weissman MM, Bland RC, Canino GJ et al. The cross-national epidemiology of obsessive-compulsive disorder. *J Clin Psychiatry* 1994; **55:** 5–10.

2. Murray CLJ, Lopex AD. *Global Burden of Disease: A Comprehensive Assessment of Mortality and Morbidity from Diseases, Injuries, and Risk Factors in 1990 and Projected to 2020*, Volume I. (World Health Organization: Havard, 1996.)

3. Greist JH, Jefferson J, Koback KA et al. Efficacy and tolerability of serotonin transport inhibitors in obsessive-compulsive disorder: a meta-analysis. *Arch Gen Psychiatry* 1995; **52:** 53–60.

4. Marks I, Behaviour therapy for obsessive-compulsive disorder: a decade of progress. *Can J Psychiatry* 1997; **42:** 1021–7.

5. Silbersweig DA, Stern E. Symptom localization in neuropsychiatry; a functional neuroimaging approach. *Ann NY Acad Sci* 1997; **835:** 410–20.

6. Cummings JL. Frontal–subcortical circuits and human behavior. *Arch Neurol* 1993; **50:** 873–80.

7. Baxter LR, Saxena S, Brody AL et al. Brain mediation of obsessive-compulsive disorder symptoms: evidence from functional brain imaging studies in the human and non-human primate. *Semin Clin Neuropsychiatry* 1996; **1:** 32–47.

8. Baxter LR, Ackermann RF, Swerdlow NR et al. Specific brain system mediation of OCD responsive to either medication or behavior therapy. In: (Goodman W, Maser J, eds) *Obsessive-Compulsive Disorder: Contemporary Issues in Treatment.* (Mahwah, NJ: Lawrence Erlbaum Associates Inc, 2000: 573–609.)

9. Rauch SL, Baxter LR. Neuroimaging of OCD and related disorders. In: (Jenike MA, Baer L, Minichiello WE, eds) *Obsessive–Compulsive Disorders: Practical Management.* (Mosby: Boston, 1998) 289–317.

10. Saxena S, Brody AL, Schwartz JM et al. Neuroimaging and frontal–subcortical circuitry in obsessive-compulsive disorder. *Br J Psychiatry* 1998; **173:** 26–38.

11. Saxena S, Rauch SL. Functional neuroimaging and the neuroanatomy of obsessive-compulsive disorder. *Psychiatr Clin N Am* 2000; **23:** 563–84.

12. Saxena S, Bota RG, Brody AL. Brain–behavior relationships in obsessive-compulsive disorder. *Semin Clin Neuropsychiatry* 2001; **6:** 82–101.

13. Insel TR, Donnelly EF, Lalakea ML et al. Neurological and neuropsychological studies of patients with obsessive-compulsive disorder. *Biol Psychiatry* 1983; **18:** 741–51.

14. Behar D, Rapoport, JL, Berg CJ et al. Computerized tomography and neuropsychological test measures in adolescents with obsessive-compulsive disorder. *Am J Psychiatry* 1984; **141:** 363–9.

15. Stein DJ, Hollander E, Chan S et al. Computed tomography and neurological soft signs in obsessive-compulsive disorder. *Psychiatry Res* 1993; **50:** 143–50.

16. Luxenberg JS, Swedo SE, Flamant MF et al. Neuroanatomical abnormalities in obsessive-compulsive disorder determined with quantitative x-ray computed tomography. *Am J Psychiatry* 1988; **145:** 1089–93.

17. Scarone S, Colombo C, Livian S et al. Increased right caudate nucleus size in obsessive-compulsive disorder: detection with magnetic resonance imaging. *Psychiatry Res* 1992; **45:** 115–21.

18. Robinson D, Wu H, Munne RA et al. Reduced caudate nucleus volume in obsessive-compulsive disorder. *Arch Gen Psychiatry* 1995; **52:** 393–8.

19. Rosenberg DR, Keshavan MS, O'Hearn KM et al. Frontostriatal measurement in treatment-naive children with obsessive-compulsive disorder. *Arch Gen Psychiatry* 1997; **54:** 824–30.

20. Kellner CH, Jolley RR, Holgate RC et al. Brain MRI in obsessive-compulsive disorder. *Psychiatry Res* 1991; **36:** 45–9.

21. Aylward EH, Harris GH, Hoehn-Saric R et al. Normal caudate nucleus in obsessive-compulsive disorder assessed by quantitative neuroimaging. *Arch Gen Psychiatry* 1996; **53:** 577–84.

22. Swedo SE, Leonard HL, Garvey M et al. Pediatric autoimmune neuropsychiatric disorders associated with streptococcal infections: clinical description of the first 50 cases. *Am Psychiatry* 1998: **155:** 262–71.

23. Giedd JN, Rapaport JL, Garvey MA et al. MRI assessment of children with obsessive-compulsive disorder or tics associated with streptococcal function. *Am J Psychiatry* 2000; **157:** 281–3.

24. Peterson BS, Leckman JF, Tucker D et al. Preliminary findings of antistreptococcal antibody titers and basal ganglia volumes in tic, obsessive-compulsive, and attention-deficit/hyperactivity disorders. *Arch Gen Psychiatry* 2000; **57:** 364–72.

25. Peterson B, Riddle MA, Cohen DJ et al. Reduced basal ganglia volumes in Tourette's syndrome using three-dimensional reconstruction techniques from magnetic resonance images. *Neurology* 1993; **43:** 941–9.

26. Hyde TM, Stacey ME, Coppola RC et al. Cerebral morphometric abnormalities in Tourette's syndrome: a quantitative MRI study in monozygotic twins. *Neurology* 1995; **45:** 1176–85.

27. Garber HJ, Ananth JV, Chiu LC et al. Nuclear magnetic resonance study of obsessive-compulsive disorder. *Am J Psychiatry* 1989; **146:** 1001–5.

28. Jenike MA, Breiter HC, Baer L et al. Cerebral structural abnormalities in obsessive-compulsive disorder: a quantitative morphometric magnetic resonance imaging study. *Arch Gen Psychiatry* 1996; **53:** 625–32.

29. Grachev I, Breiter HC, Rauch SL et al. Structural abnormalities of frontal neocortex in obsessive-compulsive disorder. *Arch Gen Psychiatry* 1998; **55:** 181–2.

30. Rosenberg DR, Keshavan MS. Toward a neurodevelopmental model of obsessive–compulsive disorder. AE Bennett Research Award. *Biol Psychiatry* 1998; **43:** 623–40.

31. Szezko PR, Robinson D, Ma J et al. Orbital frontal and amygdala volume reductions in obsessive-compulsive disorder. *Arch Gen Psychiatry* 2000; **56:** 913–19.

32. Kim J, Lee MC, Kim J et al. Grey matter abnormalities in obsessive-compulsive disorder. *Br J Psychiatry* 2001; **179:** 330–4.

33. Gilbert AR, Moore GJ, Keshavan MS et al. Decrease in thalamic volumes of pediatric patients with obsessive-compulsive disorder who are taking paroxetine. *Arch Gen Psychiatry* 2000; **57:** 449–56.

34. Rosenberg DR, Keshavan MS, Dick EL et al. Corpus callosal morphology in treatment-naive pediatric obsessive-compulsive disorder. *Prog Neuro-Psychopharmac Biol Psychiatry* 1997; **21:** 1269–83.

35. MacMaster FP, Keshavan MS, Dick EL et al. Corpus callosal signal intensity in treatment-naive pediatric obsessive-compulsive disorders. *Prog Neuro-Psychopharmac Biol Psychiatry* 1999; **23:** 601–12.

36. Rosenberg DR, Benazon NR, Gilbert A et al. Thalamic volume in pediatric obsessive-compulsive disorder patients before and after cognitive behavioral therapy. *Biol Psychiatry* 2000; **48:** 294–300.

37. Rauch SL, Kim H, Makris N et al. Volume reduction in the caudate nucleus following stereotactic placement of lesions in the anterior cingulate cortex in humans: a morphometric magnetic resonance imaging study. *J Neurosurg* 2000; **93:** 1019–25.

38. Rubin RT, Villanueva-Meyer J, Ananth J et al. Regional 133Xe cerebral blood flow and cerebral 99m-HMPAO uptake in unmedicated obsessive-compulsive disorder patients and matched normal control subjects: determination by high-resolution single-photon emission computed tomography. *Arch Gen Psychiatry* 1992; **49:** 695–702.

39. Sorenson JA, Phelps ME. *Physics in Nuclear Medicine.* (WB Saunders Co: Philadelphia, 1987.)

40. Andreasen N. *Brain Imaging: Applications in Psychiatry.* (American Psychiatric Press: Washington, DC, 1989.)

41. Maier M. In vivo magnetic resonance spectroscopy. *Br J Psychiatry* 1995; **167:** 299–306.

42. Baxter LR, Phelps ME, Mazziotta JC et al. Local cerebral glucose metabolic rates in obsessive-compulsive disorder – a comparison with rates in unipolar depression and in normal controls. *Arch Gen Psychiatry* 1985; **44:** 211–18.

43. Baxter LR, Schwartz JM, Mazziotta JC et al. Cerebral glucose metabolic rates in non-depressed obsessive-compulsives. *Am J Psychiatry* 1988; **145:** 1560–3.

44. Nordahl TE, Benkelfat C, Semple WE et al. Cerebral glucose metabolic rates in obsessive-compulsive disorder. *Neuropsychopharmacology* 1989; **2:** 23–8.

45. Swedo SE, Schapiro MG, Grady CL et al. Cerebral glucose metabolism in childhood onset obsessive-compulsive disorder. *Arch Gen Psychiatry* 1989; **46:** 518–23.

46. Sawle GV, Hymas NF, Lees AJ et al. Obsessional slowness: functional studies with positron emission tomography. *Brain* 1991; **114:** 191–202.

47. Perani D, Colombo C, Bressi S et al. [18F]-FDG PET Study in obsessive-compulsive disorder: a clinical/metabolic correlation study after treatment. *Br J Psychiatry* 1995; **166:** 244–50.

48. Saxena S, Brody AL, Ho ML et al. Cerebral metabolism in major depression and obsessive-compulsive disorder occurring separately and concurrently. *Biol Psychiatry* 2001; **50:** 159–70.

49. Martinot JL, Allilaire JF, Mazoyer BM et al. Obsessive-compulsive disorder: a clinical, neuropsychological and positron emission tomography study. *Acta Psychiatr Scand* 1990; **82:** 233–42.

50. Baxter LR, Schwartz JM, Guze BH et al. PET imaging in obsessive-compulsive disorder with and without depression. *J Clin Psychiatry* 1990; **51:** 61–9.

51. Martinot JL, Allilaire JF, Mazoyer BM et al. Left prefrontal glucose hypometabolism in the depressed state: a confirmation. *Am J Psychiatry* 1990; **147:** 1313–17.

52. Edmonstone Y, Austin MP, Prentice N et al. Uptake of 99m-Tc-exametazime shown by single photon emission computerized tomography in obsessive-compulsive

disorder compared with major depression and normal controls. *Acta Psychiatr Scand* 1994; **90:** 298–303.

53. Adams BL, Warneke LB, McEwan AJB et al. Single photon emission computerized tomography in obsessive-compulsive disorder: a preliminary study. *J Psychiatry Neurosci* 1989; **18:** 109–12.

54. Lucey JV, Costa DC, Blanes T et al. Regional cerebral blood flow in obsessive–compulsive disordered patients at rest: differential correlates with obsessive–compulsive and anxious-avoidant dimensions. *Br J Psychiatry* 1995; **167:** 629–34.

55. Lucey JV, Costa DC, Adshead G et al. Brain blood flow in anxiety disorders. OCD, panic disorder with agoraphobia, and post-traumatic stress disorder on 99mHMPAO single photon emission tomography (SPET). *Br J Psychiatry* 1997; **171:** 346–50.

56. Crespo-Facorro B, Cabranes JA, Lopez-Ibor Alcocer MI et al. Regional cerebral blood flow in obsessive-compulsive patients with and without chronic tic disorder. A SPECT study. *Eur Arch Psychiatry Clin Neurosci* 1999; **249:** 156–61.

57. Machlin SR, Harris GJ, Pearlson GD et al. Elevated medial–frontal cerebral blood flow in obsessive-compulsive patients: a SPECT study. *Am J Psychiatry* 1991; **148:** 1240–2.

58. Alptekin K, Degirmenci B, Kivircik B et al. Tc-99m HMPAO brain perfusion SPECT in drug-free obsessive-compulsive patients without depression. *Psychiatry Res: Neuroimaging* 2001; **107:** 51–6.

59. Busatto GF, Zamignani DR, Buchpiguel CA et al. A voxel-based investigation of regional cerebral blood flow abnormalities in obsessive-compulsive disorder using single photon emission computed tomography (SPECT). *Psychiatry Res: Neuroimaging* 2000; **99:** 15–27.

60. Riddle MA, Rasmussen AM, Woods SW et al. SPECT imaging of cerebral blood flow in Tourette's syndrome. In: (Chase TN, Friedhoff AJ, Cohen DJ, eds) *Advances in Neurology, Gilles de la Tourette Syndrom: Genetics Neurobiology, and Treatment*, Volume 58. (Raven Press: New York, 1992) 207–11.

61. Moriarty J, Eapen V, Costa DC et al. HMPAO SPET does not distinguish obsessive-compulsive and tic syndromes in family multiply affected with Gilles de la Tourette's syndrome. *Psychol Med* 1997; **27:** 737–40.

62. Braun AR, Stoetter B, Randolph C et al. The functional neuroanatomy of Tourette's syndrome: an FDG-PET study. I. Regional changes in cerebral glucose metabolism differentiating patients and controls. *Neuropsychopharmacology* 1993; **9:** 277–91.

63. Hall M, Costa DC, Shields J et al. Brain perfusion patterns with 99mTc-HMPAO/SPET in patients with Gilles de la Tourette syndrome. Short report. *Nucl Med Suppl* 1990; **27:** 243–5.

64. Heilman KM, Voeller KKS, Nadeau SE. A possible pathophysiological substrate of attention deficit/hyperactivity disorder. *J Child Neurol* 1991; **6 (Suppl):** S76–S81.

65. Zametkin AJ, Nordahl TE, Gross M et al. Cerebral glucose metabolism in adults with hyperactivity of childhood onset. *N Engl J Med* 1990; **323:** 1361–6.

66. Birken D, Oldendorf WH. NAA: a literature review of a compound prominent in 1H NMR spectroscopic studies of brain. *Neurosci Biobehav Rev* 1989; **13:** 23–31.

67. Ebert D, Speck O, Konig A et al. H-magnetic resonance spectroscopy in obsessive-compulsive disorder: evidence for neuronal loss in the cingulate gyrus and the right striatum. *Psychiatry Res: Neuroimaging* 1996; **74:** 173–6.

68. Bartha R, Stein MB, Williamson PC et al. A short echo ^{1}H spectroscopy and volumetric MRI study of the corpus striatum in patients with obsessive-compulsive disorder and comparison subjects. *Am J Psychiatry* 1998; **155**: 1584–91.

69. Rosenberg DR, Amponsah A, Sullivan A et al. Increased medial thalamic choline in pediatric obsessive-compulsive disorder as detected by quantitative in vivo spectroscopic imaging. *J Child Neurology* 2001; **16**: 636–41.

70. Fitzgerald KD, Moore GJ, Paulson LA et al. Proton spectroscopic imaging of the thalamus in treatment-naive pediatric obsessive-compulsive disorder. *Biol Psychiatry* 2000; **47**: 174–82.

71. Rosenberg DR, MacMaster FP, Keshavan M et al. Decrease in caudate glutamate concentrations in pediatric obsessive-compulsive disorder patients taking paroxetine. *J Am Acad Child Adolesc Psychiatry* 2000; **39**: 1096–103.

72. Baer L. Factor analysis of symptom subtypes of obsessive-compulsive disorder and their relation to personality and tic disorders. *J Clin Psychiatry* 1994; **55**: 18–23.

73. Leckman JF, Grice DE, Boardman J et al. Symptoms of obsessive-compulsive disorder. *Am J Psychiatry* 1997; **154**: 911–17.

74. Rauch SL, Dougherty DD, Shin LM et al. Neural correlates of factor-analyzed OCD symptom dimensions: a PET study. *CNS Spect* 1998; **3**: 37–43.

75. Ball SG, Baer L, Otto MW. Symptom subtypes of obsessive-compulsive disorder in behavioral treatment studies: a quantitative review. *Behav Res Ther* 1996; **34**: 47–51.

76. Benkelfat C, Nordahl TE, Semple WE et al. Local cerebral glucose metabolic rates in obsessive-compulsive disorder: patients treated with clomipramine. *Arch Gen Psychiatry* 1990; **47**: 840–8.

77. Swedo SE, Pietrini P, Leonard HL et al. Cerebral glucose metabolism in childhood-onset obsessive-compulsive disorder: revisualization during pharmacotherapy. *Arch Gen Psychiatry* 1992; **49**: 690–4.

78. Saxena S, Brody AL, Maidment KM et al. Localized orbitofrontal and subcortical metabolic changes and predictors of response to paroxetine treatment in obsessive-compulsive disorder. *Neuropsychopharmacology* 1999; **21**: 683–93.

79. Mindus P, Nyman H, Mogard J et al. Orbital and caudate glucose metabolism studied by positron emission tomography (PET) in patients undergoing capsulotomy for obsessive-compulsive disorder. In: (Jenike MA, Asberg M, eds) *Understanding Obsessive–Compulsive Disorder (OCD)*. (Hogrefe and Huber Publishers: Toronto, 1991) 52–7.

80. Baxter LR, Schwartz, JM, Bergman KS et al. Caudate glucose metabolic rate changes with both drug and behavior therapy for obsessive-compulsive disorder. *Arch Gen Psychiatry* 1992; **49**: 681–9.

81. Schwartz JM, Stoessel PW, Baxter LR et al. Systematic changes in cerebral glucose metabolic rate after successful behavior modification treatment of obsessive–compulsive disorder. *Arch Gen Psychiatry* 1996; **53**: 109–13.

82. Saxena S, Brody A, Ho ML et al. Differential cerebral metabolic changes with paroxetine treatment of obsessive-compulsive disorder versus major depression. *Arch Gen Psychiatry* 2002; **59**: 156–70.

83. Hansen ES, Hasselbach S, Law I, Bolwig TG. The caudate nucleus in obsessive–compulsive disorder. Reduced metabolism following treatment with paroxetine: a PET study. *Int J Neuropsychopharmac* 2002; **5**: 1–10.

84. Hoehn-Saric R, Pearlson GD, Harris GJ et al. Effects of fluoxetine on regional cerebral blood flow in obsessive-compulsive patients. *Am J Psychiatry* 1991; **148:** 1243–5.

85. Rubin RT, Ananth J, Villanueva-Meyer J et al. Regional ^{133}Xenon cerebral blood flow and cerebral Tc-HMPAO uptake in patients with obsessive-compulsive disorder before and after treatment. *Biol Psychiatry* 1995; **38:** 429–37.

86. Hoehn-Saric R, Schlaepfer TE, Greenberg BD et al. Cerebral blood flow in obsessive compulsive patients with major depression: effect of treatment with sertraline or desipramine on treatment responders and non-responders. *Psychiatry Res: Neuroimaging* 2001; **108:** 89–100.

87. Moore GJ, MacMaster FP, Stewart C et al. Case study: glutamatergic changes with paroxetine therapy for pediatric obsessive-compulsive disorder. *J Am Acad Child Adolesc Psychiatry* 1998; **37:** 663–7.

88. Brody AL, Saxena S, Schwartz JM et al. FDG-PET predictors of response to behavioral therapy versus pharmacotherapy in obsessive-compulsive disorder. *Psychiatry Res: Neuroimaging* 1998; **84:** 1–6.

89. Saxena S, Brody AL, Ho ML et al. Differential brain metabolic predictors of response to paroxetine in obsessive-compulsive disorder versus major depression. *Am J Psychiatry* 2003; **160:** 522–32.

90. Rauch SL, Dougherty DD, Cosgrove GR et al. Cerebral metabolic correlates as potential predictors of response to anterior cingulotomy for obsessive-compulsive disorder. *Biol Psychiatry* 2001; **50:** 659–67.

91. Rauch SL, Jenike MA, Alpert NM et al. Regional cerebral blood flow measured during symptom provocation in obsessive-compulsive disorder using oxygen 15-labeled carbon dioxide and positron emission tomography. *Arch Gen Psychiatry* 1994; **51:** 62–70.

92. McGuire PK, Bench CJ, Frith CD et al. Functional anatomy of obsessive-compulsive phenomena. *Br J Psychiatry* 1994; **164:** 459–68.

93. Cottraux J, Gerard D, Cinotti L et al. A controlled positron emission tomography study of obsessive and neutral auditory stimulation in obsessive-compulsive disorder with checking rituals. *Psychiatry Res* 1996; **60:** 101–12.

94. Breiter HC, Rauch SL, Kwong KK et al. Functional magnetic resonance imaging of symptom provocation in obsessive-compulsive disorder. *Arch Gen Psychiatry* 1996; **49:** 595–606.

95. Adler CM, McDonough-Ryan P, Sax KW et al. fMRI of neuronal activation with symptom provocation in unmedicated patients with obsessive compulsive disorder. *J Psychiatry Res* 2000; **34:** 317–24.

96. Zohar J, Insel TR. Berman KF et al. Anxiety and cerebral blood flow during behavioral challenge: dissociation of central from peripheral and subjective measures. *Arch Gen Psychiatry* 1989; **46:** 505–10.

97. Hollander E, Prohovnik I, Stein DJ. Increased cerebral blood flow during m-CPP exacerbation of obsessive-compulsive disorder. *J Neuropsychiatry Clin Neurosci* 1995; **7:** 485–90.

98. Stein DJ, Van Heerden B, Wessels C et al. Single photon emission computed tomography with Tc-99 HMPAO during sumatriptan challenge in obsessive-compulsive disorder: investigating the functional role of the serotonin autoreceptor. *Prog Neuropsychopharmac Biol Psychiatry* 1999; **23:** 1079–99.

99. Rauch SL, Savage CR, Alpert NM et al. Probing striatal function in obsessive–compulsive disorder: a PET study of implicit sequence learning. *J Neuropsychiatry Clin Neurosci* 1997; **9**: 568–73.

100. Rauch SL, Whalen PJ, Curran T et al. Probing striato-thalamic function in OCD and TS using neuroimaging methods. In: (Cohen DJ, Goetz C, Jankovic J, eds) *Tourette Syndrome and Associated Disorders*. (Lippincott, Williams & Wilkins: Philadelphia, 2001) 207–24.

101. Squire LR. Memory and the hippocampus: a synthesis of findings from rats, monkeys, and humans. *Psychol Rev* 1992; **99**: 195–231.

102. Lucey JV, Burness CE, Costa DC et al. Wisconsin Card Sorting Task (WCST) errors and cerebral blood flow in obsessive-compulsive disorder (OCD). *Br J Med Psychol* 1997; **70**: 403–11.

103. Pujol J, Torres L, Deus J et al. Functional magnetic resonance imaging study of frontal lobe activation during word generation in obsessive-compulsive disorder. *Biol Psychiatry* 1999; **45**: 891–7.

104. Alexander GE, DeLong MR, Strick PL. Parallel organization of functionally segregated circuits linking basal ganglia and cortex. *Ann Rev Neurosci* 1986; **9**: 357–81.

105. Alexander GE, Crutcher MD. Functional architecture of basal ganglia circuits: neural substrates of parallel processing. *TINS* 1990; **13**: 266–71.

106. Parent A, Hazrati L-N. Functional anatomy of the basal ganglia I. The cortico–basal ganglia–thalamo–cortico loop. *Brain Res Rev* 1995; **20**: 91–127.

107. Parent A, Hazrati L-N. Functional anatomy of the basal ganglia II. The place of subthalamic nucleus and external pallidum in basal ganglia circuitry. *Brain Res Rev* 1995; **20**: 128–54.

108. Graybiel AM. Neurotransmitters and neuromodulators in the basal ganglia. *TINS* 1990; **13**: 244–54.

109. Nauta WJH. Reciprocal links of the corpus striatum with cortex and limbic system: a common substrate for movement and thought? In: (Mueller J, ed) *Neurology and Psychiatry: A Meeting of Minds*. (Karger: New York, 1989, 43–63.)

110. Saint-Cyr JA, Taylor AE. The mobilization of procedural learning: the 'key signature' of the basal ganglia. In: (Squire LR, Butters N, eds) *Neuropsychology of Memory*, 2nd edn. (Guilford Press: New York, 1992) 188–202.

111. Shink E, Bevan MD, Bolam JP et al. The subthalamic nucleus and the external pallidum: two tightly interconnected structures that control the output of the basal ganglia in the monkey. *Neuroscience* 1996; **73**: 335–57.

112. Smith Y, Hazrati L-N, Parent A. Efferent projections of the subthalamic nucleus in the squirrel monkey as studied by the PHA-L anterograde tracing method. *J Comp Neurol* 1990; **299**: 306–23.

113. Joel D, Weiner I. The connections of the primate subthalamic nucleus: indirect pathways and the open-interconnected scheme of basal ganglia–thalamocortical circuitry. *Brain Res Rev* 1997; **23**: 63–78.

114. Mega M, Cummings JL. Frontal–subcortical circuits and neuropsychiatric disorders. *J Neuropsychiatry Clin Neurosci* 1994; **6**: 358–70.

115. Rapoport JL, Wise SP. Obsessive-compulsive disorder: is it a basal ganglia dysfunction? *Psychopharmac Bull* 1988; **24**: 380–4.

116. Insel TR. Obsessive-compulsive disorder: a neuroethological perspective. *Psychopharmac Bull* 1988; **24:** 365–69.

117. Modell JG, Mountz JM, Curtis GC et al. Neurophysiologic dysfunction in basal ganglia/limbic striatal and thalamocortical circuits as a pathogenetic mechanism of obsessive-compulsive disorder. *J Neuropsychiatry Clin Neurosci* 1989; **1:** 27–36.

118. Baxter LR, Schwartz JM, Guze BH et al. Neuroimaging in obsessive-compulsive disorder: seeking the mediating neuroanatomy. In: (Jenike MA, Baer L, Minichiello W, eds) *Obsessive–Compulsive Disorders: Theory and Management*, 2nd edn. (Year Book Medical Publishers: Chicago, 1990) 167–88.

119. Swerdlow NR, Koob GF. Dopamine, schizophrenia, mania and depression: toward a unified hypothesis of cortico–striato–pallido–thalamic function. *Behav Brain Sci* 1987; **10:** 197–245.

120. Zald DH, Kim SW. Anatomy and function of the orbital frontal cortex, I: Anatomy, neurocircuitry, and obsessive-compulsive disorder. *J Neuropsychiatry Clin Neurosci* 1996; **8:** 125–38.

121. Greenberg BD, Ziemann U, Cora-Locatelli G et al. Altered cortical excitability in obsessive-compulsive disorder. *Neurology* 2000; **54:** 142–7.

122. Desban M, Kemel ML, Glowinski J, Gaucy C. Spatial organization of patch and matrix compartments in the rat striatum. *Neuroscience* 1993; **57:** 661–71.

123. Gerfen CR. The neostriatal mosaic: multiple levels of compartmental organization in the basal ganglia. *Ann Rev Neurosci* 1992; **115:** 285–320.

124. Eblen F, Graybiel AM. Highly restricted origin of prefrontal cortical inputs to striosomes in the macaque monkey. *J Neurosci* 1995; **15:** 5999–6013.

125. Murphy TK, Goodman WK, Fudge MW et al. B lymphocyte antigen d8/17: a peripheral marker for Tourette's syndrome and childhood-onset obsessive-compulsive disorder? *Am J Psychiatry* 1997; **154:** 402–7.

126. Swedo SE. Sydenham's chorea: a model for childhood autoimmune neuropsychiatric disorders. *J Am Med Ass* **272:** 1788–91.

127. Swerdlow NR. Serotonin, obsessive-compulsive disorder, and the basal ganglia. *Int Rev Psychiatry* 1995; **7:** 115–29.

128. Insel TR. Toward a neuroanatomy of obsessive-compulsive disorder. *Arch Gen Psychiatry* 1992; **49:** 739–44.

129. Lavoie B, Parent A. Immunohistochemical study of the serotoninergic innervation of the basal ganglia in the squirrel monkey. *J Comp Neurol* 1990; **299:** 1–16.

130. Mansari ME, Bouchard C, Blier P. Alteration of serotonin release in the guinea pig orbitofrontal cortex by selective serotonin reuptake inhibitors. *Neuropsychopharmacology* 1995; **13:** 117–27.

131. Bergqvist PB, Bouchard C, Blier P. Effect of long-term administration of antidepressant treatments on serotonin release in brain regions involved in obsessive-compulsive disorder. *Biol Psychiatry* 1999; **45:** 164–74.

132. Sizer AR, Kilpatrick GJ, Roberts MHT. A post-synaptic depressant modulatory action of 5-hydroxytryptamine on excitatory amino acid responses in rat entorhinal cortex in vitro. *Neuropharmacology* 1992; **31:** 5331–9.

8. IMAGING BRAIN STRUCTURE AND FUNCTION IN SCHIZOPHRENIA: NEW TECHNIQUES ENCOUNTER OLD PROBLEMS

Rebekah AE Honey, Karl J Friston, Paul C Fletcher

Background

In the past, formulations of schizophrenia as a functional illness have implied that abnormalities accompanying the condition are unlikely to be visible on examination of the brain. This position is no longer tenable, partly as a result of advances in the sensitivity and precision of structural brain imaging techniques. These have pointed to a number of localized abnormalities – clear evidence for brain changes associated with schizophrenia. Furthermore, the newer functional brain imaging techniques offer the possibility of estimating levels of brain response to particular tasks or conditions. These have produced further evidence for regional abnormalities in living patients.

However, the brain imaging literature is full of inconsistencies. Different techniques, together with variations in experimental design, have led to different conclusions. Consider, for example, the notion that a characteristic functional neuroimaging feature of schizophrenia is resting hypofrontality (i.e. a reduced level of brain activity in the frontal lobes). This finding has been reported in many studies using different techniques to estimate regional brain activity.[1–5] However, other studies, again using a variety of techniques, have shown that frontal activity is not demonstrably reduced in patients.[6–10] Indeed, a relative increase in frontal activity in patients has also been reported.[11] Since the search for a frontal deficit has been a staple of the functional neuroimaging approach, such gross inconsistencies must invite pessimism.

In part, these inconsistencies may be attributable to heterogeneity in the condition itself. It could be that different studies are using different types of patient (e.g. some acute, some chronic, some with predominantly positive symptoms such as hallucinations, some with negative symptoms such as psychomotor poverty). It is possible, too, that different studies include representatives of different (and, possibly, yet to be identified) subgroups, inappropriately treating them as an homogenous group. In part, too, inconsistencies may arise from the different psychological tasks that are used to induce brain activity across studies.

These various sources of inconsistency may be addressed through refinements in our understanding of the nature of schizophrenia, and in the selection of subjects and of experimental tasks. However, we suggest that there is a further reason for the failure of brain imaging studies to identify an abnormality that is sufficiently consistent to be considered a hallmark of schizophrenia. It may be that the core deficit in schizophrenia lies not in the abnormal function or structure of a localized region but rather in the ways in which separate regions interact with each other. Functional neuroimaging may characterize these interactions and, if used in this way, may offer insights that cannot be gained through techniques exploring brain structure.

Introduction

With advances in structural and functional neuroimaging, remarkable power to visualize the living brain has been achieved. We are now able to quantify its structural and functional attributes with astonishing sensitivity, and to compare data across groups of patients and control subjects. The goal of such comparisons is an objective, brain-based expression of the disease state: a goal that, if achievable, will have implications for diagnosis, prognosis, therapy and even prevention. The possibilities are especially exciting in relation to schizophrenia, a condition that has been considered a functional illness, differentiating it from other organic illnesses such as dementia in which the cerebral origin is much clearer. Through early application of brain imaging, it was quickly established that structural abnormalities could be identified in schizophrenic patients,[12] helping to make this dichotomy (organic versus functional) redundant. However, subsequent, imaging studies of structural changes in schizophrenia, while they have almost invariably produced evidence for abnormalities, have not identified a core deficit and have been notable more for the lack of a consistent pattern.[13,14]

The elusiveness of a consistent structural deficit perhaps counsels in favour of a modified view of schizophrenia as a functional disorder. In this view, it is functional in the sense not that a measurable brain deficit is absent, but rather that the deficit will manifest most appreciably in the brain's dynamics rather than its structure. If this is so, then the functional neuroimaging techniques – positron emission tomography (PET) and functional magnetic resonance imaging (fMRI) – may be most appropriate to identifying core deficits. As the two techniques have developed in power and sophistication over the last decade, there has been excitement at their potential value to schizophrenia research.[15] Unhappily, however, from functional neuroimaging too, evidence for a core and reliable deficit has yet to emerge. As with structural imaging, most studies have produced some evidence for abnormal brain responses to differing situations and tasks in patient groups, but these abnormalities in functional response have proved highly variable in localization and in nature.

The marked inconsistency across structural and functional neuroimaging studies invites at least three explanations.

(1) There is no structural or functional brain abnormality that characterizes or indicates schizophrenia.

(2) There is a structural and/or functional abnormality that may be considered characteristic of schizophrenia but the nature and location of this abnormality differs across differing subtypes of the syndrome. Furthermore, with respect to functional neuroimaging studies, elucidation of any particular abnormality will depend upon the psychological state that predominates during the acquisition of the imaging data.

(3) There are functional deficits that characterize schizophrenia or its subtypes. However, these deficits are not regionally localized and will be invisible to studies that concentrate either on the anatomical characteristics of separate brain regions or on the task-induced responses of these brain regions in isolation. Rather they will be seen as abnormal regional interactions, i.e. a *disintegration* of brain function.

We do not believe that an acceptance of the first explanation is yet forced upon us. We will concentrate, instead, upon the latter two, focusing first upon the idea that the absence of a consensus from existing neuroimaging studies reflects the heterogeneity of the subject groups and, furthermore, that the large variability in findings from studies that measure task/condition-related regional brain activity arises mainly out of differences in experimental designs rather than variability in the patients that are assessed. In the final part of the chapter we address the question of whether core deficits in schizophrenia may be explored more fruitfully at the level of interacting systems rather than through characterization of functional and structural attributes of isolated brain areas.

We begin by considering some of the neuroimaging data concerned with the identification of regionally specific abnormalities accompanying schizophrenia.

The search for a regional brain abnormality

This chapter describes the theoretical limitations in the notion that schizophrenia can be 'placed' within the brain. Our position – that the search for a single schizophrenia region will prove fruitless – is an increasingly common one but should not be taken as a dismissal of the large body of neuroimaging work in which regional abnormalities have been identified. While we draw attention to inconsistencies between studies and to the unlikelihood that any single abnormality will explain or reflect schizophrenia in its entirety, we do so with due acknowledgement of two key points. First, the majority of abnormalities are reported on the basis of careful observation and/or strenuous statistical thresholding. They cannot be explained away or ignored. It is inconsistencies across studies that we wish to address rather than individual findings. Second, the elucidation of regional abnormalities is, of course, a most useful enterprise, particularly when, as is almost always the case, authors are duly cautious about the implications of their findings for the syndrome as a whole. Below, we review some of the studies implicating several brain regions in schizophrenia. We refer to structural (both gross anatomy and neuroreceptors) and functional neuroimaging separately, and then discuss some of the theoretical problems accompanying these approaches.

Structural brain imaging

Imaging brain regions

The earliest finding with respect to structural brain changes in schizophrenia was enlargement of the ventricles, reflecting a reduction in brain volume. Computerized tomography (CT) and MRI studies have shown a relatively small but consistent enlargement of lateral ventricles in schizophrenia with approximately 10% of patients showing ventricular enlargement.[13,16] In monozygotic and dizygotic twin pairs there is a consistent finding of enlarged ventricles, both in terms of the ventricle:brain ratio (VBR) and absolute size of the left lateral and third ventricles in affected twins compared to unaffected twins.[17–19]

Ventricular enlargement in patients with schizophrenia is predominantly in the lateral ventricles, with limited evidence of enlargement of the third ventricle but no evidence of fourth ventricle enlargement.[16] The weight of evidence suggests that ventricular enlargement in schizophrenia is associated with reductions in particular brain regions, rather than a reduction in whole brain volume. The majority of MRI and post-mortem studies have failed to find reduced whole brain volume in patients with schizophrenia.[13,14,16] However, a minority of studies have found an overall reduction in brain volume which may reflect a specific impairment in a subgroup of patients with schizophrenia. There is evidence that this subgroup represents those patients who suffered neurological trauma during birth. McNeil and colleagues[18] and Fannon et al[20] found an association between ventricular enlargement and perinatal complications, and there is also evidence of developmental delay in patients with ventricular enlargement. Studies finding reductions in whole brain volumes and ventricular enlargement include early-onset and first episode studies.[13,20–22] This suggests that these deficits are not progressive but may represent a developmental predisposition to developing schizophrenia.

One important observation from both MRI and post-mortem studies is a reduction of some temporal lobe regions. While the evidence for an overall reduction in temporal lobe volume is not strong, there does seem to be a reduction in the volumes of specific hippocampal regions and in other areas of the medial temporal lobes, including the amygdala and parahippocampal areas (Figure 8.2).[13,14,16,23] The observation of abnormalities in medial temporal lobe structures is intriguing. As well as being critical to memory function, which is undoubtedly impaired in schizophrenia,[24,25] these regions have been suggested to relate to symptoms of thought disorder and auditory hallucinations, which are prominent in schizophrenia. Neuroimaging studies of temporal lobes have been reviewed by Nelson et al.[26]

Cognitive deficits in schizophrenia have also led to an interest in the role of the frontal lobes in the disorder. Patients with schizophrenia exhibit deficits on executive tasks, often performing similarly to patients with frontal lesions.[27–29] However, while there is some evidence of reduced frontal lobe volume, this effect is weak and has not always been replicated.[13,14,16] One possible reason for the lack of structural abnormality in the frontal lobes, in spite of impaired performance on frontal tasks, is that the task difficulties experienced by such patients arises not from an abnormality of frontal structure but rather from aberrant connections of this region with other brain areas. We will return to this possibility later.

Other cortical regions have not been investigated in great detail: studies investigating the volume of the parietal and occipital lobes have failed to find a consistent reduction in these regions, and subcortical structures have also been neglected although they are receiving increasing attention. There is evidence for structural abnormalities in the thalamus, corpus callosum, and basal ganglia,[16] though this must, at present, be considered preliminary.

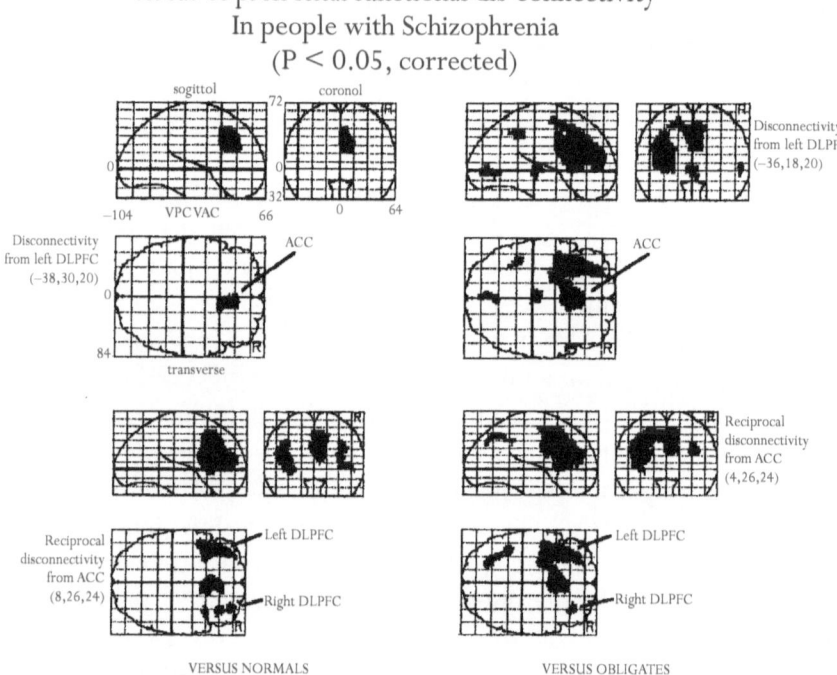

Areas of prefrontal functional dis-connectivity
In people with Schizophrenia
(P < 0.05, corrected)

People with schizophrenia exhibit a relative functional dis–connectivity between left DLPFC and ACC
compared with both other groups

Figure 8.1 *Brain areas exhibiting reduced functional connectivity with the left dorsolateral prefrontal cortex (DLPFC) in people with schizophrenia relative to normal controls (upper left) and obligate carriers (upper right). Below are the reciprocal analyses, showing disconnectivity from the anterior cingulate cortex (ACC) in patients relative to normals (lower left) and obligate carriers (lower right). These diagrams show statistical parametric maps thresholded for display purposes at* P < 0.05 *(corrected for multiple comparisons). On all comparisons, patients exhibit reduced connectivity between the ACC and left DLPFC. (Reproduced from Spence et al. Functional anatomy of verbal fluency in people with schizophrenia and those at genetic risk: focal dysfunction and distributed disconnectivity re-appraised. Br J Psychiatry 2000;* **176:** *52–60 with permission from The Royal College of Psychiatrists.)*

One potentially useful approach to structural imaging in schizophrenia lies in the observation of an association between abnormalities in brain regions and particular symptoms. This has offered a way of making sense of conflicting findings by reducing the heterogeneity of schizophrenic samples. That is, by acknowledging the variability of the symptom patterns across individuals, we may introduce a valuable piece of information into the analysis and, thus, identify within-group differences that might otherwise be treated as noise in the data. So, for example, structural abnormalities in the superior temporal gyrus have been associated with symptoms of formal thought disorder, although there is also some evidence of an association with auditory hallucinations and delusions.[13] Abnormalities in the medial temporal lobe are associated with positive symptoms as a whole with some suggestion that they may be specifically related to auditory hallucinations. Although there is some evidence of an association between structural

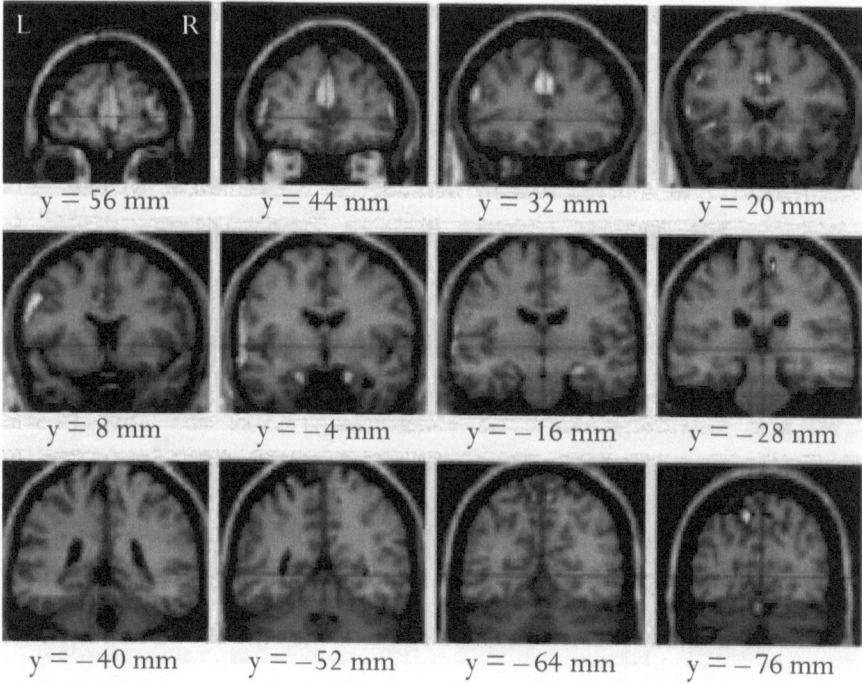

Figure 8.2 *Regional grey matter changes in patients with schizoprenia. Areas with significantly reduced and increased grey matter in patients with schizophrenia compared with controls were rendered onto coronal slices of the normal template magnetic resonance images, shown in yellow and blue/white, respectively. (Reproduced from Suzuki et al. Schizophrenia Res 2002; **55**: 41–54[23] with permission from Elsevier.)*

abnormalities in the medial temporal region and negative symptoms.[30] There have been very few studies investigating the association between structural changes to the frontal lobes and schizophrenic symptoms. However, there is some evidence of an association between reduction in prefrontal white matter volume and negative symptoms.[31,32]

Imaging neurotransmitter receptors

Unlike structural imaging, which measures brain volume, or functional imaging, which measures cerebral blood flow, receptor imaging focuses on neuroreceptors. Receptor imaging is primarily used to assess neurochemical theories of schizophrenia. Studies have generally focused on three groups of receptors: dopamine receptors, serotonin receptors and gamma-aminobutyric acid (GABA) receptors.[33]

The dopamine hypothesis posits that there is an excess of activity of dopamine systems in patients with schizophrenia. This is largely based on the efficacy of dopamine antagonists in treating schizophrenic symptoms.[34] However, contrary to this theory, there is a lack of strong evidence for a major abnormality of dopamine in schizophrenia. There may be subtle differences in striatal and temporal D2 receptors in patients with schizophrenia, e.g. male patients with schizophrenia show increased D2 asymmetry[33,35,36] and post-mortem studies show disruptions to D2 receptors in the temporal cortex.[37] There is some evidence of reduced D1 receptors in the frontal cortex in patients with schizophrenia.[38,39] However, this effect has also been shown in patients with bipolar disorder and so this may not be specific to schizophrenia.[33] While there is not strong evidence for a specific increase in dopamine activity in schizophrenia, there is increasing evidence of poor regulation of dopamine in these patients. Patients given an acute administration of amphetamine show increased striatal dopamine, and this increase is associated with the activation of psychotic symptoms.[40-42] This may reflect dopamine disregulation rather than a simple increase in dopamine levels in patients with schizophrenia. Evidence from dopamine-based treatments of schizophrenia support the theory that these patients exhibit disregulation of dopamine, particularly D2. Atypical medications for the treatment of schizophrenia target the D2 receptor and are associated with significant clinical improvement.[43,44] Clinical improvement following these treatments is associated with the degree of D2-receptor occupancy with greater D2 occupancy predicting improved clinical outcome.[45]

Serotonin lacks a selective radioligand so there have been few receptor imaging studies of serotonin levels in schizophrenia. However, studies investigating serotonin occupancy induced by atypical neuroleptic medication, in particular clozapine, have shown a high occupancy of serotonin receptors in patients with schizophrenia.[46] This finding has also been extended to neuroleptic-naïve patients with schizophrenia.[47] This may reflect an excess of serotonin in patients with schizophrenia.[33] Finally, there is some weak evidence of reduced GABA receptor binding in schizophrenia, especially in relation to positive symptoms,[48] although this has not been found consistently.[49] The inconsistent results may be due to reduced GABA receptor binding being specific to a subset of patients showing cognitive deficits.[50]

Some more recent studies have investigated other neuroreceptors, such as cholinergic and glutamate receptors, in patients with schizophrenia and there is some suggestion that these receptors may be involved in schizophrenia. For example, receptor binding is reduced at cholinergic receptors in the prefrontal cortex in patients with schizophrenia.[51] Similarly, reduced receptor binding at prefrontal, hippocampal and thalamic sites has been found at glutamate receptors in patients with schizophrenia.[52–54]

Functional imaging

Functional imaging techniques have had a major impact upon neuroscience within the last decade or so. They offer spatially precise, *in vivo* methods of exploring responses in the living brain. The two main techniques are PET and fMRI. A technical discussion of these two approaches is beyond the scope of this chapter but a key thing to remember is that each provides an estimation of the level of brain activity (from region to region) that occurs in association with a specific mental state. The extent to which this activity is interpretable is largely dependent upon the extent to which we can define and manipulate the subject's mental state. This has connotations for experimental design and interpretability, as will be discussed below.

The earliest studies, attempting to identify brain regions associated with abnormal functioning in schizophrenia, explored brain activity while patients were at rest. A number of studies showed reduced activation in the frontal cortex in patients with schizophrenia compared to controls. However, a larger number of studies failed to find reduced frontal activity (so-called hypofrontality) in these patients. In an early review of the emerging literature, Chua and McKenna[13] suggested that hypofrontality may relate to negative symptoms in schizophrenia – an early indication that the clinical

233

heterogeneity may obfuscate results of such studies. Furthermore, imaging studies of patients at rest are inherently problematic, as will be discussed further below.

An alternative to the resting state study is the activation study in which subjects are required to perform a cognitive task. We are then able to evaluate the way in which each brain region changes its activity in response to the demands of this task and, crucially, to elucidate abnormalities in these regional responses associated with disease states. In such cases, the level of regional activity provoked by this task may be compared across groups in order to identify brain areas that are failing to increase their activity in response to the task demands. It has been suggested that the hypofrontality of schizophrenia may best be understood in terms of reduced task-invoked frontal activation rather than a simple reduction in resting activity. With this in mind, a number of studies have explored frontal responses in schizophrenia to a variety of tasks. However, as with resting studies, findings have proved inconsistent, with some studies showing task-related hypofrontality and some not. For example, it has been shown that the Wisconsin Card Sorting Task (WCST; a test of frontal function that requires subjects to identify the rules that govern the division of cards and to change the rule that they use periodically) provokes less lateral frontal activity in schizophrenic patients than in control subjects.[55–57] In the Tower of London task (a task that requires the planning of a series of moves in order to reach a specified goal) an underactivation of a more medial part of the frontal lobe has been shown.[58] In other studies, e.g. of language production, lateral frontal activity in patients has been indistinguishable from that in controls,[59] while medial frontal activation has been reduced.[60] However, in contrast to this, it has also been shown that lateral frontal activity in response to language tasks is indeed reduced.[61]

Other tasks, particularly those involving memory, planning and problem-solving, have been associated with abnormalities in activation, particularly in the frontal lobe[62–65] and hippocampus.[66] A key problem to interpreting such findings, however, is that when the patients are unable to perform the task, these failures of brain activity could reflect this failed performance (e.g. if the patient becomes bored or frustrated) rather than an intrinsic abnormality in that region. It has been suggested, and shown, that when tasks are changed so that patients with schizophrenia perform at the same level as control subjects, there is no longer evidence of hypofrontality in these patients.[13,67,68]

Imaging studies using tasks involving attention and inhibitory processes have also produced evidence for abnormalities in patients with schizophrenia. These include reduced frontal and cingulate activation with tasks that require a high degree of attention.[69-71] There is also evidence that, when confronted with certain types of tasks, patients show abnormal activity in regions associated with a phenomenon that has been referred to as monitoring.[72,73] Temporal lobe abnormalities have also been shown, especially in tasks that engage memory processes.[74,75]

Just from this very brief and limited review, it is obvious that, while promising much, functional imaging techniques have delivered no clearer idea of the locus of brain abnormality in schizophrenia than have the structural techniques. In the next section, we put forward a number of explanations for this disappointing state of affairs.

Theoretical considerations in studies of regional abnormalities

The majority of studies attempting to identify regional structural or functional abnormalities in schizophrenia have adopted a case-control approach. Scans or images from groups of subjects falling into the diagnostic category are compared with those from subjects falling into a separate category or deemed to be healthy. The extent to which the group differences identified by such studies may be considered as plausible markers for schizophrenic pathology is dependent upon the thoroughness with which the groups are balanced. In the perfect study, the patient and the control groups would be identical in every physical, emotional, social, economic and cognitive way. In such a case, only the presence of the illness could be invoked to explain the imaging differences. This is an unachievable goal and we must, of course, work within the constraints of this admission.

Another factor contributing to ambiguity in understanding the group differences is the validity of the diagnostic category and the extent to which a group of subjects meeting diagnostic criteria may be considered homogenous. Clearly, this is a consideration that arises in any case-control study, but it is perhaps particularly relevant in schizophrenia in which the very existence of the disease as a valid nosological entity is frequently called into question.[76-78] As an explanation for inconsistencies in the imaging findings, the uncertainty surrounding the notion of schizophrenia as a unitary illness must be taken into account. It should be remembered that this is by no means a problem that is unique to neuroimaging but one that arises in any study of schizophrenia that relies upon this broad diagnostic grouping. Of course, this will remain a prominent obstacle to the interpretation of such studies until schizophrenia is more clearly understood with respect to the extent and nature of its heterogeneity. Meanwhile, unless neuroimaging research works within the constraints of this incomplete understanding, apparent inconsistency is likely to predominate.

The points raised above are relevant to all imaging techniques. However, with the development and increasing use of functional imaging techniques comes a new set of problems: these are raised and discussed below.

In distinction to structural imaging techniques, functional neuorimaging techniques are state dependent, i.e. the brain activity that they measure is considered to be reflective of the mental state that predominates during the measurement. This has important implications with respect to interpreting the findings from such studies. To begin with, we must choose the state in which the measurement is to be made. Many early studies measured brain activity at rest. However, since 'rest' is a highly underspecified condition, a brain activity measurement acquired in association with it is likely to be highly variable. The resting scan is usually preceded by an instruction to lie still and try to empty their minds. Anecdotally, healthy subjects have reported variable mental states, e.g. they may engage in a train of thoughts comprised of associated memories, they may make plans, they may fall asleep. One colleague reports the case of a subject who became preoccupied with the worry that they may have left their gas turned on. Added to this variability in healthy subjects is the possibility of highly different subjective experiences of rest in the patient groups. In the latter case, rest may be an anxious state accompanied by unpleasant hallucinations. Alternatively, in those with predominantly negative symptoms, it may be a highly impover-ished cognitive state. Thus, resting brain activity in schizophrenia is very difficult to interpret whether it is accompanied by hypo- or hyperfrontality.

The alternative to the resting state study is the activation study in which subjects are required to perform a cognitive task. In such cases, the level of regional activity provoked by this task may be compared across groups in order to identify brain areas that are failing to increase their activity in response to the task demands. As described above, it has been suggested that the hypofrontality of schizophrenia may best be understood in terms of reduced task-invoked frontal activation rather than a simple reduction in resting activity. However, as with resting state studies, and despite their attempts to evaluate brain activity in the setting of more specific psychological tasks, activation studies have not produced a clear consensus with respect to frontal function in schizophrenia. Once again, attention should be drawn to the theoretical ambiguities that accompany such studies. As with resting studies, these arise from the state-related measurements that are the hallmark of functional imaging. In activation studies, the task-related activity is measured by comparison to a baseline, e.g. rest or the performance of some undemanding cognitive task. If the baseline systematically differs across groups of patients and their controls, then any activation difference observed across groups is ambiguous. Furthermore, since activation tasks are often of interest because schizophrenic patients have difficulty in performing them, one must take this into account in assessing task-related activation. Could it be that underactivation in the patients reflects the fact that they are not performing the task properly? Fletcher et al,[67] for example, observed that patients show normal levels of frontal activation when performing a memory task that has been tailored to their capabilities but that activation falls away when the demands of the task are further increased. This is in contrast to control subjects whose frontal response to increasing demands was a further increase in activity. This study, though consistent with other work,[79] must be viewed in the light of other studies with apparently contradictory findings.[80] The critical point is that whether a cognitive activation study or a resting study is used, many inconsistencies are likely to arise because of the difficulties in defining the mental state that predominates at the time of scanning. Since this is likely to differ across different subject groups (and, indeed, will differ within one group at different times), the idea of a localized functional imaging abnormality that characterizes schizophrenia may be fanciful.

These cautionary points are raised both to explain the inconsistencies across the imaging literature on schizophrenia and as a pointer to likely directions for future searches for localized structural or functional pathology in schizophrenia. With respect to the latter, we suggest that the key issues will lie in identifying patient groups and, in the setting of functional neuroimaging studies, in specifying the psychological state in which the measurements are made. We will discuss, briefly, each of these areas below.

Identifying the patient group

It has been suggested (and the inconsistent neuroimaging literature indirectly testifies) that schizophrenia exists as a constellation of loosely grouped symptoms whose existence as a unitary phenomenon has yet to be established. In view of this, perhaps we should design neuroimaging studies in a way that speaks more directly to the heterogeneity that exists under the rubric of schizophrenia. If we focus, for example, upon how different symptoms such as hallucinations or delusions may be associated with structural or functional brain abnormalities, data may be much cleaner. Such an approach has been taken in the past. For example, Frith et al[59] divided patients with schizophrenia, all performing a language-production task, into three groups with differing symptomatology showing that an abnormality of blood flow in the temporal cortex was common to all three groups, a finding that perhaps speaks in favour of schizophrenia as a meaningful construct. Liddle et al,[81] on the other hand, showed varying patterns of resting activity across groups of schizophrenic patients divided according to a predominance of positive symptoms (such as delusions and hallucinations), a predominance of negative symptoms or a predominance of thought disorder. These findings were echoed by Kaplan et al.[82]

An alternative, though related, approach is to explore the imaging correlates of the symptoms themselves, and to establish the extent to which, say, hallucinations occurring within the diagnosis of schizophrenia compare and contrast (in terms of the associated imaging findings) with experientially similar phenomena in the setting, e.g. of depression. This is technically difficult in functional imaging since subjects must be scanned during the occurrence of the phenomenon of interest and during a baseline condition in which this phenomenon is absent or reduced. Nevertheless, ingenious approaches have been used to image brain changes associated with auditory hallucinations.[83–86] Furthermore, cognitive task-related activations have been studied in patients with highly specific symptoms such as paranoid delusions[87] and delusions of alien control.[88] Such studies will be ultimately important in determining the extent to which behaviourally similar states may be associated with differing patterns of brain activity across differing diagnostic categories. Alternatively, it may turn out that auditory hallucinations, say, are neurobiologically indistinguishable across schizophrenia and bipolar disorder.

A further exciting development is in the introduction of genetic information to brain imaging. Such information provides objective evidence for within-group homogeneity and heterogeneity. Thus, it may be used to identify and validate subgroupings, and these subgroupings may then be explored at the level of brain structure and function. While this approach is in its early stages, it has already proved possible to explore the brain morphological correlates of genetic information.[89] Furthermore, it has proven possible to observe genetic influences upon cognitive function and upon brain activation, a finding that may be directly relevant to schizophrenia. For example, the COMT genotype, which regulates dopamine activity, has been found to account for 4% of the perseverative errors on the WCST in a sample including patients with schizophrenia, their unaffected siblings and control participants.[90,91] This uniting of differing levels of subgrouping from the genetic to the behavioural to the imaging may prove enormously powerful with respect to clarifying the extent to which heterogeneity in patient groups produces variability in imaging observations.

Thus, neuroimaging studies may be used with greater precision in order to establish the particular relationship between brain regions and schizophrenia. There is the possibility too that the techniques will contribute to, rather than depend upon, our understanding of schizophrenia as a syndrome. Since neuroimaging presents an objective measure of the ways in which the schizophrenic patient differs from the control or the patient with affective disorder, perhaps the techniques may form an important part of validation of the diagnosis. Alternatively, they may play a part in the dissolution of the categorical notion of diagnosis in favour of a view that emphasizes the heterogeneity of the condition.

Specifying the psychological setting in which functional neuroimaging measurements are made

The most important feature of functional neuroimaging techniques lies in their state dependence. While a structural scan may be assessed in almost complete isolation from the mental state that accompanied its acquisition, a functional scan is meaningless without a precise view of what the subject was doing during this time. Furthermore, many functional images express brain activity relative to baseline scans, in which subjects are carrying out tasks designed to 'subtract out' the more general brain activity related to moving, speaking, seeing, etc. This means that our interpretation of functional brain images is entirely dependent upon the extent to which we can specify the cognitive processes that occur. Any degree of uncertainty (and some degree of uncertainty is inevitable) will affect interpretation. This effect is further complicated by issues surrounding task performance and baseline measures in schizophrenic patients. After all, if two groups of subjects are performing tasks differently, we would predict differing patterns of brain activity even in the absence of any illness.

While it has been argued that the cognitive opacity of most tasks and conditions renders attempts to 'map' the human brain ultimately intractable,[92] we suggest that there is still much to be learned about the nature of schizophrenia from brain activation studies. Even if it appears unlikely that the identification of a core, regionally localized abnormality will be achievable, functional neuroimaging is likely to provide anatomical clues that may be taken up in the application of other techniques, e.g. microscopic anatomical analyses. Furthermore, we believe that functional imaging activation studies may find an important niche through the use of an alternative approach. A major strength is that PET and fMRI provide a measure of cognitive processing that may be, under certain circumstances, more sensitive and powerful than existing behavioural measures. Thus, for example, tasks exist on which schizophrenic patients achieve behavioural performance that is indistinguishable from that seen in control subjects. A key question is whether the apparently normal performance is achieved in a 'normal' way. More specifically, does a patient successfully performing, say, a language-production task, activate the same system of brain regions (and to the same extent) as a control subject who, to an external observer, is performing the task identically? Functional neuroimaging offers increasingly powerful and sensitive ways to answer this question. Frith et al[59] identified a superior temporal abnormality existing in three groups of schizophrenic patients, each of whom were performing the language task in a way that matched that of control subjects. While this finding has been called into question with respect to its validity as a trait marker for schizophrenia,[93] the approach clearly offers potential insights. Alternatively, one might identify whether the functional neuroanatomical underpinnings of task performance differ within subjects depending upon whether they are in the acute stages of the illness or in remission. Spence et al,[94] for example, have shown that task-related hypofrontality is specific to the acute state even though task performance was not measurably impaired.

Summary – a regional abnormality in schizophrenia?
Many difficulties attend the search for core structural and functional abnormalities in schizophrenia. These are rooted in an incomplete understanding of the illness itself and the extent to which it may be considered a unitary phenomenon. This uncertainty may account for a good deal of the inconsistency surrounding structural and functional imaging findings in schizophrenia. Furthermore, studies of brain function carry with them additional uncertainties surrounding the extent to which chosen 'activation' tasks may succeed in isolating and manipulating the cognitive processes of interest. These uncertainties are compounded when the same tasks are carried

out by schizophrenic people since unequal performance levels introduce further ambiguity and even matched performance may be achievable through activation of different brain systems. Nevertheless, careful group selection, informed perhaps by more specific subgrouping on the basis of both phenotypic and genotypic features, is likely to have a major impact, particularly when combined with improved models of cognitive function. In this setting the techniques may realize an exciting potential. This potential, however, addresses only one aspect of structure–function relations in the brain: that of functional segregation. A functionally segregated view of the brain is based upon the notion that different functions and processes are carried out in different parts of the brain. As a partial description of brain organization, this is indisputable. It is not, however, complete. An understanding of brain function (and dysfunction) must also acknowledge the enormous degree of interregional connectivity and the compelling likelihood that separable regions, while showing functional specialization, must act as parts of integrated systems. This description of brain organization, i.e. in terms of functional integration, will be discussed in the final section with particular emphasis on its disruption as a key feature of schizophrenia. We will examine, furthermore, the peculiar advantages of the functional neuroimaging techniques to evaluating brain function in terms of interregional integration.

Schizophrenia: a disorder of brain integration?

Since brain function may be fully characterized only with reference both to regional specialization of function and to the integration of brain regions with differing functions, we must consider the possibility that the core disturbance in schizophrenia is a distributed one. Does schizophrenia exist as a disconnection syndrome?[95]

Before considering the insights that may be offered by high-resolution, whole brain functional neuroimaging, it is important to clarify what is meant by the term disconnection in the current formulation. We are referring specifically to a *functional* disconnection. The existence of such a disconnection does not necessarily depend upon a gross disturbance of white matter tracts (i.e. an *anatomical* disconnection). That is not to say that there is no infrastructural marker for the functional disconnection (e.g. at the synaptic level) but we wish to confine our discussion to a disconnection expressed in terms of abnormal functional interactions between brain regions. We suggest that such deficits may be invoked to explain the symptoms of schizophrenia more adequately than the idea of schizophrenia as a localized brain impairment.

Before considering the contribution of functional neuroimaging (specifically that of fMRI) to this theoretical position, it is worth identifying some of the key pieces of evidence that point towards schizophrenia as a disconnection syndrome. One important observation was the degree of symptomatic overlap between schizophrenia and metachromatic leukodystrophy, a condition accompanied by disruptions in white matter tracts (i.e. anatomical disconnectivity), and features of psychosis that, to some extent, mimic acute schizophrenia.[96] While this is not to suggest that identical deficits underlie the two conditions, the anatomical disconnection as a partial model of schizophrenia may be informative. Furthermore, chemical disconnection produced by the acute administration of phencyclidine (a NMDA [N-methyl-D-aspartate] receptor antagonist) also produces symptoms that compellingly mimic schizophrenia.[97] This re-emerging viewpoint of schizophrenia as a disconnection disorder is lent support by consideration of the condition within the field of connectionist modelling[98,99] and by suggestions that a core (but distributed) deficit in schizophrenia lies in an abnormal neuronal plasticity.[100] The significance of this latter observation is that interregional functional connectivity is, to a large extent, dependent upon synaptic changes that occur in response to experience. Abnormalities in these changes are likely to produce abnormal connections.

A further observation lending indirect weight to the notion of schizophrenia as a disconnection lies in the nature of the symptomatology. The term itself refers to a splitting of mental functions,[101] and it is difficult to explain the experiences and behaviour without recourse to a consideration of the relations and integration between cognitive processes (see Frith[102] for full discussion). For example, an auditory hallucination may be explained in terms of a misattribution of internal speech to the outside world (one's inner voice is 'heard' as an external person). This may be construed as a failure to integrate a process with the attribution of the origin of that process. An analogous explanation may be invoked to account for passivity phenomena, e.g. when someone makes a movement but does not recognize themselves as having generated that movement, attributing it instead to some unseen force or tormentor. Thus, the nature of much of the schizophrenic psychopathology demands an explanation in terms of disintegration of separate functions rather than in specific and well-circumscribed cognitive domains.

So how might these observations and this theoretical stance inform neuroimaging experimentation, and how might the findings from imaging experiments be formulated in terms of a search for interregional disintegration rather than intraregional deficits? The suitability of PET and fMRI in addressing brain integration was recognized early in their development.[103] It seems likely that, of the functional neuroimaging techniques that offer high spatial resolution, fMRI is most suitable to an assessment of functional connectivity, as such analysis demands a great deal of data (scans) to be acquired as rapidly as possible and PET is very limited in these respects. It should also be admitted that, since fMRI is dependent upon the very sluggish blood flow response to neuronal activity, this technique too has many limitations and perhaps, ultimately, will best be combined with techniques that offer millisecond level temporal resolution. Bearing these constraints in mind, we will nevertheless consider how fMRI may be used to gain an understanding of task-related brain integration/connectivity and the extent to which disconnectivity may be characteristic of schizophrenia.

The key to understanding functional imaging evaluations of brain integration is the observation that if two brain regions are connected (in the sense that their functions are integrated), the activity of one may correlate with that of the other. This correlation may be negative or positive. Thus, for example, across many different tasks, activity of the anterior cingulate cortex and lateral prefrontal cortex has been observed to show a high correlation. The two regions, on this basis, may be asserted to be functionally connected. (Interestingly, evidence has emerged that this functional connection may be weakened in obligate carriers of schizophrenia.[104]) This idea of the correlation between regions as a marker of functional connectivity is not, in itself, of great theoretical value. While it does encourage a systems-based view of brain function, rather than overemphasizing separate anatomical regions, it does not carry much explanatory power. The activity in any two regions may correlate strongly (and they may thus be deemed as functionally connected) even though they do not function as part of a system. Rather their co-activation may be driven by the influence of a third region – one that drives activity in each of them separately.

So while we may observe functional connectivity between brain regions using fMRI and characterize, with great specificity, the extent to which such connectivity/correlation is specific to particular cognitive tasks or conditions, such analysis carries no information about the influential relationship between brain regions that show such connectivity. Rather it refers simply to a statistical connection. If regions A and B are observed to be so connected, it could be that activity in A causes activity in B, that activity in B causes activity in A or that activity in a third region, C, causes activity in A and B separately.

In order to have a clearer idea of how A and B relate to each other, we must introduce an analysis of *effective connectivity*.[105] This refers to the causal relationship that exists between regions. To say that A is effectively connected to B carries with it an assertion that A has an influence upon B. Effective connectivity may be postulated upon the basis of a rather more complex analysis of the imaging data, one that requires a system of inter-locking regression analyses within an a priori model of the brain regions of interest. Such a model must include regions with hypothesized, direction-ally specified connections and this is applied to the actual observations (scans) so that the extent to which it fits the data may be assessed. This approach has proved fruitful, for example, in identifying how interregional connections may change as a function of experience in fMRI learning experiments.[106–108]

There are reasons, therefore, to suppose that assessments of interregional correlations may have a growing impact upon the nature and analysis of functional neuroimaging studies. As the field gains a more thorough under-standing of brain connectivity, there is likely to be a growth in the use of this approach to identify deficits in schizophrenia. Already, a number of sugges-tions have been made about likely candidates for 'disconnected' regions. We outline these below.

Functional neuroimaging and the schizophrenia disconnection

Prefrontal–thalamic–cerebellar disconnectivity?

Andreasen et al[109] have suggested that a common neurodevelopmental pathophysiology links the apparently diverse subtypes of schizophrenia. A feature of this pathophysiology is held to lie in aberrant connectivity in the neuronal circuit that links the prefrontal cortex to the thalamus to the cerebellum and back to the cortex. Having amassed evidence in favour of this position on the basis of regionally localized abnormalities in these components of the putatively abnormal circuit,[15,110] the group recently carried out a more direct test of the hypothesis on the basis of inter-regional correlation.[111] They showed that, in the setting of simple motor task (e.g. finger-tapping), schizophrenia is indeed characterized by abnormal connectivity between regions within this circuitry. In addition, they showed that this disconnectivity was 'normalized' when the schizophrenic people were treated with olanzapine. The prospect of exploring the condition in terms of interregional disconnectivity and then characterizing how these disconnections are modified by drugs with specific neuromodulatory actions is a rich and exciting one.

Prefrontal–temporal disconnectivity?

Friston and Frith[95] suggested that a feature of schizophrenia may the abnormal interaction between the lateral prefrontal and superior temporal cortices. This is consistent with a number of studies showing that while control subjects tend to show a reciprocal relationship between left prefrontal cortex and superior temporal gyrus activity, this relationship is lost (and even reversed) in schizophrenia.[59,112] Interestingly, this is not an effect of medication, since the subjects studied by Fletcher et al[112] were unmedicated. Furthermore, Frith et al[59] observed the phenomenon across three different subgroups of schizophrenia, suggesting that it may provide a general marker for the condition. One further observation emerging from this early work was that when a dopamine agonist (apomorphine) was administered, the prefronto–temporal pattern of activity became more 'normal'. While this finding in itself is ambiguous, it is certainly interesting to note that the disconnectivity is sensitive to a dopaminergic perturbation.

This idea of disconnectivity was tested more formally (through a functional connectivity analysis of PET data) by Friston and Frith,[95] who showed that patterns of prefronto–temporal correlation are indeed abnormal in patient groups. A more powerful approach, using fMRI, has produced further evidence for a disturbance in the fronto–temporal relationship in schizophrenia.[113]

Lateral prefrontal–cingulate disconnectivity?

On the basis of a PET study on language production in obligate carriers of schizophrenia, Spence et al[104] challenged the notion that an abnormal prefronto–temporal relationship is a trait marker for schizophrenia. They observed that this group of subjects was characterized by an abnormally weak connectivity between the lateral prefrontal cortex and the anterior cingulate cortex (see Figure 8.1). While this does not exclude the validity of prefronto–temporal disconnectivity as a core feature in acute schizophrenia, it certainly does damage to any simplistic notion that schizophrenia may be explained by an ever-present deficit of this sort.

One interesting piece of evidence linking the hypotheses of Friston and Frith[95] and of Spence et al[104] is the idea that prefronto–temporal connectivity is dependent upon the anterior cingulate cortex. An early observation by Dolan and colleagues[60,112] of a regional deficit in task-related anterior cingulate cortex activity was accompanied by the finding that apomorphine produced an augmentation in this activity; furthermore, in the setting of this 'normalized' cingulate response, prefronto–temporal connectivity also became more normal in schizophrenia.[112] Dolan and colleagues[60,112] suggested a slightly more complex account of disconnectivity, acknowledging the central importance of an anterior cingulate deficit but implying both an abnormality of regional function and of connectivity: 'in schizophrenia, there is a dysregulation in the dopaminergic modulation of cingulate neuronal activity [i.e. a localized abnormality] with a consequent impairment in the functional integration of more remote, but anatomically connected, cortical regions'. More recently, this suggestion has been formally tested through a connectivity analysis of PET data acquired during a memory task. Fletcher et al[114] showed that in control subjects, prefronto–temporal connectivity is stronger when anterior cingulate activity is greater. This modulatory effect of cingulate activity was not found in schizophrenia.

So, the crop of more recent connectivity studies of schizophrenia has identified abnormalities in a number of circuits – prefronto–temporal, prefronto–cingulate, prefronto–cingulo–temporal and prefronto–thalamo–cerebellar. Perhaps, therefore, we might conclude that the search for a distributed deficit has, so far, produced results that are as inconsistent as the search for a regional deficit. This would be, in our view, unnecessarily pessimistic: if disconnectivity of function (rather than an anatomical disconnection arising from disruption in specific white matter tracts) is a feature of schizophrenia then we would expect it to be protean. It would appear in different ways in different situations, depending upon the nature of the task. Thus, for example, in studies of word production, which tend to engage the prefrontal and temporal cortices, we might expect to identify abnormalities in connectivity relationships between these regions. In a task emphasizing, say, motor output (such as that referred to above[111]), the disintegration of thalamic and cerebellar integration would likely stand out, whereas prefronto–temporal connectivity might not be demonstrably abnormal. In brief, the notion of a disintegration of function is a general one and may not be amenable to a simple regionally based exploration.

Summary – schizophrenia and functional disintegration

Functional-imaging-based assessments of brain integration are not immune to the problems of group selection and task design described earlier in the chapter. They do, however, offer a view of normal and abnormal brain function that complements ideas of regional specialization of function. Moreover, a picture of schizophrenia as arising from a fragmentation of functions captures more fully the nature of the symptoms.

Using neuroimaging to evaluate and characterize brain connectivity is, however, difficult. Such analyses are complex and prone to errors since they are dependent upon a priori notions of the nature of brain systems. In addition, since PET and fMRI carry information about second to second changes, whereas the temporal domain of brain function is at the millisecond level, it is important to acknowledge their imprecision with respect to causal interactions between brain regions. Nevertheless, they enable the acquisition of spatially precise data from each brain region, almost simultaneously. We are thus able to use them to determine the behaviour of entire systems: a capability that may be very suited to understanding schizophrenia.

Conclusions

Critics of imaging have pointed to large inconsistencies in the findings from structural and functional studies. These inconsistencies, however, currently say rather more about the uncertainties surrounding schizophrenia as a unitary syndrome than they do about the limitations of the neuroimaging techniques. In order to maximize the potential of both structural and functional neuroimaging, a much clearer understanding is needed of the constellation of subsyndromes that come under the heading of schizophrenia. Strenuous efforts will need to be made in order to ensure that we are not carrying out studies in which we are comparing 'one group of people who, in all probability, have nothing in common with another group of people who also probably have nothing in common'.[77] One option is to select groupings on the basis of symptom profiles, another on the basis of genetic markers. Whatever criteria are used, an ultimate goal will be to establish the extent to which differing groups show similar structural and functional brain attributes. With this information, we may be able to modify ideas about the extent to which, at the neurobiological level, schizophrenia as a meaningful diagnosis may be justifiable.

As well as contributing to a refinement of our ideas about the validity of schizophrenia at the neurobiological level, imaging may also provide insights into the nature of the brain changes that characterize schizophrenia or its subsyndromes. It is possible that core, localized abnormalities in function may be identified and such findings may provide valuable regional information with respect to the application of other, more structurally sensitive, techniques. Further insights may arise from assessments of interregional communication, as estimated by the degree to which anatomically separate brain regions correlate in their activity. This is particularly exciting with respect to a fundamental understanding of the symptoms of schizophrenia in terms of a failure to integrate and unite separate functions – an understanding that, perhaps, gets close to the core deficit.

Summary

- The application of brain imaging techniques offers the potential for understanding mental illnesses such as schizophrenia in terms of localized abnormalities in brain structure and behaviour.
- However, the literature so far is full of inconsistencies and no single region is consistently found to be abnormal.
- These inconsistencies likely reflect variability in schizophrenia itself and perhaps point to the fact that it is not a unitary illness. If this is so, then perhaps the imaging techniques may play a part in telling us the best ways in which it may be subdivided.
- Furthermore, it seems likely that, even with a fuller understanding into the nature of the illness, it is unlikely to be explained in terms of the abnormal structure or function of a single brain region. Rather, we suggest that the techniques should be used to identify abnormalities in the ways in which different brain regions interact with each other, formulating schizophrenia as a disorder of brain integration.
- The functional neuroimaging techniques offer ways of exploring brain integration and disintegration. They may, therefore, be especially well suited to exploring a complex functional illness such as schizophrenia.

References

1. Buchsbaum MS, Ingvar DH, Kessler R et al. Cerebral glucography with positron tomography. Use in normal subjects and in patients with schizophrenia. *Arch Gen Psychiatry* 1982; **39:** 251–9.

2. Ariel RN, Golden CJ, Berg RA et al. Regional cerebral blood flow in schizophrenics. Tests using the xenon Xe 133 inhalation method. *Arch Gen Psychiatry* 1983; **40:** 258–63.

3. Wolkin A, Angrist B, Wolf A et al. Low frontal glucose utilization in chronic schizophrenia: a replication study. *Am J Psychiatry* 1988; **145:** 251–3.

4. Paulman RG, Devous Sr MD, Gregory RR et al. Hypofrontality and cognitive impairment in schizophrenia: dynamic single-photon tomography and neuropsychological assessment of schizophrenic brain function. *Biol Psychiatry* 1990; **27:** 377–99.

5. Andreasen NC, O'Leary DS, Flaum M et al. Hypofrontality in schizophrenia: distributed dysfunctional circuits in neuroleptic-naive patients. *Lancet* 1997; **349:** 1730–4.

6. Sheppard G, Gruzelier J, Manchanda R et al. 15O positron emission tomographic scanning in predominantly never-treated acute schizophrenic patients. *Lancet* 1983; **2:** 1448–52.

7. Gur RE, Resnick SM, Alavi A et al. Regional brain function in schizophrenia. I. A positron emission tomography study. *Arch Gen Psychiatry* 1987; **44:** 119–25.

8. Gur RE, Gur RC, Skolnick BE et al. Brain function in psychiatric disorders. III. Regional cerebral blood flow in unmedicated schizophrenics. *Arch Gen Psychiatry* 1985; **42:** 329–34.

9. Gur RE, Skolnick BE, Gur RC et al. Brain function in psychiatric disorders. I. Regional cerebral blood flow in medicated schizophrenics. *Arch Gen Psychiatry* 1983; **40:** 1250–4.

10. Early TS, Reiman EM, Raichle ME, Spitznagel EL. Left globus pallidus abnormality in never-medicated patients with schizophrenia. *Proc Natl Acad Sci USA* 1987; **84:** 561–3.

11. Cleghorn JM, Garnett ES, Nahmias C et al. Increased frontal and reduced parietal glucose metabolism in acute untreated schizophrenia. *Psychiatry Res* 1989; **28:** 119–33.

12. Johnstone EC, Crow TJ, Frith CD et al. Cerebral ventricular size and cognitive impairment in chronic schizophrenics. *Lancet* 1976; **2:** 924–6.

13. Chua SE, McKenna PJ. Schizophrenia – a brain disease? A critical review of structural and functional cerebral abnormality in the disorder. *Br J Psych* 1995; **166:** 563–82.

14. Wright IC, Rabe-Hesketh S, Woodruff PWR et al. Regional brain structure in schizophrenia: a meta-analysis of volumetric MRI studies. *Am J Psychiatry* 2000; **157:** 16–25.

15. Andreasen NC. Pieces of the schizophrenia puzzle fall into place. *Neuron* 1996; **16:** 697–700.

16. McCarley RW, Wible CG, Frumin M et al. MRI anatomy of schizophrenia. *Biol Psychiatry* 1999; **45:** 1099–119.

17. Baare WFC, van Oel CJ, Hulshoff HE et al. Volumes of brain structures in twins discordant for schizophrenia. *Arch Gen Psychiatry* 2001; **58:** 33–40.

18. McNeil TF, Cantor-Graae E, Weinberger DR. Relationship of obstetric complications and differences in size of brain structures in monozygotic twin pairs discordant for schizophrenia. *Am J Psychiatry* 2000; **157:** 203–12.

19. Ohara K, Xu HD, Matsunaga T et al. Cerebral ventricle–brain ratio in monozygotic twins discordant and concordant for schizophrenia. *Prog Neuropsychopharmac Biol Psychiatry* 1998; **22:** 1043–50.

20. Fannon D, Tennakoon L, Sumich A et al. Third ventricle enlargement and developmental delay in first-episode psychosis: preliminary findings. *Br J Psychiatry* 2000; **177:** 354–9.

21. Matsumoto H, Simmons A, Williams S, Pipe R, Murray R, Frangou S. Structural magnetic imaging of the hippocampus in early onset schizophrenia. *Biol Psychiatry* 2001; **49:** 824–31.

22. Matsumoto H, Simmons A, Williams S et al. Superior temporal gyrus abnormalities in early-onset schizophrenia: similarities and differences with adult-onset schizophrenia. *Am J Psychiatry* 2001; **158:** 1299–304.

23. Suzuki M, Nohara S, Hagino H et al. Regional changes in brain gray and white matter in patients with schizophrenia demonstrated with voxel-based analysis of MRI. *Schizophrenia Res* 2002; **55:** 41–54.

24. McKenna PJ, Tamlyn D, Lund CE, Mortimer AM, Hammond S, Baddeley AD. Amnesic syndrome in schizophrenia. *Psychol Med* 1990; **20:** 967–72.

25. Tamlyn D, McKenna PJ, Mortimer AM, Lund CE, Hammond S, Baddeley AD. Memory impairment in schizophrenia: its extent, affiliations and neuropsychological character. *Psychol Med* 1992; **22:** 101–15.

26. Nelson MD, Saykin AJ, Flashman LA, Riordan HJ. Hippocampal volume reduction in schizophrenia as assessed by magnetic resonance imaging: a meta-analytic study. *Arch Gen Psychiatry* 1998; **55:** 433–40.

27. Mahurin RK, Velligan DI, Miller AL. Executive–frontal lobe cognitive dysfunction in schizophrenia: a symptom subtype analysis. *Psychiatry Res* 1998; **79:** 139–49.

28. Morice R, Delahunty A. Frontal/executive impairments in schizophrenia. *Schizophrenia Bull* 1996; **22:** 125–37.

29. McGrath J, Scheldt S, Welham J, Clair A. Performance on tests sensitive to impaired executive ability in schizophrenia, mania and well controls: acute and subacute phases. *Schizophrenia Res* 1997; **26:** 127–37.

30. Foong J, Symms MR, Barker GJ et al. Neuropathological abnormalities in schizophrenia: evidence from magnetization transfer imaging. *Brain* 2001; **124:** 882–92.

31. Sanfilipo M, Lafargue T, Rusinck H et al. Volumetric measure of the frontal and temporal lobe regions in schizophrenia. *Arch Gen Psychiatry* 2000; **57:** 471–80.

32. Sigmundsson T, Suckling J, Maier M et al. Structural abnormalities in frontal, temporal, and limbic regions and interconnecting white matter tracts in schizophrenic patients with prominent negative symptoms. *Am J Psychiatry* 2001; **158:** 234–43.

33. Bigliani V, Pilowsky LS. *In vivo* neuropharmacology of schizophrenia. *Br J Psychiatry* 1999; **174:** 23–33.

34. Krystal JH, Abi-Dargham A, Laruelle M, Moghaddam B. Pharmacologic models of psychoses. In: (Charney DS, Nestler EJ, Bunney BS, eds) *Neurobiology of Mental Illness.* (Oxford University Press: New York, 1999) 214–24.

35. Schroder J, Bubeck B, Silvestri S, Demisch S, Sauer H. Gender differences in D2 dopamine receptor binding in drug-naive patients with schizophrenia: an [123I]iodobenzamide single photon emission computed tomography study. *Psychiatry Res* 1997; **75:** 115–23.

36. Tibbo P, Silverstone PH, McEwan AJ, Scott J, Joshua A, Golberg K. A single photon emission computed tomography scan study of striatal dopamine D2 receptor binding with 123I-epidepride in patients with schizophrenia and controls. *J Psychiatry Neurosci* 1997; **22:** 39–45.

37. Goldsmith SK, Shapiro RM, Joyce JN. Disrupted pattern of D2 dopamine receptors in the temporal lobe in schizophrenia: a postmortem study. *Arch Gen Psychiatry* 1997; **54:** 649–58.

38. Domyo T, Kurumaji A, Toru M. An increase in [3H]SCH23390 binding in the cerebral cortex of postmortem brains of chronic schizophrenics. *J Neural Trans* 2001; **108:** 1475–84.

39. Karlsson P, Farde L, Halldin C, Sedvall G. PET study of D(1) dopamine receptor binding in neuroleptic-naive patients with schizophrenia. *Am J Psychiatry* 2002; **159:** 761–7.

40. Abi-Dargham A, Gil R, Krystal J et al. Increased striatal dopamine transmission in schizophrenia: confirmation in a second cohort. *Am J Psychiatry* 1998; **155:** 761–7.

41. Laruelle M, Abi-Dargham A. Dopamine as the wind of the psychotic fire: new evidence from brain imaging studies. *J Psychopharmac* 1999; **13:** 358–71.

42. Laruelle M, Abi-Dargham A, Gil R, Kegeles L, Innis R. Increased dopamine transmission in schizophrenia: relationship to illness phases. *Biol Psychiatry* 1999; **46:** 56–72.

43. Kapur S, Roy P, Daskalakis J, Remington G, Zipursky R. Increased dopamine d(2) receptor occupancy and elevated prolactin level associated with addition of halo-peridol to clozapine. *Am J Psychiatry* 2001; **158:** 311–14.

44. Raskin S, Durst R, Katz G, Zislin J. Olanzapine and sulpiride: a preliminary study of combination/augmentation in patients with treatment-resistant schizophrenia. *J Clin Psychopharmac* 2000; **20:** 500–3.

45. Kapur S, Zipursky R, Jones C, Remington G, Houle, S. Relationship between dopamine D(2) occupancy, clinical response, and side effects: a double-blind PET study of first-episode schizophrenia. *Am J Psychiatry* 2000; **157:** 514–20.

46. Okubo Y, Suhara T, Suzuki K et al. Serotonin 5-HT2 receptors in schizophrenic patients studied by positron emission tomography. *Life Sci* 2000; **66:** 2455–64.

47. Ngan ET, Yatham LN, Ruth TJ, Liddle PF. Decreased serotonin 2A receptor densities in neuroleptic-naive patients with schizophrenia: a PET study using [(18)F]setoperone. *Am J Psychiatry* 2000; **157:** 1016–18.

48. Busatto GF, Pilowsky LS, Costa DC et al. Correlation between reduced in vivo benzo-diazepine receptor binding and severity of psychotic symptoms in schizophrenia. *Am J Psychiatry* 1997; **154:** 56–63.

49. Abi-Dargham A, Laruelle M, Krystal J et al. No evidnece of altered in vivo benzo-diazepine receptor binding in schizophrenia. *Neuropsychopharmacology* 1999; **20:** 650–61.

50. Ball S, Busatto GF, David AS et al. Cognitive functioning and GABAA/benzo-diazepine receptor binding in schizophrenia: a 123I-iomazenil SPET study. *Biol Psychiatry* 1998; **43**: 107–17.

51. Crook JM, Tomaskovic-Crook E, Copolov DL, Dean B. Low muscarinic receptor binding in prefrontal cortex from subjects with schizophrenia: a study of Brodmann's areas 8, 9, 10, and 46 and the effects of neuroleptic drug treatment. *Am J Psychiatry* 2001; **158**: 918–25.

52. Gao XM, Sakai K, Roberts RC, Conley RR, Dean B, Tamminga CA. Ionotropic glutamate receptors and expression of N-methyl-D-aspartate receptor subunits in subregions of human hippocampus: effects of schizophrenia. *Am J Psychiatry* 2000; **157**: 1141–9.

53. Ibrahim HM, Hogg AJ, Healy DJ, Haroutunian V, Davis KL, Meador-Woodruff JH. Ionotropic glutamate receptor binding and subunit mRNA expression in thalamic nuclei in schizophrenia. *Am J Psychiatry* 2000; **157**: 1811–23.

54. Meador-Woodruff JH, Davis KL, Haroutunian V. Abnormal kainate receptor expression in prefrontal cortex in schizophrenia. *Neuropsychopharmacology* 2001; **24**: 545–52.

55. Weinberger DR, Berman KF, Zec RF. Physiologic dysfunction of dorsolateral pre-frontal cortex in schizophrenia. I. Regional cerebral blood flow evidence. *Arch Gen Psychiatry* 1986; **43**: 114–24.

56. Berman KF, Ostrem JL, Randolph C et al. Physiological activation of a cortical network during performance of the Wisconsin Card Sorting Test: a positron emission tomography study. *Neuropsychologia* 1995; **33**: 1027–46.

57. Volz HP, Gaser C, Hager F et al. Brain activation during cognitive stimulation with the Wisconsin Card Sorting Test – a functional MRI study on healthy volunteers and schizophrenics. *Psychiatry Res* 1997; **75**: 145–57.

58. Andreasen NC, Rezai K, Alliger R et al. Hypofrontality in neuroleptic-naive patients and in patients with chronic schizophrenia. Assessment with xenon 133 single-photon emission computed tomography and the Tower of London. *Arch Gen Psychiatry* 1992; **49**: 943–58.

59. Frith CD, Friston KJ, Herold S et al. Regional brain activity in chronic schizophrenic patients during the performance of a verbal working memory task. *Br J Psychiatry* 1995; **167**: 343–9.

60. Dolan RJ, Fletcher PC, Frith CD, Friston KJ, Frackowiak RSJ, Grasby PM. Dopaminergic modulation of impaired cognitive activation in the anterior cingulate cortex in schizophrenia. *Nature* 1995; **378**: 180–2.

61. Yurgelun Todd DA, Waternaux CM, Cohen BM, Gruber SA, English CD, Renshaw PF. Functional magnetic resonance imaging of schizophrenic patients and comparison subjects during word production. *Am J Psychiatry* 1996; **153**: 200–5.

62. Callicott JH, Ramsey NF, Tallent K et al. Functional magnetic resonance imaging brain mapping in psychiatry: methodological issues illustrated in a study of working memory in schizophrenia. *Neuropsychopharmacology* 1998; **18**: 186–96.

63. Carter CS, Braver TS, Barch DM, Botvinick MM, Noll D, Cohen JD. Anterior cingulate cortex, error detection, and the online monitoring of performance. 1998; **280**: 747–9.

64. Curtis VA, Bullmore ET, Brammer MJ et al. Attenuated frontal activation during a verbal fluency task in patients with schizophrenia. *Am J Psychiatry* 1998; **155:** 1056–63.

65. Menon V, Anagnoson RT, Mathalon DH, Glover GH, Pfefferbaum A. Functional neuroanatomy of auditory working memory in schizophrenia: relation to positive and negative symptoms. *Neuroimage* 2001; **13:** 433–46.

66. Heckers S, Rauch SL, Goff D et al. Impaired recruitment of the hippocampus during conscious recollection in schizophrenia. *Nature Neurosci* 1998; **1:** 318–23.

67. Fletcher PC, McKenna PJ, Frith CD, Grasby PM, Friston KJ, Dolan RJ. Brain activations in schizophrenia during a graded memory task studied with functional neuroimaging. *Arch Gen Psychiatry* 1998; **55:** 1001–8.

68. Manoach DS, Gollub RL, Benson ES et al. Schizophrenic subjects show aberrant fMRI activation of dorsolateral prefrontal cortex and basal ganglia during working memory performance. *Biol Psychiatry* 2000; **48:** 99–109.

69. Cohen RM, Nordahl TE, Semple WE, Andreason P, Pickar D. Abnormalities in the distributed network of sustained attention predict neuroleptic treatment response in schizophrenia. *Neuropsychopharmacology* 1998; **19:** 36–47.

70. Fallgatter AJ, Strik WK. Reduced frontal functional asymmetry in schizophrenia during a cued continuous performance test assessed with near-infrared spectroscopy. *Schizophrenia Bull* 2000; **26:** 913–19.

71. Yucel M, Pantelis C, Stuart GW et al. Anterior cingulate activation during Stroop task performance: a PET to MRI coregistration study of individual patients with schizophrenia. *Am J Psychiatry* 2002; **159:** 251–4.

72. Menon RR, Barta PE, Aylward EH et al. Posterior superior temporal gyrus in schizophrenia: grey matter changes and clinical correlates. *Schizophrenia Res* 1995; **16:** 127–35.

73. McGuire PK, Quested DJ, Spence SA, Murray RM, Frith CD, Liddle PF. Pathophysiology of 'positive' thought disorder in schizophrenia. *Br J Psychiatry* 1998; **173:** 231–5.

74. Shenton ME, Kikinis R, Jolesz FA et al. Abnormalities of the left temporal lobe and thought disorder in schizophrenia: a quantitative magnetic resonance imaging study. *N Engl J Med* 1992; **327:** 604–12.

75. Zorrilla LTE, Jeste DV, Brown GG. Functional MRI and novel picture-learning among older patients with chronic schizophrenia: abnormal correlations between recognition memory and medial temporal brain response. *Am J Geriatr Psychiatry* 2002; **10:** 52–61.

76. Bentall R. Deconstructing the concept of schizophrenia. *J Ment Health* 1993; **2:** 223–38.

77. Bentall RP, Jackson HF, Pilgrim D. Abandoning the concept of 'schizophrenia': some implications of validity arguments psychological research into psychotic phenomena. *Br J Clin Psychol* 1988; **27:** 303–24.

78. Bentall RP, Jackson HF, Pilgrim D. The concept of schizophrenia is dead: long live the concept of schizophrenia? *Br J Clin Psychol* 1988; **27:** 329–31.

79. Carter CS, Perlstein W, Ganguli R, Brar J, Mintun M, Cohen JD. Functional hypofrontality and working memory dysfunction in schizophrenia. *Am J Psychiatry* 1998; **155:** 1285–7.

80. Ganguli R, Carter C, Mintun M et al. PET brain mapping study of auditory verbal supraspan memory versus visual fixation in schizophrenia. *Biol Psychiatry* 1997; **41:** 33–42.

81. Liddle PF, Friston KJ, Frith CD, Frackowiak RS. Cerebral blood flow and mental processes in schizophrenia. *J Roy Soc Med* 1992; **85:** 224–7.

82. Kaplan RD, Szechtman H, Franco S et al. Three clinical syndromes of schizophrenia in untreated subjects: relation to brain glucose activity measured by positron emission tomography (PET). *Schizophrenia Res* 1993; **11:** 47–54.

83. Cleghorn JM, Franco S, Szechtman B et al. Toward a brain map of auditory hallucinations. *Am J Psychiatry* 1992; **149:** 1062–9.

84. McGuire PK, Shah GM, Murray RM. Increased blood flow in Broca's area during auditory hallucinations in schizophrenia. *Lancet* 1993; **342:** 703–6.

85. Silbersweig DA, Stern E, Frith C et al. A functional neuroanatomy of hallucinations in schizophrenia. *Nature* 1995; **378:** 176–9.

86. Shergill SS, Brammer MJ, Williams SC, Murray RM, McGuire PK. Mapping auditory hallucinations in schizophrenia using functional magnetic resonance imaging. *Arch Gen Psychiatry* 2000; **57:** 1033–8.

87. Blackwood NJ, Howard RJ, Ffytche DH, Simmons A, Bentall RP, Murray RM. Imaging attentional and attributional bias: an fMRI approach to the paranoid delusion. *Psychol Med* 2000; **30:** 873–83.

88. Spence SA, Brooks DJ, Hirsch SR, Liddle PF, Meehan J, Grasby PM. A PET study of voluntary movement in schizophrenic patients experiencing passivity phenomena (delusions of alien control). *Brain* 1997; **120:** 1997–2011.

89. Baare WF, Pol HE, Boomsma DI et al. Quantitative genetic modeling of variation in human brain morphology. *Cereb Cortex* 2001; **11:** 816–24.

90. Egan MF, Goldberg TE, Kolachana BS et al. Effect of COMT Val108/158 Met genotype on frontal lobe function and risk for schizophrenia. *Proc Natl Acad Sci USA* 2001; **98:** 6917–22.

91. Weinberger DR, Egan MF, Bertolino A et al. Prefrontal neurons and the genetics of schizophrenia. *Biol Psychiatry* 2001; **50:** 825–44.

92. Uttal WR. *The New Phrenology: The Limits of Localizing Cognitive Processes in the Brain.* (MIT Press: Cambridge, MA, 2001.)

93. Dye SM, Spence SA, Bench CJ et al. No evidence for left superior temporal dysfunction in asymptomatic schizophrenia and bipolar disorder. PET study of verbal fluency. *Br J Psychiatry* 1999; **175:** 367–74.

94. Spence SA, Hirsch SR, Brooks DJ, Grasby PM. Prefrontal cortex activity in people with schizophrenia and control subjects. Evidence from positron emission tomography for remission of 'hypofrontality' with recovery from acute schizophrenia. *Br J Psychiatry* 1998; **172:** 316–23.

95. Friston K, Frith CD. Schizophrenia: a disconnection syndrome? *Clin Neurosci* 1995; **3:** 89–97.

96. Hyde TM, Ziegler JC, Weinberger DR. Psychiatric disturbances in metachromatic leukodystrophy. Insights into the neurobiology of psychosis. *Arch Neurol* 1992; **49:** 401–6.

97. Allen RM, Young SJ. Phencyclidine-induced psychosis. *Am J Psychiatry* 1978; **135**: 1081–4.

98. Cohen JD, Servan Schreiber D. Context, cortex, and dopamine: a connectionist approach to behavior and biology in schizophrenia. *Psychol Rev* 1992; **99**: 45–77.

99. Hoffman RE, McGlashan TH. Parallel distributed processing and the emergence of schizophrenic symptoms. *Schizophrenia Bull* 1993; **19**: 119–40.

100. Haracz JL. Neural plasticity in schizophrenia. *Schizophrenia Bull* 1985; **11**: 191–229.

101. Bleuler E. *Dementia Praecox or the Group of Schizophrenias* [English Translation]. (International Universities Press: New York, 1961.)

102. Frith CD. *The Cognitive Neuropsychology of Schizophrenia*. (Lawrence Earlbaum Associates: Hove, Sussex, 1992.)

103. Mcintosh AR, Gonzales-Lima F. Structural equation modelling and its application to network analysis in functional brain imaging. *Hum Brain Mapping* 1994; **2**: 2–22.

104. Spence SA, Liddle PF, Stefan MD et al. Functional anatomy of verbal fluency in people with schizophrenia and those at genetic risk. Focal dysfunction and distributed disconnectivity reappraised. *Br J Psychiatry* 2000; **176**: 52–60.

105. Friston KJ, Frith CD, Frackowiak RSJ. Time-dependent changes in effective connectivity measured with PET. *Hum Brain Mapping* 1993; **1**: 69–79.

106. McIntosh AR, Grady CL, Haxby JV, Ungerleider LG, Horwitz B. Changes in limbic and prefrontal functional interactions in a working memory task for faces. *Cereb Cortex* 1996; **6**: 571–84.

107. Buchel C, Friston KJ. Dynamic changes in effective connectivity characterized by variable parameter regression and Kalman filtering. *Hum Brain Mapp* 1998; **6**: 403–8.

108. Fletcher PC, Buchel C, Josephs O, Friston KJ, Dolan RJ. Learning-related neuronal responses in prefrontal cortex studied with functional neuroimaging. *Cereb Cortex* 1999; **9**: 168–78.

109. Andreasen NC, Nopoulos P, O'Leary DS, Miller DD, Wassink T, Flaum M. Defining the phenotype of schizophrenia: cognitive dysmetria and its neural mechanisms. *Biol Psychiatry* 1999; **46**: 908–20.

110. Andreasen NC, Arndt S, Swayze 2nd, V et al. Thalamic abnormalities in schizophrenia visualized through magnetic resonance image averaging. *Science* 1994; **266**: 294–8.

111. Stephan KE, Magnotta VA, White T et al. Effects of olanzapine on cerebellar functional connectivity in schizophrenia measured by fMRI during a simple motor task. *Psychol Med* 2001; **31**: 1065–78.

112. Fletcher PC, Frith CD, Grasby PM, Friston KJ, Dolan RJ. Local and distributed effects of apomorphine on fronto–temporal function in acute unmedicated schizophrenia. *J Neurosci* 1996; **16**: 7055–62.

113. Meyer Lindenberg A, Poline JB, Kohn PD et al. Evidence for abnormal cortical functional connectivity during working memory in schizophrenia. *Am J Psychiatry* 2001; **158**: 1809–17.

114. Fletcher PC, McKenna PJ, Friston KJ, Frith CD, Dolan RJ. Abnormal cingulate modulation of fronto–temporal connectivity in schizophrenia. *Neuroimage* 1999; **9**: 337–42.

9. Functional Imaging Studies of Psychopathy, Antisocial Personality Disorder (APD) and Related Psychological Processes

Nigel Tunstall, Thomas Fahy, Philip McGuire

Diagnostic concepts

Attempts to define a personality profile of individuals disposed principally to self-serving and antisocial behaviour can be traced at least as far back as Pinel's concept of 'manie sans delire'.[1] Rush[2] relabelled it as 'moral alienation of the mind', and contributed strongly to the Anglo-American conception of psychopathy as predominantly antisocial. Prichard[3] concerned himself with the question of antisocial actions under the control of the will, and stimulated a debate that shaped the concept of criminal responsibility, though his term 'moral insanity' had a limited lifespan. Subsequently, Partridge[4] suggested the designation 'sociopathy' for personality disturbances whose outstanding feature is antisocial behaviour. Cleckley,[5] in his monograph *The Mask of Sanity*, proposed the use of the term 'psychopathy' (which had been coined by Koch,[6] in 1891) for individuals showing lifelong maladaptive behaviour not caused by neurosis, psychosis or mental handicap. Cleckley's definitions were developed in the diagnostic and statistical manual of mental disorders (DSM) and International Classification of Diseases (ICD) schemes.

The current diagnoses most frequently used for research purposes are the antisocial personality disorder (APD) category of DSM-IV[7] and the psychopathy concept as defined by Hare et al's[8] psychopathy checklist (PCL). The different criteria for these diagnoses reflect overlapping conceptual models, differing in the relative emphasis given to putative psychological attributes or to social deviance.

APD is applied to individuals who have displayed some symptoms of conduct disorder before 15 years of age, and who demonstrate a persistent disregard for the wishes, rights or feelings of others, and for the law. They are characterized in this scheme as frequently manipulative and deceitful, impulsive, remorseless, and liable to irritability and aggression not restricted to acts of self-defence. Also emphasized are reckless disregard for the safety of others and themselves, evidenced in a range of high-risk behaviours and lack of responsibility in the areas of relationships, employment, finance and support of dependents. To fulfill the criteria, three or more items from a list of seven must be met (see Box 9.1 for full criteria). Psychological features, including lack of empathy, callousness, inflated and arrogant self-appraisal, and superficial charm, are identified as 'associated features' and described as more

---

Box 9.1 Diagnostic criteria for 301.7 antisocial personality disorder (APD) DSM-IV

(1) There is a pervasive pattern of disregard for and violation of the rights of others occurring since 15 years of age, as indicated by three (or more) of the following:
   (a) failure to conform to social norms with respect to lawful behaviours as indicated by repeatedly performing acts that are grounds for arrest;
   (b) deceitfulness, as indicated by repeated lying, use of aliases or conning of others for personal profit or pleasure;
   (c) impulsivity or failure to plan ahead;
   (d) irritability and aggressiveness, as indicated by repeated physical fights or assaults;
   (e) reckless disregard for the safety of others;
   (f) consistent irresponsibility, as indicated by repeated failure to sustain consistent work behaviour or honour financial obligations;
   (g) lack of remorse, as indicated by being indifferent to or rationalizing having hurt, mistreated or stolen from another.

(2) The individual is at least 18 years of age.

(3) There is evidence of conduct disorder with onset before 15 years of age.

(4) The occurrence of antisocial behaviour is not exclusively during the course of schizophrenia or a manic episode.

common in APD samples in prison or forensic settings. Hence, it is possible to meet DSM-IV criteria for APD on the basis of behaviour that is reckless, irresponsible and impulsive, but not necessarily manipulative and deceitful.

The ICD 10 category F60.2, dissocial personality disorder,[9] identifies a clinical syndrome resembling APD as operationalized in DSM-IV; it adds the criterion of showing inability to profit from experience (see Box 9.2).

Psychopathy, as defined by the PCL, derives directly from Cleckely's[5] clinical description, and therefore places central importance on identifying the emotional deficit. Developed in Canada by Hare et al,[8] the PCL comprises 20 items, including glibness or superficial charm, pathological lying and deception, lack of remorse or guilt, and failure to accept responsibility for actions. Each item is scored on a scale of 0 (not present) to 2 (definitely present). The cut-off point for a case-level diagnosis of psychopathy is 30 in North America and 25 in the UK. The PCL may be administered by means of either a chart (case note) review or an interview (see Box 9.3 for a complete list of items).

Box 9.2 F60.2 Dissocial personality disorder

Personality disorder, usually coming to attention because of a gross disparity between behaviour and the prevailing social norms, is characterized by:
(1) callous unconcern for the feelings of others;
(2) gross and persistent attitudes of irresponsibility and disregard for social norms, rules and obligations;
(3) incapacity to maintain enduring relationships, though having no difficulty in establishing them;
(4) very low tolerance to frustration and a low threshold for discharge of aggression, including violence;
(5) incapacity to experience guilt and to profit from experience, particularly punishment;
(6) marked proneness to blame others, or to offer plausible rationalizations, for the behaviour that has brought the patient into conflict with society.

There may also be persistent irritability as an associated feature. Conduct disorder during childhood and adolescence, though not invariably present, may further support the diagnosis.

Box 9.3 Revised psychopathy checklist (PCL)

(1) Glibness/superficial charm

(2) Grandiose sense of self-worth

(3) Need for stimulation/proneness to boredom

(4) Pathological lying

(5) Conning/manipulative

(6) Lack of remorse or guilt

(7) Shallow affect

(8) Callous/lack of empathy

(9) Parasitic lifestyle

(10) Poor behavioural controls

(11) Promiscuous sexual behaviour

(12) Early behavioural problems

(13) Lack of realistic, long-term goals

(14) Impulsivity

(15) Irresponsibility

(16) Failure to accept responsibility for actions

(17) Many short-term marital relationships

(18) Juvenile delinquency

(19) Revocation of conditional release

(20) Criminal versatility

In summary, there is significant overlap in clinical features between DSM-IV APD and PCL psychopathy. Samples of people with APD will contain individuals who also fulfill PCL criteria for psychopathy. Criteria shared between the two diagnoses include: superficial charm, deceitfulness, manipulative behaviour, instrumental aggression, lack of empathy, guilt or remorse, impulsivity and lack of planning, and irresponsibility. This cluster of abnormalities suggests that the underlying abnormality has both cognitive and emotional components. (A detailed analysis of the relationship between psychopathy and APD is beyond the scope of this review; relevant recent studies include those of Verona et al[10] and Windle[11].)

This review explores the possible neural basis for the abnormalities observed in individuals with psychopathy and APD. It surveys evidence from neuropsychology, neurophysiology, and structural imaging studies of psychopathy, APD and individuals with acquired brain lesions; and from functional imaging studies of decision-making, mentalizing abilities, conditioning and emotional processing, either in individuals with psychopathy/APD or unaffected subjects.

What is the neural basis of antisocial personality disorder (APD)/psychopathy?

Psychological and neurophysiological functioning

Several areas of cognitive and emotional functioning have been investigated in samples of individuals with psychopathy and/or APD. On an advanced theory of mind task, the performance of psychopaths is comparable to that of non-psychopathic controls, and superior to that of high-functioning autistics.[12] Psychopaths show no deficits in recognition of emotional facial expressions[13] and no impairment on social cognition tests, with the exception of a task designed to test whether the subject can distinguish moral from conventional transgressions.[14] Both subjects with APD and psychopathy show impairment on neuropsychological measures of orbitofrontal–ventromedial functioning, such as a visual go/no-go task[15] and the Porteus Maze task,[16] in comparison to controls; but no deficits on a range of tasks thought to engage other frontal regions.[17] The only data available on decision-making in subjects with APD[18] are difficult to interpret as evidence of disadvantageous decision-making in this group due to the potentially confounding effects of heavy alcohol use and low IQ.

Psychopaths are quantifiably less emotional than non-psychopaths.[19] In addition, they also show differences on various indices of autonomic functioning, e.g. they have low resting skin conductance,[20] fail to show normal potentiation of the startle reflex during imagery of unpleasant and fearful experiences,[21] show reduced fear conditioning relative to non-psychopaths,[22] and autonomic hyporesponsiveness to sad and fearful faces.[23,24]

Structural magnetic resonance imaging (MRI) studies

There are two published structural MRI studies of psychopathy/APD. In the first of these, prefrontal grey and white matter volumes were derived from MRI of subjects with DSM-IV APD and three control groups.[25] PCL scores were obtained on all subjects, and skin conductance and heart rate measurements made while each subject read aloud a prepared speech about his faults. The APD group showed an 11% reduction in prefrontal grey matter volume and reduced autonomic activity during the stressor. The APD, substance-dependence and 'healthy' groups included in the study were found to have rates of psychopathy of 28.5, 20.1 and 14.2%, respectively. The prefrontal grey matter decrements were suggested by the authors to underlie the autonomic abnormalities and clinical characteristics of individuals with psychopathy/APD. However, interpretation of the results is not straightforward: 66.7% of the APD group was reported to be dependent on cocaine, compared with 30.8% in the substance-dependent group; and the data demonstrated higher rates of stimulant dependence and abuse, and higher rates of polysubstance abuse and other drug abuse in the APD group. Raine[26] produced a further analysis showing the absence of any correlation between drug use (for cocaine or other drugs) and prefrontal volume loss. Nevertheless, the APD label may conceal diagnostic heterogeneity due to the inclusion of individuals with behavioural abnormalities secondary to the effects of drugs or alcohol.

A second structural MRI study examined a sample of violent offenders with APD and comorbid alcoholism.[27] Negative correlations (up to −0.79) were found between PCL psychopathy scores and volume of the posterior hippocampus, estimated from manual image analysis. However, the sample size was small and the generalizability of the findings was limited by the comorbid alcoholism of the individuals in the sample.

Studies of individuals with 'acquired' sociopathy

An alternative approach to understanding the neural basis of psychopathy/APD has been to build models of social cognition based on the study of individuals who have developed behaviour resembling the syndrome after sustaining brain injury. EVR was a successful businessman until he began to suffer severe headaches, a symptom of an orbitofrontal meningioma.[28] Following surgical removal of his tumour, he appeared superficially undamaged, but he was unable to hold down a job. Subsequently, he was twice divorced and went bankrupt. EVR exhibited normal/superior performance on tasks measuring the ability to generate response options to social situations and consider future consequences of pursuing specific response options, as well as predict the likely outcome of a particular configuration of social stimuli, and performed at an advanced developmental level on moral reasoning tests. However, on the gambling task,[29] he performed at subnormal levels, and failed to developed anticipatory skin conductance responses before risky choices.[29] The task involves the subject gambling on two decks of cards, one of which is a high-reward deck and the other a low-reward deck. The subject does not know the rules in advance and must form an impression of the relative worth of each deck EVR showed a preference for the high-risk deck, whereas control subjects tend to select only from the low-risk deck after about 30 rounds, ensuring net wins.

Damasio[30] proposed the somatic marker hypothesis to account for certain aspects of decision-making in the context of punishments/rewards. This states that emotionally related knowledge biases decision-making by assigning value to alternative actions and their predicted consequences. This is proposed to occur both automatically, through effects on attention and working memory, and overtly, through the conscious evaluation of alternative responses. In this model, the integration of emotional responses with high level (abstract) reasoning is posited to occur in the ventromedial prefrontal cortex. Thus, in the case of EVR, access to covert, emotionally significant information was disrupted, resulting in catastrophic impairment of decision-making in real social situations.

In a single case study with contrasting findings, Blair et al[24] examined the cognitive functioning of a patient (JS) with behavioural problems, including marked reactive aggression, following trauma to the right orbitofrontal cortex (OFC). JS showed unimpaired performance on the four-pack card-playing task, indicating preserved decision-making in the context of punishments/rewards, but had severe difficulty in recognizing angry and disgusted facial expressions. Additionally, he showed impaired autonomic responses to these expressions but not to other stimuli.

Anderson et al[31] studied two individuals with severely impaired social behaviour, including instrumental violence and criminality, following prefrontal damage before 16 months of age. The first subject had bilateral prefrontal lesions involving the poles and ventromedial prefrontal cortex. The second subject had a unilateral lesion in the right frontal pole. Despite normal intelligence and basic cognitive abilities, both subjects showed impaired performance on the gambling task, defective autonomic responses to punishment, and impairment on tests of moral and social reasoning.

Some conclusions can be reached from studies of individuals with acquired brain lesions. Antisocial behaviour in subjects with frontal brain lesions acquired in adulthood (termed 'acquired sociopathy' by Damasio[30]) appears to be reactive, i.e. it reflects impaired frustration tolerance, rather than instrumental. Furthermore, it occurs despite intact factual knowledge of moral and social rules. Impairment of decision-making in subjects with acquired sociopathy appears to vary, depending on the extent to which emotionally related retrieval of social information is impaired. In contrast, subjects with early prefrontal lesions display instrumental aggression and antisocial behaviour, and show impairment of both emotionally related and factual modes of information retrieval.

Functional imaging studies of antisocial personality disorder (APD), psychopathy and related psychological processes

To date, relatively few functional imaging (FI) studies of psychopathy/APD have been reported. They have utilized classical conditioning and emotional processing paradigms, approaches clearly suggested by the findings from neurophysiology studies of psychopaths and the clinical phenotype of the disorders, respectively. The foregoing account of brain lesion studies suggests that decision-making in the context of punishment/reward might be a further promising approach to the study of these populations; hence, FI studies of decision-making are reviewed in this section. Since traits such as pathological lying, manipulativeness, lack of empathy and shallow affect are characteristic of psychopathy, also considered here are FI studies of social cognition and deception, and FI studies of emotional processing in psychopaths.

Decision-making

The brain lesion studies reviewed previously suggest that the defective social reasoning of some individuals who have suffered orbitofrontal damage is due to impaired access to emotionally related information, and is reflected in aberrant patterns of performance on neuropsychological tests of decision-making. Psychopathy is associated with an emotional deficit at the clinical level and autonomic deficits at the level of neurophysiology. An important empirical question arising from these observations is whether psychopaths also show an aberrant pattern of performance on decision-making tasks, as would be predicted from the somatic marker hypothesis. So far, there has been no adequate experimental study of decision-making in the context of punishment/reward in psychopaths. However, FI data on decision-making in healthy individuals, or other individuals without gross brain lesions, provide a basis for designing FI studies of decision-making in psychopaths and making predictions about what they will show.

Ernst et al[32] measured regional cerebral blood flow (rCBF) in 20 healthy adult subjects using positron emission tomography (PET) while they performed a computerized risk-taking test resembling the Bechara gambling task. This was contrasted with a control condition, which resembled the risk-taking task with the exception of the decision-making component. The comparison was associated with activation in a predominantly right-lateralized neural network comprising the OFC, dorsolateral prefrontal cortex, ventrolateral prefrontal cortex, anterior cingulate, insula, parietal cortex, thalamus and cerebellum. Analysis of the component processes of the task showed that informed decision-making engaged a network that included areas subserving memory (the hippocampus and posterior cingulate) and motor control (the striatum and cerebellum), whereas un-informed decision-making was associated with activation of left-sided sensory–motor associative areas and the amygdala.

In another study, Critchley et al[33] used functional magnetic resonance imaging (fMRI) to investigate the pattern of brain activity associated with anticipation of feedback following decision-making. Subjects were asked to decide whether a series of as-yet unseen playing cards would be higher or lower in value than a corresponding series of cue cards. The degree of uncer-tainty associated with the predictions varied, according to the face values of the cards: if the face value was one, for example, there was a 100% chance that the feedback card would be higher, whereas for a value of 5, a prediction of the feedback card being higher was associated with a 44% chance of being wrong. Correct or incorrect decisions were associated with monetary gain or loss, respectively. fMRI was used to measure neural activity during the period between presentation of cue and feedback cards; anticipatory arousal was indexed by galvanic skin conductance (GSR). The main effect during the anticipatory period was widespread bilateral activation of the ventral and medial prefrontal cortices, lateral and anterior temporal lobes, right dorso-lateral prefrontal cortex and inferior parietal lobe, with the most significant effect evident bilaterally in inferior prefrontal regions, including the OFC. Uncertainty and arousal (indexed by GSR) were shown by conjunction analysis to be conjointly associated with increased activity in regions of the anterior cingulate cortex bilaterally. A separate analysis determined that neural activity in the right dorsolateral prefrontal cortex and right anterior cingulate cortex increased as a function of arousal.

These studies provide FI evidence of a distributed neural network associ-ated with decision-making. The finding that anterior cingulate cortex ac-tivity correlates with anticipatory arousal points to a role for this region in integrating cognitive processing of uncertainty with representations of changes in bodily state, and raises the question of whether psychopaths' abnormally low arousal levels might produce a different patterns of neural activation during decision-making – a hypothesis that could be tested in future FI studies.

Social cognition and deception

FI studies of social cognitive skills, including the ability to represent the mental states of the self and others, suggest a further possible approach to investigating the neural basis of psychopaths' deviant social behaviour. Such studies of social cognition have focused on metarepresentation (in which the subjects monitor and report on their own mental states) and mentalization, or theory of mind (other people's mental states). fMRI studies of metarepresentation and theory of mind have shown medial prefrontal cortex activation to be common to both processes.[34,35] Theory of mind has additionally been associated with increased neural activity in the left temporopolar cortex and anterior cingulate cortex, and metarepresentation with increased activity in the right temporoparietal junction and anterior cingulate.[36]

The process of empathy, which may be defined as projecting oneself into the object of a perception, has an emotional component in addition to a cognitive mentalization component. Absent or deficient empathy is a core feature of psychopathy. Its neural basis has been explored using fMRI by Farrow et al,[37] who scanned 10 healthy subjects while they performed the following tasks: (1) a task designed to elicit empathy; (2) one in which they judged the forgivability of another's crimes; and (3) a high-level, social reasoning (control) task. Both empathic and forgivability judgements activated the left superior frontal gyrus, orbitofrontal gyrus and precuneus. Empathic judgements also activated the left anterior middle temporal and left inferior frontal gyri, while forgivability judgements activated the posterior cingulate gyrus.

Two fMRI studies have recently been reported that attempt to pin down the pattern of neural activation associated with deception,[38,39] an ability unimpaired, and possibly enhanced, in psychopathy. Spence et al[38] scanned 10 healthy subjects with fMRI who were instructed either to lie or answer truthfully in response to computer-administered questions (in a counter-balanced design). Lying was associated with increased activity in the bilateral ventrolateral prefrontal cortices relative to telling the truth. Langleben et al[39] used a different experimental model of deception, the guilty knowledge test (GKT), to test 18 healthy subjects during fMRI scanning. Increased activations associated with deceptive responses occurred in the anterior cingulate cortex, superior frontal gyrus (SFG), and left premotor, motor

Table 9.1 Activation maps: summary of functional imaging studies of processes impaired, or possibly impaired, in psychopathy/antisocial personality disorder (unless otherwise indicated, results refer to studies of healthy subjects)

Author and year (ref)	Paradigm	Anatomic region	Coordinates (x, y, z) (mm)	Z value/ †T peak
Farrow et al, 2001 (37)	Empathy	Left middle temporal gyrus	−57, −3, 18	6.36
		Left inferior frontal gyrus	−53, 25, −6	5.38
Kiehl et al, 2001 (42)	Affective memory Control versus Psychopath	Rostral anterior cingulate	0, 38, 8	4.55
		Caudal anterior cingulate	−8, 22, 20	5.35
		Left inferior frontal gyrus parietal lobe	−38, 41, −8	7.38
		Posterior cingulate gyrus	−8, −38, 16	8.30
		Right amygdala/hippocampus	34, −12, −20	7.57
Critchley et al, 2001 (33)	Anticipation of feedback following decision-making	Right orbitofrontal cortex/anterior insula	42, 34, −14	7.70
		Right orbitofrontal cortex	−48, 40, −12	7.47
		Left inferior frontal gyrus/anterior insula	−54, 20, 10	6.88
		Right middle temporal gyrus	56, −28, −12	6.86
		Left temporal pole	−36, 8, −34	6.42
Ernst et al, 2002 (32)*	Guessing	Left amygdala	−28, 2, −26	3.81†
		Left middle frontal gyrus	−26, 6, 58	3.51†
		Left posterior inferior parietal cortex	−32, −66, 44	3.37†
	Informed decision-making	Right cingulate gyrus	6, −58, 16	3.13†
		Left cingulate gyrus	−4, −52, 6	2.94†
		Left caudate nucleus	−14, 10, 0	3.96†
		Left globus pallidus	−12, 2, −6	2.91†
		Right caudate nucleus	22, 20, 8	3.26†

* Positron emission tomography study.

and anterior parietal cortices. The anatomical distribution of deception-related activity in this latter study indicates that deception involves suppression of truthful responses. The emotional deficit associated with psychopathy suggests that such suppression is performed relatively effortlessly by psychopaths and may be predicted to be associated with differential neural activity, such as might be measured by future fMRI studies of deception in psychopaths.

Table 9.2 Activation maps: summary of functional magnetic resonance imaging studies utilizing processes unimpaired or enhanced in psychopathy/antisocial personality disorder (unless otherwise specified (results refer to studies of healthy subjects)

Author and year (ref)	Paradigm	Anatomic region	Coordinates (x, y, z) (mm)	Z value
Spence et al, 2001 (38)	Deception			
	Visual task	Right ventrolateral prefrontal cortex	56, 16, –8	5.29
		Left ventrolateral prefrontal cortex	–52, 18, –8	5.30
		Medial premotor cortex	0, 18, 54	5.52
	Auditory task	Right ventrolateral prefrontal cortex	56, 18, –6	5.66
		Left ventrolateral prefrontal cortex	–52, 18, –6	5.00
Langleben et al, 2002 (39)	Deception	Anterior cingulate gyrus	–1, 16, 29	3.8
		Right superior frontal gyrus	3, 28, 43	3.17
		Superior frontal gyrus	0, 24, 52	3.15
Gallagher et al, 2000 (35)	Theory of mind stories	Medial prefrontal gyrus	–8, 50, 10	3.86
		Left temporal pole	–48, 14, 10	4.15
		Right temporal pole	54, 12, –44	3.66
		Left temporoparietal junction	–46, –56, 26	4.04
		Right temporoparietal junction	66, –52, 8	
Vogeley et al, 2001 (36)	Taking self-perspective	Right temporoparietal junction	58, –56, 12	6.27
		Right anterior cingulate gyrus	6, 54, –4	5.93
		Right premotor cortex	22, 2, 68	5.78
		Right motor cortex	60, –12, 42	5.70
		Left precuneus	–10, –48, 64	5.61

Classical conditioning

The pattern of neural activation associated with the most basic form of emotional learning – aversive classical conditioning – has been investigated in psychopaths using fMRI. Schneider et al[40] employed a differential conditioning paradigm previously used in a study of social phobia.[41] They selected 12 right-handed male subjects who scored above cut-off on the PCL and who also fulfilled DSM-IV criteria for APD, and 12 controls matched for handedness. Aversive and neutral odours (produced by rotten yeast and unmodified air, respectively) were employed as the unconditioned stimuli, and photographs of emotionally neutral, though nonetheless distinguishable, faces as conditioned stimuli. Subjects were scanned during the habituation, acquisition and extinction phases. During the habituation phase, the stimuli were presented separately to each subject; during the acquisition phase, subjects received randomly paired trials of unconditioned stimulus and conditional stimuli, and were scanned during 10 exposures to each pairing. In both groups, subjective ratings of emotional valence indicated that behavioural conditioning had occurred.

Between-group differences in neural activation associated with conditioning were found. During habituation, presentation of the aversive stimulus compared with the neutral stimulus in controls was associated with activation of the amygdala, whereas psychopathic individuals showed amygdalar deactivation. During acquisition, psychopaths demonstrated activations in the amygdala and dorsolateral prefrontal cortex, as well as a trend toward signal increase in the orbitofrontal region; the controls showed deactivation. The authors hypothesized that the observed signal increases in psychopaths resulted from compensatory recruitment of wider neural networks, which was necessary to form negative emotional associations.

Emotional processing in memory and language

Further data concerning the neural basis of emotional behaviour in psychopaths comes from a study in which the pattern of neural activation during performance of an affective memory task was investigated with fMRI.[42] In comparison with criminal non-psychopaths and non-criminal controls, criminal psychopaths showed diminished activation in the amygdala/hippocampal formation, parahippocampal gyrus, ventral striatum, and anterior and posterior cingulate gyri; but bilaterally increased activation in the frontotemporal cortex. A single functional imaging study of affective language processing in psychopaths, using single position emission computed tomography (SPECT), has also been reported.[43] Eight male PCL-psychopaths and nine controls performed a modified version of a lexical decision task. Subjects were presented with blocks of either neutral or emotional words (the order of presentation being counterbalanced across subjects). Relative to controls, psychopaths showed greater activation for emotional words in frontotemporal regions bilaterally. Although the sample

269

was small, the authors suggested that, in psychopaths, lexical decisions involving words with emotional connotations place greater demands on brain regions required for such processing.

Conclusions

Few fMRI studies of subjects with case-level diagnoses of psychopathy/APD have so far been reported. An adequate neurobiological account of psychopathy/APD must explain the following findings: deceitfulness and instrumental aggression; incapacity to make the moral/conventional distinction, but otherwise preserved social knowledge; preserved basic cognitive abilities and theory of mind, but possible ventromedial–orbitofrontal cortex neuropsychological impairment; and a range of abnormalities of autonomic functioning, including reduced startle reflex and fear conditioning, and autonomic hyporesponsiveness to sad and fearful faces. None of the individual case reports of patients with acquired frontal lesions exactly parallels the known findings in psychopathy/APD, although they suggest the existence of interactions between cognitive and emotional processes that are crucial to the adaptive negotiation of complex social situations.

The ventromedial–orbitofrontal cortex appears to play a central role in decision-making, independent of other high-level cognitive skills. Although further behavioural data are needed on patterns of decision making in psychopathy/APD, the existing neuroimaging data are consistent with the notion that these disorders involve dysfunction in this region. Other frontal areas, including the anterior cingulate cortex, superior frontal gyrus and ventrolateral prefrontal cortex, have been implicated by fMRI studies in the inhibition of truthful responses or generation of lies. These networks might be predicted to function normally, or at a superior level, in psychopaths, since impaired retrieval of emotionally related knowledge would tend facilitate inhibition of truthful responses. In contrast, components of the neural circuitry underlying empathic responding, which include the left middle temporal and left inferior frontal gyri, may be dysfunctional in psychopathy.

There is preliminary evidence that psychopaths show differential patterns of neural activity during aversive conditioning compared with non-psychopaths. These differences are relevant to cognitive and emotional processing, and cannot be explained purely in terms of differential learning. Reduced activation in the amygdala and related structures in psychopaths, compared with non-psychopaths, and increased activation bilaterally in the frontotemporal cortex, during an affective memory task, further point to dysfunction in low-level emotional processing regions such as the amygdala, and compensatory increased frontotemporal activity.

Future FI studies of psychopathy/APD are likely to employ a broad array of paradigms. The clinical phenotype(s) of psychopathy/APD is complex and heterogeneous, but includes core deficits in emotional and social behaviour. Still missing are FI data on the patterns of neural activity associated with basic emotional states, particularly fear, sadness and anger, and conditioning to a range of stimuli. Such data might be acquired, in part, through studies of emotional face processing. FI studies of complex cognitive–emotional tasks, such as deception and empathic judgement, are also indicated.

A related line of enquiry is likely to stem from the role of emotion in guiding strategic behaviour, particularly in conditions of relative uncertainty. Decision-making has been investigated successfully in complex FI designs incorporating measures of arousal and perceived risk, and these could be extended to the study of psychopaths. Such studies might focus on the pattern of neural activity associated with relatively uninformed decision-making, since this might be expected to differ from that observed in healthy individuals, in view of the deviant profile of autonomic responding seen in psychopaths. FI paradigms could be further modified to yield neurochemical data relevant to APD/psychopathy by combining FI with pharmacological challenges (e.g. tryptophan depletion). Such designs would permit the artificial manipulation of emotional responses and the provocation of impulsive responding, thereby facilitating the experimental study of these mercurial phenomena, and advancing our understanding of their role in psychopathy and APD.

References

1. Pinel P. *Traité Médico-Philosophique sur l'Aliénation Mentale ou la La Manie*. Richard Caille et Ravier: Paris, 1801.
2. Rush B. *Medical Inquiries and Observations, Upon the Diseases of the Mind*. (Kimber and Richardson: Philadelphia, 1812.)
3. Prichard JC. *A Treatise on Insanity and Other Disorders Affecting the Mind*. (Sherwood: London, 1835.)
4. Partridge GE. Current conceptions of psychopathic personality. *Am J Psychiatry* 1930; **10:** 53–9.

5. Cleckley H. *The Mask of Sanity*. (CV Mosby: St Louis, 1941.)

6. Koch JLA. *Die psychopathischen minderwertigkeiten*. (Maier: Ravensburg, 1891.)

7. American Psychiatric Association. *American Psychiatric Association Diagnostic and Statistical Manual of Mental Disorders*. (American Psychiatric Association: Washington, DC, 1994.)

8. Hare RD, Hart SD, Harpur TJ. Psychopathy and the DSM-IV criteria for antisocial personality disorder. *J Abnorm Psychol* 1991; **100:** 391–8.

9. World Health Organization (WHO). *The ICD-10 Classification of Mental and Behavioural Disorders*. (WHO: Geneva, 1992.)

10. Verona E, Patrick CJ, Joiner TE. Psychopathy, antisocial personality, and suicide risk. *J Abnorm Psychol* 2001; **110:** 462–70.

11. Windle M. Psychopathy and antisocial personality disorder among alcoholic inpatients. *J Studies Alcohol* 1999; **60:** 330–6.

12. Blair RJ, Sellers C, Strickland I et al. Theory of mind in the psychopath. *J Forensic Psychiatry* 1996; **7:** 15–25.

13. Blair RJ, Cipolotti L. Impaired social response reversal. A case of 'acquired sociopathy'. *Brain* 2000; **123:** 1122–41.

14. Blair RJ. A cognitive developmental approach to mortality: investigating the psychopath. *Cognition* 1995; **57:** 1–29.

15. Lapierre D, Braun, Hodgins S. Ventral frontal deficits in psychopathy: neuropsychological test findings. *Neuropsychologia* 1995; **33:** 139–51.

16. Dinn WM, Harris CL. Neurocognitive function in antisocial personality disorder. *Psychiatry Res* 2000; **27:** 173–90.

17. Hare RD. Performance of psychopaths on cognitive tasks related to frontal lobe function. *J Abnorm Psychol* 1984; **93:** 133–40.

18. Mazas CA, Finn PR, Steinmetz JE. Decision-making biases, antisocial personality, and early-onset alcoholism. *Alcohol Clin Exp Res* 2000; **24:** 1036–40.

19. Day R, Wong S. Anomalous perceptual asymmetries for negative emotional stimuli in the psychopath. *J Abnorm Psychol* 1996; **105:** 648–52.

20. Hare RD, Quinn MJ. Psychopathy and autonomic conditioning. *J Abnorm Psychol* 1971; **77:** 223–35.

21. Patrick CJ. Emotion and psychopathy: startling new insights. *Psychophysiology* 1994; **31:** 319–30.

22. Hare RD. Psychopathy and physiological activity during anticipation of an adversive stimulus in a distraction paradigm. *Psychophysiology* 1982; **19:** 266–71.

23. Anskiewicz AS. Autonomic components of vicarious conditioning and psychopathy. *J Clin Psychol* 1979; **35:** 60–7.

24. Blair RJ, Jones L, Clark F, Smith M. The psychopathic individual: a lack of responsiveness to distress cues? *Psychophysiology* 1997; **34:** 192–8.

25. Raine A, Lencz T, Bihrle S et al. Reduced prefrontal gray matter volume and reduced autonomic activity in antisocial personality disorder. *Arch Gen Psychiatry* 2000; **57:** 119–27.

26. Raine A. Is prefrontal cortex thinning specific to antisocial personality disorder? *Arch Gen Psychiatry* 2001; **58:** 402–3.

27. Laakso MP, Vaurio O, Koivisto E et al. Psychopathy and the posterior hippocampus. *Behav Brain Res* 2001; **118:** 187–93.

28. Saver JL, Damasio AR. Preserved access and processing of social knowledge in a patient with acquired sociopathy due to ventromedial frontal damage. *Neuropsychologia* 1991; **29:** 1241–9.

29. Bechara A, Damasio H, Tranel D, Damasio AR. Deciding advantageously before knowing the advantageous strategy. *Science* 1997; **275:** 1293–5.

30. Damasio AR. The somatic marker hypothesis and the possible functions of the prefrontal cortex. *Phil Trans Roy Soc Lond Series B: Biol Sci* 1996; **351:** 1413–20.

31. Anderson SW, Bechara A, Damasio H et al. Impairment of social and moral behavior related to early damage in human prefrontal cortex. *Nature Neurosci* 1999; **2:** 1032–7.

32. Ernst M, Bolla K, Mouratidis M et al. Decision-making in a risk-taking task. A PET study. *Neuropsychopharmacology* 2002; **26:** 682–91.

33. Critchley HD, Mathias, Dolan RJ. Neural activity in the human brain relating to uncertainty and arousal during anticipation. *Neuron* 2001; **29:** 537–45.

34. McGuire PK, Paulesu E, Frackowiak RS, Frith CD. Brain activity during stimulus independent thought. *Neuroreport* 1996; **7:** 2095–9.

35. Gallagher HL, Happe F, Brunswick N et al. Reading the mind in cartoons and stories: an fMRI study of 'theory of mind' in verbal and nonverbal tasks. *Neuropsychologia* 2000; **38:** 11–21.

36. Vogeley K, Bussfield P, Newen A. Mind reading: neural mechanisms of theory of mind and self-perspective. *Neuroimage* 2001; **14:** 170–81.

37. Farrow TF, Zheng Y, Wilkinson ID et al. Investigating the functional anatomy of empathy and forgiveness. *Neuroreport* 2001; **12:** 2433–8.

38. Spence SA, Farrow TF, Herford AE et al. Behavioural and functional anatomical correlates of deception in humans. *Neuroreport* 2001; **17:** 2849–53.

39. Langleben DD, Schroeder L, Maldjian JA et al. Brain activity during simulated deception: an event-related functional magnetic resonance study. *Neuroimage* 2002; **15:** 727–32.

40. Schneider F, Habel U, Kessler C et al. Functional imaging of conditioned aversive emotional responses in antisocial personality disorder. *Neuropsychobiology* 2000; **42:** 192–201.

41. Schneider F, Weiss U, Kessler C et al. Subcortical correlates of differential classical conditioning of aversive emotional reactions in social phobia. *Biol Psychiatry* 1990; **45:** 863–71.

42. Kiehl KA, Smith AM, Hare RD et al. Limbic abnormalities in affective processing by criminal psychopaths as revealed by functional magnetic resonance imaging. *Biol Psychiatry* 2001; **50:** 677–84.

43. Intrator J, Hare R, Stritzke P et al. A brain imaging (single photon emission computerized tomography) study of semantic and affective processing in psychopaths. *Biol Psychiatry* 1997; **42:** 96–103.

INDEX